Radiographic Techniques and Image Evaluation

Radiographic Techniques and Image Evaluation

Elizabeth M. Unett DCR(R), BSc (HONS), FAETC, SRR

Clinical Teacher
Department of Radiographic Studies
Keele University
UK

and

Amanda J. Royle DCR(R), BSc (HONS), FAETC, CT CERT, SRR

Diagnostic Imaging Department Manager
The Grosvenor Nuffield Hospital
Chester
UK

Consultant Editor: Jo Campling

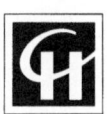 SPRINGER-SCIENCE+BUSINESS MEDIA, B.V.

ISBN 978-1-56593-442-9   ISBN 978-1-4899-2997-6 (eBook)
DOI 10.1007/978-1-4899-2997-6

First edition 1997

Typeset in 10/12 pt Palatino by Type Study, Scarborough

A catalogue record for this book is available from the British Library

Library of Congress Catalog Card Number: 96-85957

∞ Printed on permanent acid-free text paper, manufactured in
accordance with ANSI/NISO Z39.48–1992 and ANSI/NISO Z39.48–1984
(Permanence of Paper).

To Sean and Ian for being there; and to
William and Alexandra for being themselves

Contents

Foreword

I welcome this book on behalf of radiographic practitioners everywhere. It arrives at a time of rapid change within the world of medical imaging where advancing technology and changes in employment conditions are having a major effect on the everyday working practices of those who physically and clinically direct radiation.

The development of radiography as a graduate profession within the United Kingdom provides the opportunity for role extension and role fulfilment for radiographers. Moves toward standardized quality assurance and quality control programmes in radiography and radiology include not only the audit of equipment but also working practices. The science and art of image production form the cornerstone for these working practices where radiographic skills and image quality lead to the provision of a caring, quality service. This book will help the development and continuation of this programme by affording detailed information on a wide range of imaging procedures for radiographers, including positioning and procedural protocols, as well as image acceptance criteria. A major feature of this book is the systematic chronological presentation of its content which makes it a boon to both the new and experienced practitioner as well as those studying for a radiography degree or involved in the first year of the FRCR examination.

Elizabeth Unett and Amanda Royle are experienced radiographers and educationists in imaging sciences. They have both played a major role in the development of clinical education programmes for diploma and undergraduate radiography students. Amanda Royle is now a Clinical Superintendent in Chester, Elizabeth Unett a Clinical Teacher at the Department of Radiographic Studies, Keele University. I applaud them for this book and I am confident that it will prove to be a great asset and friend to all those who use it.

Dr Richard W. DeCann. MSc PhD TDCR SRR
Principal (Continuing Education)
North Staffordshire Health Authority
Department of Radiographic Studies
Keele University
UK

Acknowledgements

The authors would like to thank the following people: the teaching staff, secretaries and students of the Department of Radiographic Studies, Keele University, for their interest and support during the writing of this book; the staff of the Imaging Departments of the Royal Shrewsbury and North Staffordshire Hospitals and the Department of Oral Surgery, North Staffordshire Hospital, for the use of equipment; Siemens UK for permission to use equipment in photography; John Payne for his patient and hard work in producing the photographs; Ian Simcock, Alexandra Unett and Ann Pepper for their cooperation while modelling; IGE Ltd for the provision of photographs for the mammography section; Mike Head of Heads; Susan Taberner and Dr Sylvia Aldridge for invaluable work on the barium enema and venography sections; the radiographers at the North Staffordshire Hospital, Royal Shrewsbury Hospital and Hanley Breast Screening Unit, Stoke on Trent, for their comments on the chapter on mammography; Anne Shaw, Tim Reynolds, Paul Ashcroft and Paul Renton; Pam Brown for her encouragement; Jo Campling for her infectious enthusiasm and support; Paul Kingston, Keele University; John and Sheila Copeland; Sean Royle, Ian Unett and our families for their patience and understanding.

Glossary of terms

Terms used for radiography of the skull are included in the relevant chapter.

Abduct/abduction
To move a limb away from the midline

Adduct/adduction
To move a limb towards the midline

Anterior
Relates to the front of the body/body part

Anteroposterior
Describes the direction of the X-ray beam travelling through the body from front to back

Anterior oblique
The anterior aspect of the patient is towards the cassette or bucky, with rotation to the left or right. A right anterior oblique has the right side nearest the cassette and a left anterior oblique has the left side nearest the cassette

Axial
Describes the direction of the X-ray beam travelling through the body from above to below, or vice versa.

Buccal/labial
On outer side of the dental arch, between the teeth and cheeks or lips. Used in dental radiography

Caudal
Towards the lower body, usually describing beam angulation towards the feet

Coronal plane
An imaginary plane, at 90° to the MSP, dividing the front and back of the body

Cranial
Towards the head. Often used to describe beam angulation towards the head

Craniocaudal
Describes the direction of the X-ray beam travelling from the upper to the lower aspect of the body (mainly used in mammography)

Decubitus
The patient is lying down with the cassette supported vertically and the X-ray beam horizontal

Distal
(a) Away from the trunk
(b) Following the dental arch in a posterior direction, outwards and away from the MSP

Dorsipalmar
Describes the direction of the X-ray beam travelling through the hand from the back to the palm

Dorsiplantar
Describes the direction of the X-ray beam travelling through the foot from the top to the sole

Dorsum
The posterior aspect of the hand or upper surface of the foot.

Erect
The patient is upright, sitting or standing

Extension
(a) The straightening of a joint
(b) Bending backwards with reference to the vertebral column

External
(a) Outside the body
(b) Outside/lateral, referring to rotation of a limb

Flexion
(a) Bending of a joint
(b) Bending forwards with reference to the vertebral column

Inferior
Below/under

Inferosuperior
Describes the direction of the X-ray beam travelling from the lower to the upper aspect of the area under examination

Internal
(a) Inside the body
(b) Inwards/medial, referring to rotation of a limb

Labial
See Buccal

Lateral
(a) The outer side of the body or limb
(b) Away from median sagittal plane
(c) External rotation of a limb

Lateromedial
Describes the direction of the X-ray beam travelling from the lateral to the medial aspect of the body part

Lingual/palatal
On the inner side of the dental arch, between the teeth and tongue. Used in dental radiography

Lordosis/lordotic
Leaning backwards

Medial
(a) Towards the median sagittal plane
(b) Internal rotation of a limb
(c) Inner side of a limb

Median sagittal plane
An imaginary plane which divides the body vertically into the left and right halves

Mediolateral
Describes the direction of the X-ray beam travelling from the medial to the lateral aspect of the body part

Mesial
Following the dental arch in an anterior direction, inwards and towards the MSP

Midaxillary line
An imaginary line midway between the anterior and posterior aspects of the thorax, coincident with the axilla

Midclavicular line
An imaginary line travelling down the trunk coincident with the midpoint of the clavicle.

Oblique
The body or limb is rotated to some degree

Occlusal planes
Upper: An imaginary line lying parallel to, and 4 cm below, the line adjoining the tragus of the ear and the ala of the nose. Often referred to as THE occlusal plane
Lower: In the open mouth, an imaginary line lying parallel to, and 2 cm below, the line adjoining the tragus of the ear and the corner of the mouth. The lower occlusal plane will coincide with the upper occlusal plane when the lips and teeth are closed

Palatal
See lingual

Palmar
Relates to the palm of the hand

Plantar
Relates to the sole of the foot

Posterior
Refers to the back of the body/body part
Posteroanterior
Describes the direction of the X-ray beam travelling through the body from back to front
Posterior oblique
The posterior aspect of the patient is towards the cassette or bucky, with rotation to the left or right. A right posterior oblique has the right side nearest the cassette and a left posterior oblique has the left side nearest the cassette
Pronation/pronated
Used in reference to the upper limb when the forearm is internally rotated to bring the palm of the hand and anterior aspect of the limb into contact with the table or cassette
Prone
The patient is lying face down
Proximal
Towards the trunk
Screening
Fluoroscopy
Superior
Above
Superoinferior
Describes the direction of the X-ray beam travelling from the upper to the lower aspect of the area under examination
Supination
Used in reference to the upper limb, when the forearm is externally rotated to bring the dorsum of the hand and posterior aspect of the limb into contact with the table or cassette
Supine
The patient is lying on their back

Abbreviations

A-C	Acromioclavicular
AFM	After fatty meal
AP	Anteroposterior
ASIS	Anterior, superior, iliac spine(s)
A-O	Atlanto-occipital
BDA	British Dental Association
C1–7	Cervical vertebra(e) 1–7
CC	Craniocaudal
cm	Centimetre(s)
DP	Dorsiplantar/dorsipalmar
DPO	Dorsiplantar/palmar oblique
EAM	External auditory meatus/meati
EOP	External occipital protuberance
FFD	Focus–film distance
FOD	Focus–object distance
FB	Foreign body
FO	Fronto-occipital
G	Gauge
I	Iodine
IOFB	Intraocular foreign body
IAM	Internal auditory meatus/meati
kg	Kilogram(s)
KUB	Kidneys, ureters and bladder
kVp	Kilovoltage peak
L1–5	Lumbar vertebra(e) 1–5
LAO	Left anterior oblique
LPO	Left posterior oblique
mAs	Milliampere-seconds
mg	Milligram(s)
ml	Millilitre(s)
mm	Millimetre(s)

MSP	Median sagittal plane
μmol	Micromole(s)
NRPB	National Radiological Protection Board
OFD	Object–film distance
OF	Occipitofrontal
OM	Occipitomental
OMBL	Orbitomeatal baseline
OPT/OPG	Orthopantomography
PA	Posteroanterior
PSIS	Posterior, superior, iliac spine(s)
RAO	Right anterior oblique
RPO	Right posterior oblique
SMV	Submentovertical
S-C	Sternoclavicular
S-I	Sacroiliac
SIJ	Sacroiliac joint
T1–12	Thoracic vertebra(e) 1–12
TMJ	Temporomandibular joint(s)

Introduction

AIMS OF THIS BOOK

The main aim of this book is to provide a user-friendly text which will give both instruction for radiographic examination of patients and reference for evaluation of the image produced. Although the idea of an 'instruction manual' may appear at odds with the evaluative philosophy of an honours degree, this text will at times consider and evaluate techniques in order to encourage synthesis and evaluation. An additional comment might be that students in particular need to be introduced to the skills of radiographic technique before they can undertake any form of evaluation.

The method used for technique descriptions has been selected as a logical approach to the skills of the radiographer, breaking tasks down into one-step instructions and making it relevant to actual practice, e.g. the suggestion for masking off cassettes in order to include multiple projections on one film, which is frequently carried out but never documented. Students using this book as reading material prior to clinical practice may find this approach advantageous. This style has been chosen as a result of discussion with student radiographers, who comment that, although they have access to texts or course notes on radiographic technique, descriptions of action required fail to mention essential preparatory steps, such as centring an X-ray tube to a bucky, or seldom offer tips for successful practice. Of course qualified radiographers will always pass on useful hints for successful practice, but a reliable text which offers information of this type will ensure that the information is available to all.

EXAMINATIONS INCLUDED

Routine radiographic examinations of the skeleton and viscera are included, with the addition of some contrast examinations. The topics selected are intended to reflect those examinations which require the radiographer to actually position the patient and make the radiographic exposure. This explains why the sialogram is included but the angiogram is not: radiographers position the patient for sialographic images but are more involved with procedures which assist the radiologist for arteriography, although this assistance does require a highly skilled contribution. Specialist areas (CT, MRI, RNI, ultrasound) have not been included since excellent texts, by recognized authors in the relevant field, are available. These are also areas which are not practised by students in such great depth as general radiographic procedures. However, as the frequency of use of CT and MRI continue to increase, they surely will eventually be considered 'mainstream' in the future.

One area selected for inclusion which can be considered to be 'specialist' is mammography. This has been included, with an introductory approach to the skill, after discussions with radiographers showed that many radiographers undertook this examination on symptomatic women, although they were less frequently involved in breast screening programmes. The barium enema and venogram examinations may also be deemed 'specialized' but have been included, again with an introductory approach, as examinations which are increasingly being carried out by radiographers; to omit them would have outdated this book before its publication.

IMAGE EVALUATION

As far as the authors are aware, all aspects of image evaluation have not been covered thoroughly by any text to date. Since evaluation is necessary for every image produced and is considered to be an important part of reject film analysis, it seems strange that it appears to be almost totally ignored in texts covering quality assurance in radiography. Indeed, the transmission of required information on image evaluation seems to rely almost exclusively on verbal communication between radiographers and students or lecturer and students. It is, however, more specifically referred to by the WHO document on Quality Criteria for Radiographic Images (1990), but only with regard to the chest, cranium, lumbar spine, urinary tract and breast.

The image evaluation sections in this book will be of value to all within the profession, whether student, radiographer or radiology registrar, being particularly useful for setting of image standard criteria for use in conjunction with reject film analysis. Those involved in mentorship schemes will find it to be a useful and consistent reference. It should be mentioned that evaluation lists provide information regarding the 'perfect' image, and patient condition, reasons for examination request and radiation protection considerations will affect the decision to accept or reject a slightly less than perfect film.

RADIATION PROTECTION

Radiation protection is referred to wherever relevant, whether it be the application of a lead–rubber waist apron or carrying out a projection in a position which aims to reduce the absorbed dose to radiosensitive organs, e.g. using occipitofrontal skull projections wherever possible. Lead–rubber gonad protection is conventionally applied to the body facing the X-ray tube and primary beam.

Individual departments may vary from this convention, in particular with respect to radiography of the chest. In this instance, an alternative school of thought believes that the greater radiation hazard comes from the scattered radiation reflected back from the equipment, e.g. chest stand, and striking the aspect of the body facing away from the X-ray tube. To this end, instructions for the application of lead–rubber gonad protection do not specify which aspect of the body they are to cover; this will be dependent on individual department practice.

OTHER PRACTICAL METHODS FOR RADIATION PROTECTION

1. Selection of the fastest film/screen combination available to adequately demonstrate the area under examination.
2. Use of the highest possible mA in conjunction with the shortest possible exposure time. This will reduce the chance of patient movement/breathing during exposure, and therefore the necessity for repeat exposures. If the patient is restless, increasing the kVp by 10 will allow the (mAs), and therefore exposure time, to be halved.
3. Explaining the procedure to the patient will ensure their cooperation and have the same effect as above.
4. Collimating strictly to the area under examination. With the exception of a few extremity projections, the primary beam should never fall outside the area of the cassette. In those cases where it does, owing to the centring point in relation to the body part, lead–rubber sheeting should be used to absorb the excess primary radiation.

EXPOSURE FACTORS

The exposure factors selected by the radiographer – kVp, mA, time (seconds) – affect the quality of the radiograph produced. When assessing a radiograph for correct exposure the radiographer is actually checking that the X-ray beam has adequately penetrated the body part and that sufficient radiation has reached the film, so producing the required image density. Beam penetration is governed by kVp – higher kVp = greater penetration – and image density/blackening is dependent on mAs – higher mAs = 'blacker' image. The optimum values of both kVp and mAs, with respect to the area under examination and patient size, must be selected if a diagnostic image is to be produced. A radiographic image is made up of innumerable shades of grey, ranging from white-grey at one end of the scale to black-grey at the opposite end. The mAs value will dictate where the range of greys included on a particular image are located on this white-black grey scale, and the kVp will dictate the width of the band of greys to be included within the image. The effects of kVp on the image are caused by the differential absorption of X-radiation by different structures (bone, soft tissue, muscle, fluid etc.) within the body. Higher kVp values will reduce this differential absorption and therefore image contrast (difference between the dark and light areas), and will allow a wider range of densities, e.g. bone and soft tissue detail, to be demonstrated on a single image. The resultant image will be 'flat' with an overall 'greyness'. Lower kVp values will enhance this differential absorption and increase the image contrast, demonstrating a narrower range of densities (greys) on the image, e.g. soft tissues alone. The resultant image will be more black/white than grey.

GENERAL GUIDE TO EXPOSURE FAULTS

Dark image   – overall grey = kVp too high
             – overall black = mAs too high.

Light image   – outline of structures visible, i.e.
              adequate penetration = mAs too low
              – outline of structures not visible, i.e.
              inadequate penetration = kVp too low.

This is a very simplistic guide and it must be remembered that incorrect exposure is often due to a combination of the above points.

When X-raying a patient through a plaster cast, a cause of severe image artefacts, the radiographer has two options:

1. Use a detailed film/screen combination so as to maximize image definition. This 'slower' system will require a significant increase in the exposure factors used when the body part is not in plaster.
2. Use a fast film/screen combination, as the loss of image definition due to the speed of the system will only add a little to that caused by the plaster cast. This 'faster' system will allow a reduction in the exposure factors, maybe even below those used to X-ray the part when not in plaster.

RADIOGRAPHY ON THE WARD AND IN THEATRE

Mobile radiography should only be carried out when the patient's condition will not allow them to be moved from the ward. To this end the most common examination carried out on the ward is the chest X-ray and, with regard to radiation protection and direction of the X-ray beam, any other mobile examination should be actively discouraged. Where mobile radiography is required, the techniques used are a variation on those used in the radiography department.

Radiography in the operating theatre has been described for peroperative cholangiography only. Orthopaedic techniques require the radiographer to adapt basic projectional knowledge into a fluoroscopic examination and cannot be concisely described in this text. The key to successful performance in the operating theatre is personal confidence and a skin thick enough to deflect any remarks from those who always seem to know exactly how to do your job better than you do.

TOMOGRAPHY

With the advent of CT and MR scanners the demand for conventional tomography has almost disappeared, although it is often still used for IVU patients (Chapter 11). For this reason it has not been included as a separate chapter within this text, but has been discussed, where appropriate, within individual chapters.

FOREIGN BODY DEMONSTRATION

The commonest imaging technique for demonstration of possible foreign bodies is still that of conventional X-ray examination. This is mainly due to the fact that most cases will present via the emergency department, needing early or immediate examination. Since the general rule is to produce two projections at 90° to one another, positioning usually requires PA/AP and lateral projections of the region and thus renders the examination to be relatively 'simple'.

A radio-opaque indicator should be included within the primary beam, in alignment with any visible puncture site, so that the relative position of any opacity may be assessed. It should be noted that a foreign body will, however, not necessarily be located adjacent to the wound, its position being dependent on speed and direction of entry.

A high-definition film/screen combination must be used, with scrupulously clean intensifying screens, in order that small artefacts can be demonstrated and not confused with artefacts found inside dirty cassettes. As image quality is of paramount importance, exposure factors should be carefully selected in order to demonstrate the foreign body in contrast to the surrounding body tissues. Examinations which merit special reference are included in the relevant chapters, for example intraocular foreign body appears with radiographic technique for the orbits, and ingestion/inhalation of foreign bodies is found in the chapter on the abdomen.

Upper limb

1

FINGERS

RADIOGRAPHIC TECHNIQUE

Posteroanterior – all fingers

The patient sits with the affected side next to the table. For radiation protection purposes the legs must not be placed under the table and a lead–rubber sheet is applied to the lower abdomen and upper thighs. An 18×24 cm cassette is masked off lengthwise with lead–rubber in order to use the film for two projections. The forearm is pronated with the palmar aspect of the hand in contact with the cassette and the proximal interphalangeal joint of the finger under examination coincident with the centre of the unmasked area of cassette. The long axis of the finger is parallel to the long axis of the cassette. The fingers are extended and slightly separated (Figure 1.5a demonstrates the pronated hand and fingers as used in this projection, but does not illustrate specific position of the cassette or centring).

> CENTRING: A vertical central ray, at 90° to the cassette, is centred over the proximal interphalangeal joint of the finger under examination.

Collimate to include phalanges, head of associated metacarpal and surrounding soft tissues. Apply an AP anatomical marker within the primary beam.

Lateral

The lead–rubber sheet is moved on to the exposed half of the cassette.

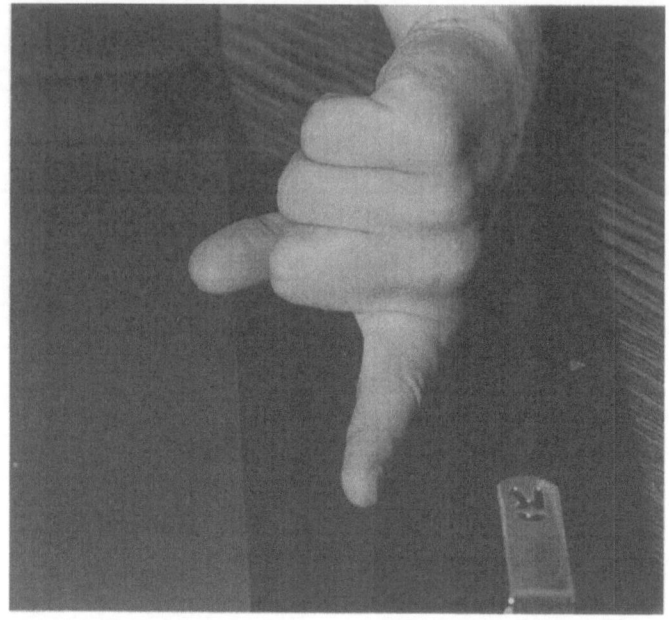

(a)

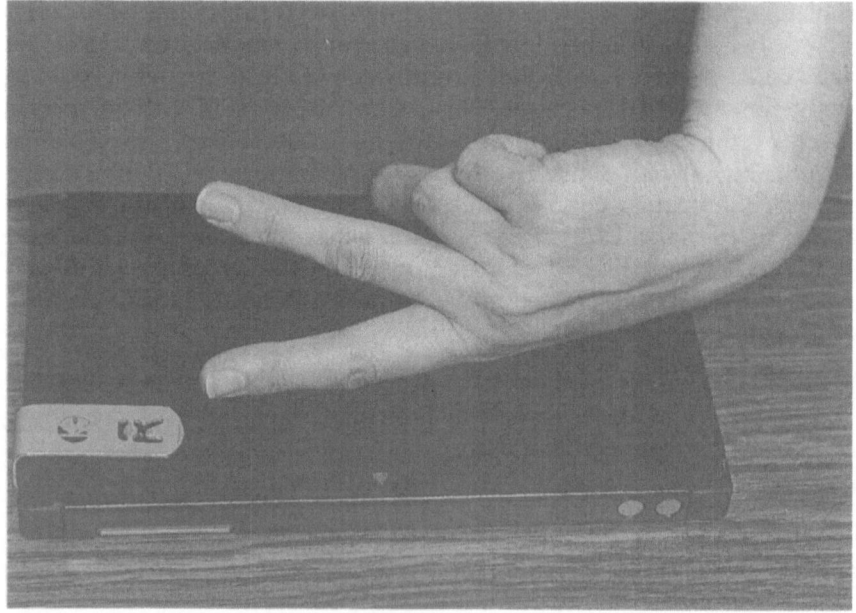

(b)

Figure 1.1 (a) Lateral index finger. (b) Lateral second finger.

Index finger (Fig. 1.1a)

The patient flexes the other fingers into the palm of the hand, immobilizing by folding the thumb across them. The lateral aspect of the index finger is placed in contact with the unmasked portion of the cassette.

Middle finger (Fig. 1.1b)

The patient flexes the ring and little finger into the palm of the hand, immobilizing by folding the thumb across them. The lateral aspect of the second metacarpal is placed in contact with the cassette and the middle finger supported on a radiolucent pad to ensure that it is parallel to the cassette.

Ring finger (Fig. 1.2a)

It is more difficult to clear the other fingers from the ring finger when undertaking a lateral projection. Some patients are able to clasp the flexed fingers as for the index finger. Alternatively, the patient should 'fan out' all four fingers and maintain separation by using radiolucent pads between them. When adequate separation has been achieved, the medial aspect of the hand is placed in contact with the cassette and the ring finger supported on a radiolucent pad to ensure that it is parallel to the cassette.

Little finger (Fig. 1.2b)

The medial aspect of the hand is placed in contact with the cassette and the little finger extended. The remaining fingers are folded into the palm of the hand and held there by the thumb. Alternatively, dorsiflexion of the other fingers and thumb will improve visualization of the proximal phalanx and metacarpophalangeal joint.

The proximal interphalangeal joint is placed over the centre of the available area of cassette, with the long axis of the finger coincident with the long axis of the cassette.

    CENTRING: A vertical central ray, at 90° to the cassette, is directed over the proximal interphalangeal joint of the finger under examination.

Collimate to include phalanges, head of associated metacarpal and surrounding soft tissues. Apply an AP anatomical marker within the primary beam if not included on the PA projection.

IMAGE EVALUATION

Correct patient identification and anatomical marker included on the radiograph.

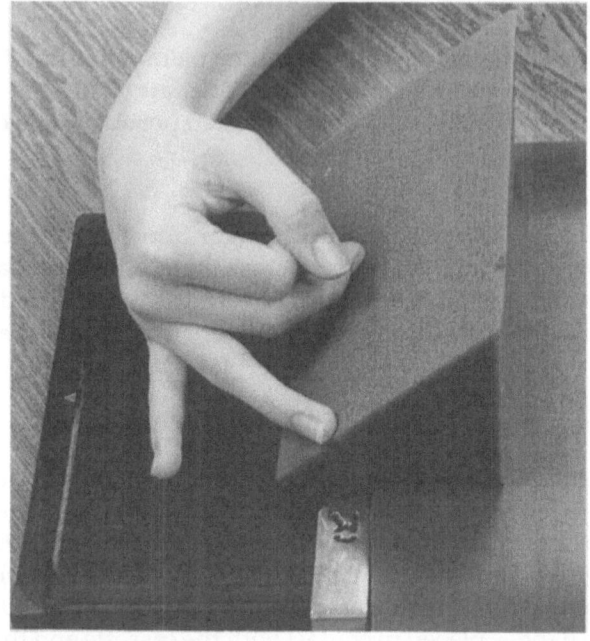

(a)

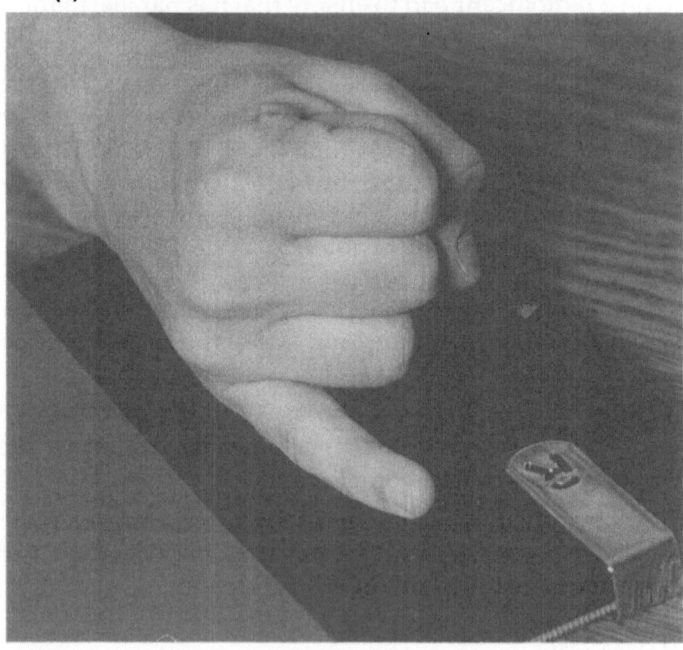

(b)

Figure 1.2 (a) Lateral ring finger. (b) Lateral little finger.

Area of interest

Posteroanterior and lateral

Head of metacarpal, distant phalanx and soft tissue outlines.

Projection

Posteroanterior

• Symmetry of medial and lateral aspects of heads and bases of phalanges.
• Separation of heads of metacarpals.

Lateral

• Superimposition of condyles of heads of phalanges.
• Superimposition of heads of metacarpals.

Posteroanterior and lateral

• Metacarpophalangeal and interphalangeal joints clearly demonstrated.
• Adjacent fingers separated from finger under examination, particularly in the LATERAL in order to demonstrate base of proximal phalanx.

Exposure factors

• kVp sufficient to demonstrate bony trabeculae and any sesamoid bones below heads of metacarpals in the PA projection, maintaining contrast between bony and soft tissue structures.
• mAs to provide adequate image density to demonstrate bony detail in contrast to the surrounding soft tissues.

No evidence of patient movement.
No artefacts present on the image.

THUMB

RADIOGRAPHIC TECHNIQUE

Lateral (Fig. 1.3a)

The patient sits with the affected side next to the table. For radiation protection purposes the legs must not be placed under the table and a lead–rubber sheet is applied to the lower abdomen and upper thighs. An

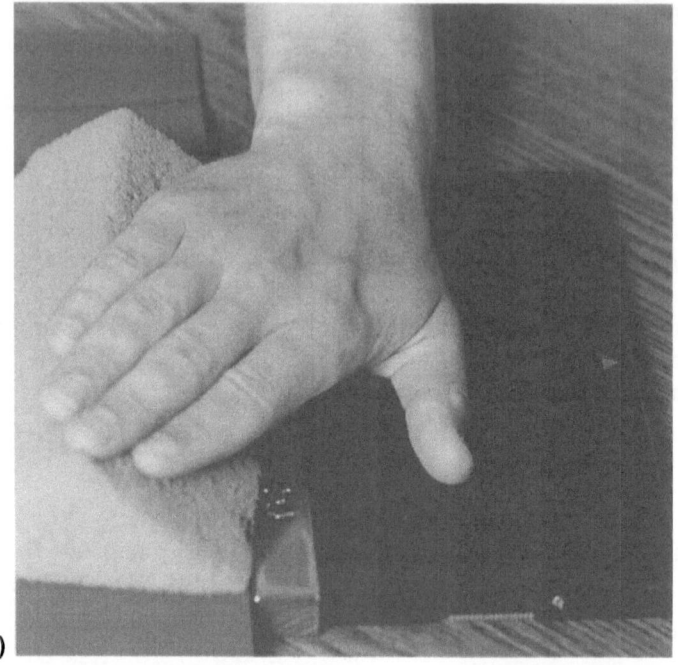

(a)

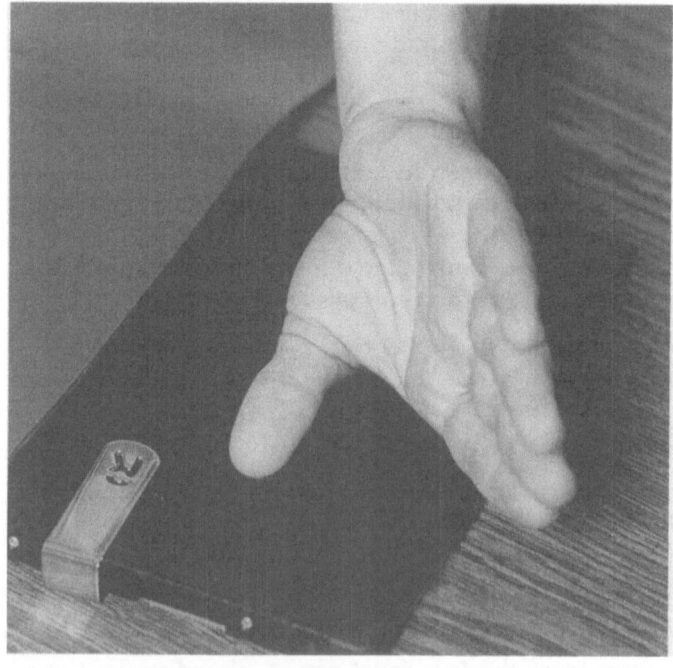

(b)

Figure 1.3 (a) Lateral thumb. (b) AP thumb.

18×24 cm cassette is masked off lengthwise with lead–rubber in order to use the film for two projections. The hand is pronated with the first metacarpophalangeal joint coincident with the midpoint of the un-exposed side of the cassette. The long axis of the thumb is coincident with the long axis of the cassette. The fingers are separated from the thumb and the forearm is internally rotated to lift the palm of the hand away from the cassette, thus bringing the thumb into a lateral position. Immobiliz-ation is achieved with a radiolucent pad placed under the palmar aspect of the hand.

CENTRING: A vertical central ray, at 90° to the cassette, is directed over the first metacarpophalangeal joint.

Collimate to include phalanges, first metacarpal, trapezium and sur-rounding soft tissues. Apply an AP anatomical marker within the primary beam.

Anteroposterior (Fig 1.3b)

The lead–rubber sheet is moved on to the exposed half of the cassette. This projection is most easily achieved with the patient sitting with their back to the table. A lead–rubber apron is applied behind the patient's lower abdomen as radiation protection. The affected arm is extended backwards over the table. The arm is internally rotated and the posterior aspect of the thumb brought into contact with the unmasked half of the cassette. The fingers and second–fifth metacarpals are cleared from the thumb and first metacarpal. The first metacarpophalangeal joint is coincident with the centre of the available area of cassette, the long axis of the thumb parallel to the long axis of the cassette.

CENTRING: A vertical central ray, at 90° to the cassette, is directed over the first metacarpophalangeal joint.

Collimate to include phalanges, metacarpal, trapezium and surrounding soft tissues. Apply an AP anatomical marker within the primary beam if not included on the lateral projection.

Posteroanterior

May be used when the patient is in a plaster cast, or when injury prevents positioning for the routine AP projection.

The patient sits with the affected side next to the table as for the lateral projection. The lead–rubber sheet is moved on to the exposed half of the cassette. The forearm is externally rotated until the palm of the hand is at 90° to the cassette, and the medial aspect of the hand and little finger in contact with it. The thumb is moved clear of the palm of the hand, its long

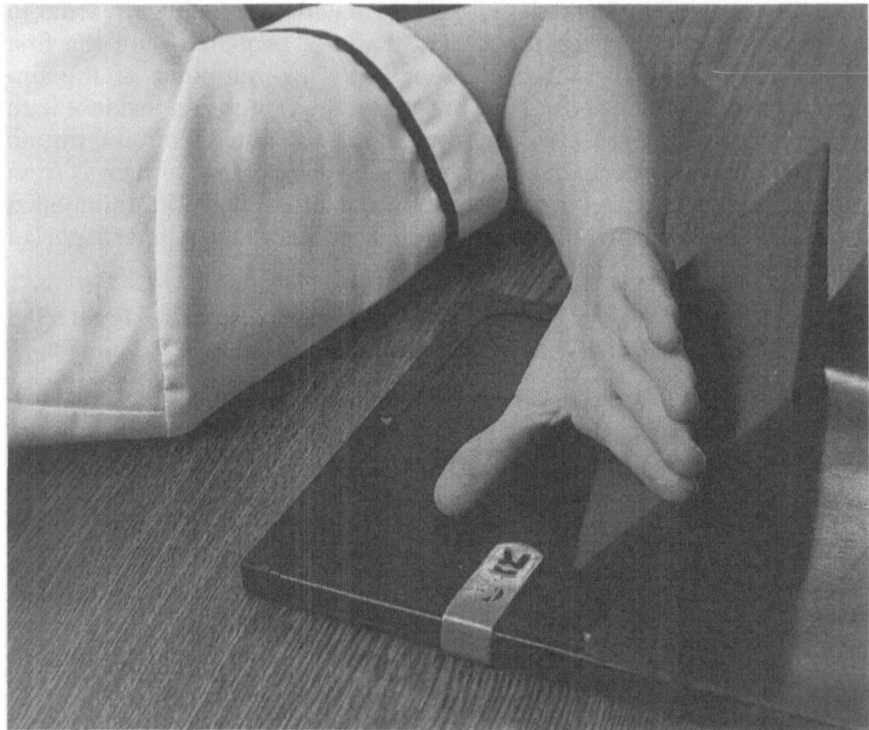

Figure 1.4 Patient supine to achieve AP thumb projection.

axis parallel to the long axis of the cassette. The middle of the available area of cassette is coincident with the first metacarpophalangeal joint. A radiolucent pad placed under the thumb and thenar eminence will aid immobilization.

CENTRING: A vertical central ray, at 90° to the cassette, is directed over the first metacarpophalangeal joint.

Collimate to include phalanges, metacarpal, trapezium and surrounding soft tissues. Although this is a PA projection it is customary to apply an AP anatomical marker within the primary beam if not included on the lateral projection.

Obtaining and maintaining patient position for the AP projection described can be difficult with the elderly or injured, and the PA may be considered unacceptable owing to image magnification and unsharpness (although this can be reduced with an increase in FFD). There is also an element of hypothenar shadowing, which partially obscures the base of the first metacarpal in the AP or PA projections.

One solution to the problem of hypothenar shadowing is to position the thumb as for the AP projection described above, but with a vertical central ray directed 10–15° along the long axis of the thumb, towards the wrist, over the first metacarpophalangeal joint (Lewis, 1988).

Many patients find the AP position difficult to achieve and in these circumstances an adaptation of the method described by Richmond (1995) may be considered:

AP thumb – patient supine (Fig 1.4)

The patient lies supine on the table. A lead–rubber sheet is applied to the thorax as radiation protection. An 18×24 cm cassette rests on the table top, level with the patient's head and on the affected side. The cassette is moved across the table as far from the head as possible. The affected arm is flexed at the elbow and the forearm rotated until the dorsum of the thumb comes into contact with the cassette. The thumb and fingers are separated and immobilization achieved with a radiolucent pad placed beneath the dorsum of the hand. The first metacarpophalangeal joint is over the centre of the cassette, the long axis of the thumb parallel to the long axis of the cassette. The head is turned away from the side under examination.

CENTRING: A vertical central ray is directed over the first metacarpophalangeal joint.

Collimation and marker as for the routine AP projection.

Richmond's original description has the patient erect with the thumb positioned against a vertical cassette. The authors describe the technique here with the patient supine, as they feel that immobilization of the limb is more certain. The possibility of increased dose to radiosensitive organs of the head and thorax is considered by Richmond, and experiments using a phantom show a negligible effect.

IMAGE EVALUATION

Correct patient identification and anatomical marker included on the radiograph.

Area of interest

Distal phalanx, metacarpal, trapezium and soft tissue outlines.

Projection

Lateral

• Superimposition of medial and lateral aspects of heads of phalanges and metacarpal.

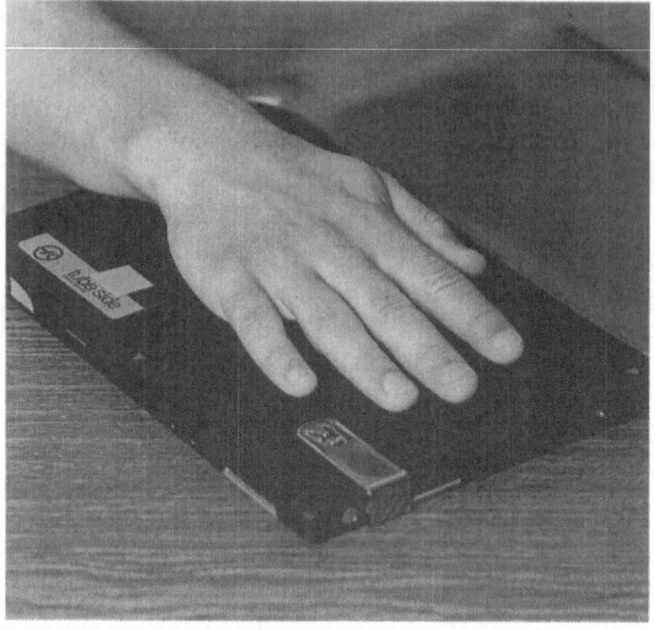

(a)

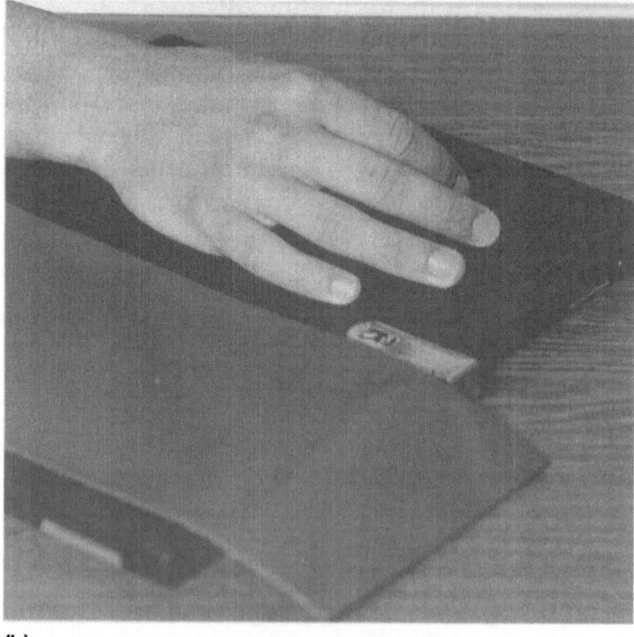

(b)

Figure 1.5 (a) Dorsipalmar hand and fingers. (b) Dorsipalmar oblique hand.

- Base of metacarpal and carpometacarpal joint clearly visualized, with no overlapping of base of second metacarpal.

Anteroposterior/posteroanterior

- Symmetry of medial and lateral aspects of heads of phalanges.
- Metacarpophalangeal and interphalangeal joint spaces clearly demonstrated.
- Clear carpometacarpal joint space, with no foreshortening of the image of metacarpal.

Exposure factors

- kVp sufficient to demonstrate bony trabeculae and any sesamoid bones below the head of metacarpal in the AP/PA projection, maintaining contrast between the bones and surrounding soft tissues.
- mAs to provide adequate image density to demonstrate bony detail in contrast to the joint spaces and soft tissues.

No evidence of patient movement.
No artefacts present on the image.

HAND

RADIOGRAPHIC TECHNIQUE

Dorsipalmar (Fig. 1.5a)

The patient is seated with the affected side next to the table. For radiation protection purposes the legs must not be placed under the table and a lead–rubber sheet is applied to the lower abdomen and upper thighs. A 24×30 cm cassette is masked off widthways with lead–rubber in order that two projections may be included on one film. The palmar aspect of the affected hand is placed in contact with the cassette, the head of the third metacarpal coincident with the centre of the unmasked area, the long axis of the cassette parallel to the long axis of the third metacarpal and forearm. The fingers are extended and slightly separated.

CENTRING: A vertical central ray, at 90° to the cassette, is directed over the head of the 3rd metacarpal.

Collimate to include phalanges, metacarpals, wrist joint and surrounding soft tissues. Apply an AP anatomical marker within the primary beam.

An alteration to the almost universally accepted positioning for the DP hand – that of the whole of the plantar aspect being in contact with the cassette – has been considered. A hand placed in this position will actually cause obliquity over the thumb and increasing obliquity from the second to fifth metacarpals (Lewis, 1988). Lewis suggests slight elevation of the medial aspect of the hand on to a radiolucent pad to rectify this, and this method can be considered to be an excellent alternative, with the disadvantage being the slight increase in OFD over the raised area of the hand. Since radiologists are most familiar with the appearances found on the traditional method, this is the one described in this text.

Dorsipalmar oblique (Fig. 1.5b)

The lead–rubber sheet is moved onto the exposed half of the cassette. From the DP position the hand and wrist are externally rotated through 45°. The medial aspect of the hand is in contact with the cassette and the lateral aspect supported by a radiolucent pad. The fingers are separated and relaxed. The head of the third metacarpal is coincident with the middle of the unexposed half of the cassette, the long axis of the cassette parallel to the long axis of the third metacarpal and forearm.

CENTRING: 1. A vertical central ray, at 90° to the cassette, is centred over the head of the third metacarpal.
  2. A vertical central ray is directed over the head of the fifth metacarpal and then angled across the hand, towards the thumb, until centred over the head of the third metacarpal.

Collimate to include phalanges, metacarpals, wrist joint and surrounding soft tissues. Apply an AP anatomical marker within the primary beam if not included on the DP projection.

Centring for the DPO has traditionally varied from text to text, mainly being the use of a vertical central ray over the head of the fifth metacarpal (Bell & Finlay, 1986), or the angled ray over the head of the third metacarpal (Swallow *et al.*, 1986). When centred over the fifth metacarpal, the oblique rays around the vertical central ray supposedly avoid superimposition of the images of adjacent metacarpals. Unfortunately, this method does not allow stringent collimation to the medial margin of the hand. Centring over the head of the fifth metacarpal and angling to the third will ensure stricter collimation, yet employ the geometry of the angle to separate the images of the metacarpals. However, it should be noted that the long axis of the hand must be at right-angles to the plane of angulation of the X-ray tube, otherwise the direction of angulation will not be correct, leading to some degree of image distortion. Since the actual amount of tube angulation, when using an FFD of 100 cm, can be calculated mathematically to approximately 2°, the validity of its use should be questioned; accurate selection of 2° tube angulation is almost impossible on general X-ray units and, since 2° will have little or no

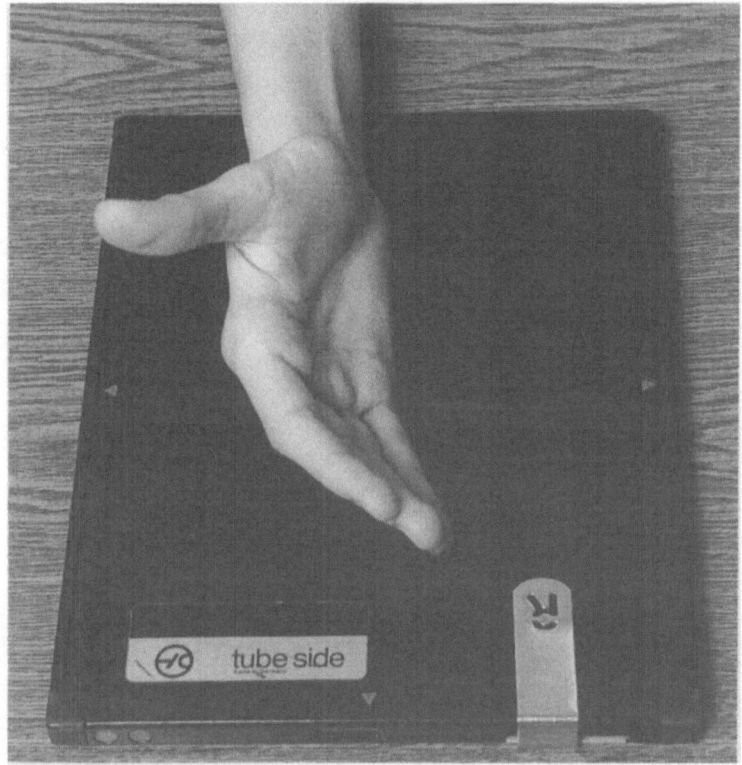

Figure 1.6 Lateral oblique hand – fifth metacarpal fracture displacement demonstration.

perceivable effect on the image, the use of a vertical central ray over the head of the third metacarpal would seem more practical.

In his series of articles on the hand, Lewis highlights his question on the value of the traditional DPO in the demonstration of a **boxer's fracture** of the fifth metacarpal. The metacarpal is seen to be superimposed in part by the fourth metacarpal, and the degree of displacement is difficult to assess. The suggested alternative is as follows:

An 18×24 cm cassette is selected. From the DP position the hand is externally rotated through 95° until the radial and ulnar styloid processes are superimposed. A further 5° external rotation is applied to clear the thenar eminence from the fifth metacarpal and the thumb fully abducted and extended. The head of the fifth metacarpal is coincident with the centre of the cassette, the long axis of the hand parallel to the long axis of the cassette. The palm of the hand is relaxed slightly. A radiolucent pad and sandbag are placed behind the dorsal aspect of the hand to aid immobilization (Fig. 1.6).

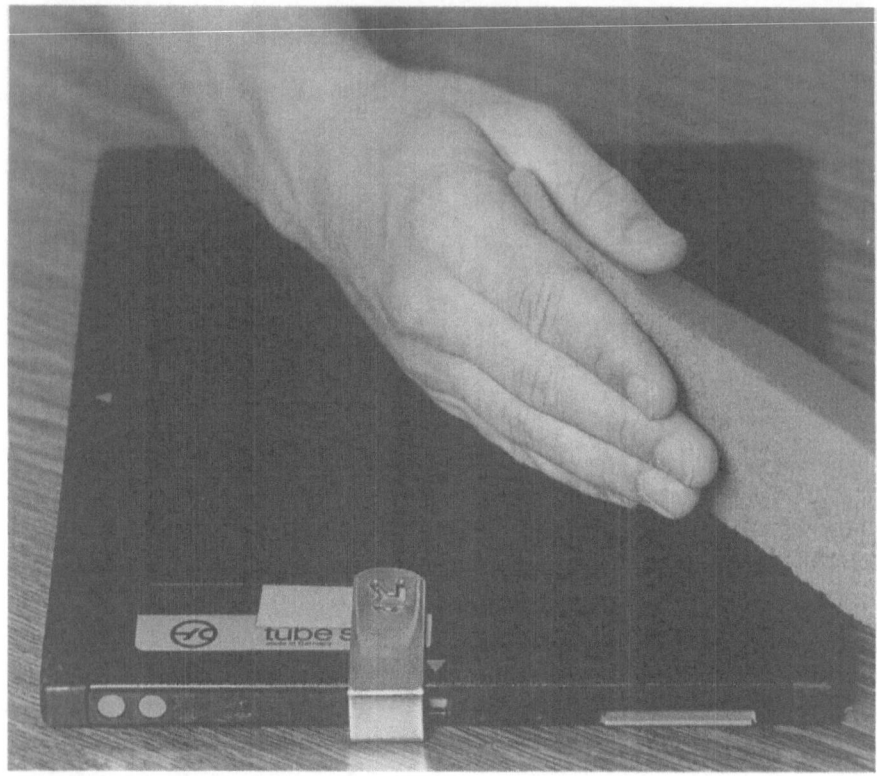

Figure 1.7   Lateral hand.

> CENTRING: A vertical central ray is angled parallel to the long axis of
> the thumb and directed to the middle of the shaft of the
> fifth metacarpal.

Collimate to include phalanges, metacarpals, wrist joint and surrounding
soft tissues. Apply an AP anatomical marker within the primary beam.

Lateral (Fig. 1.7)

This projection is used in addition to the dorsipalmar and dorsipalmar
oblique projections to demonstrate anterior or posterior displacement of
bone fragments in the presence of a fracture. For demonstration of a
foreign body it is used in addition to the DP and instead of the DPO.

An 18×24 cm cassette is selected. From the DP position the hand is
externally rotated through 90° until the medial aspects of hand and forearm
are in contact with the table/cassette. The fingers are extended and the
thumb slightly abducted to prevent its superimposition over the
second–fifth metacarpals and proximal phalanges. The thumb is

supported on a radiolucent pad. The head of the second metacarpal is coincident with the centre of the cassette, the long axis of the hand parallel to the long axis of the cassette. (The cassette may be used diagonally if the patient has large hands.)

> CENTRING: A vertical central ray, at 90° to the cassette and coincident with the line of superimposition of the metacarpals, is centred over the head of the second metacarpal.

Collimate to include phalanges, metacarpals, wrist joint, thumb and surrounding soft tissues. Apply an AP anatomical marker within the primary beam.

When selecting exposure factors for the lateral projection of the hand, the DP/DPO factors should be altered by doubling the mAs and adding approximately 5 kVp.

Rheumatoid arthritis

In this instance it is common practice to irradiate both hands simultaneously on one film. The hands are slightly separated and placed in the DP position with the tips of corresponding fingers level. The vertical X-ray beam is directed midway between the heads of the second metacarpals.

IMAGE EVALUATION

Correct patient identification and anatomical marker included on the radiograph.

Area of interest

Distal radius and ulna, terminal phalanges and soft tissue outlines.

Projection

Dorsipalmar

- Symmetry of medial and lateral aspects of heads of metacarpals 2–4.
- Slight external obliquity of fifth metacarpal and phalanges.
- Metacarpophalangeal and interphalangeal joints clearly demonstrated.
- Separation of adjacent metacarpals and phalanges.
- Oblique projection of thumb.

Dorsipalmar oblique

- Fingers slightly flexed without clear visualization of metacarpophalangeal or interphalangeal joint spaces.

- Separation of shafts of adjacent metacarpals, with slight overlap at heads and bases.
- Separation of adjacent phalanges and soft tissues outlines of fingers.
- Overlap of adjacent carpal bones.

Lateral

- Superimposition of shafts of metacarpals and phalanges 2–5.
- Superimposition of distal radius and ulna.
- First metacarpal and phalanges projected clear of those of fingers 2–5.

Exposure factors

- kVp sufficient to demonstrate bony trabeculae, sesamoid bones below the heads of metacarpals and areas of bony overlap at the bases of metacarpals and within the carpus, with visualization of each individual metacarpal in the LATERAL projection. Contrast is maintained between the bones and surrounding soft tissues of the hand.
- mAs to provide adequate image density to demonstrate bony detail in contrast to soft tissue structures.

No evidence of patient movement.
No artefacts present on the image.

WRIST

RADIOGRAPHIC TECHNIQUE

Posteroanterior (Fig. 1.8a)

An 18×24 cm cassette is masked off widthways with lead–rubber in order that two projections may be included on one film. The patient is seated with the affected side next to the table. For radiation protection purposes the legs must not be placed under the table, and a lead–rubber sheet is applied to the lower abdomen and upper thighs. The elbow is flexed to 90° and the forearm pronated with the anterior aspect of the wrist in contact with the cassette. The midpoint between the radial and ulnar styloid processes is coincident with the centre of the unmasked area of cassette, the long axis of the cassette parallel to the long axis of the forearm. The radial and ulnar styloid processes are equidistant from the cassette. The fingers are slightly flexed to bring the anterior aspect of the wrist into close contact with the cassette.

> CENTRING: A vertical central ray, at 90° to the cassette, is directed to a point midway between the radial and ulnar styloid processes.

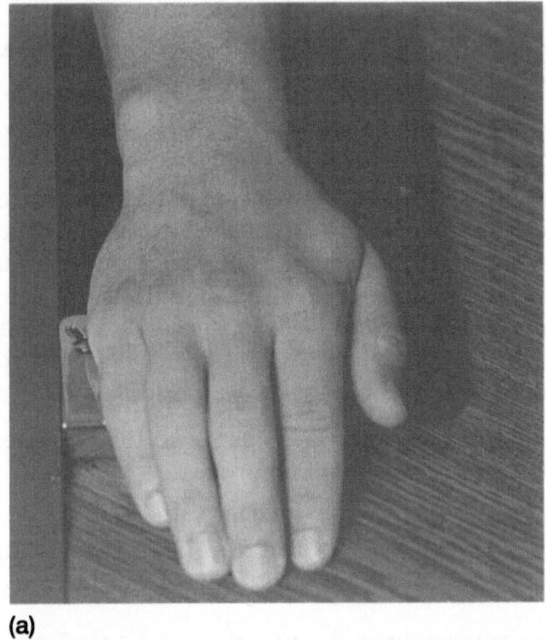

(a)

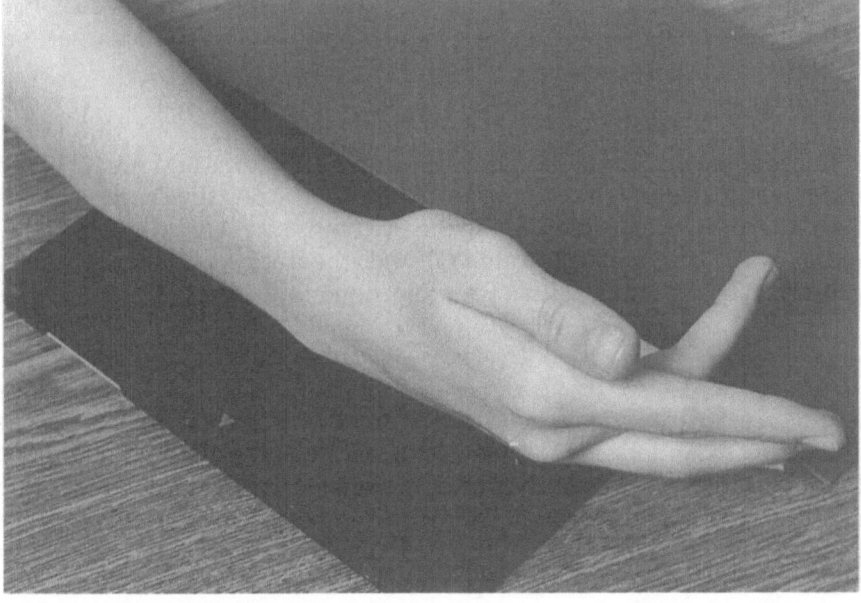

(b)

Figure 1.8 (a) PA wrist. (b) Lateral wrist.

Collimate to include proximal third of metacarpals, wrist joint, lower third of radius and ulna and surrounding soft tissues. Apply an AP anatomical marker within the primary beam.

Lateral (Fig. 1.8b)

The lead–rubber sheet is moved on to the exposed half of the cassette. The arm is abducted, extended at the elbow and externally rotated through 90°. The medial aspect of the forearm and wrist are in contact with the unexposed half of the cassette, the midpoint of this area coincident with the ulnar styloid process, the long axis of the cassette parallel to the long axis of the forearm. The fingers are extended and the wrist adjusted until the radial and ulnar styloid processes are superimposed.

CENTRING: A vertical central ray, at 90° to the cassette, is directed over the radial styloid process.

Collimate to include proximal third of metacarpals, wrist joint, lower third of radius and ulna and surrounding soft tissues. Apply an AP anatomical marker within the primary beam if not included on the PA projection.

As an additional check when positioning for the lateral wrist, instruct the patient to flex the middle finger slightly. If the finger lies parallel to the cassette the radial and ulnar styloid processes will be superimposed. This is not an accurate method of assessment for patients whose wrists are set in plaster in radial or ulnar deviation.

When selecting exposure factors for the lateral projection of the wrist, the PA factors should be altered by doubling the mAs.

In order to produce lateral projections of both radius and ulna the arm must be fully extended at the elbow. If the elbow remains bent, as in the PA projection, the position of the ulna remains unchanged and only the radius will have rotated through 90°, i.e. the image will show a lateral projection of the radius with a PA projection of the ulna.

Posteroanterior oblique (Fig. 1.9.)

An 18×24 cm cassette is selected. From the PA position the arm is abducted, extended at the elbow and externally rotated through 45°. Immobilization is achieved with a radiolucent pad placed under the anterior aspect of the forearm. The centre of the cassette is coincident with the midpoint between the radial and ulnar styloid processes, the long axis of the cassette parallel to the long axis of the forearm.

CENTRING: A vertical central ray, at 90° to the cassette, is directed to a point midway between the radial and ulnar styloid processes.

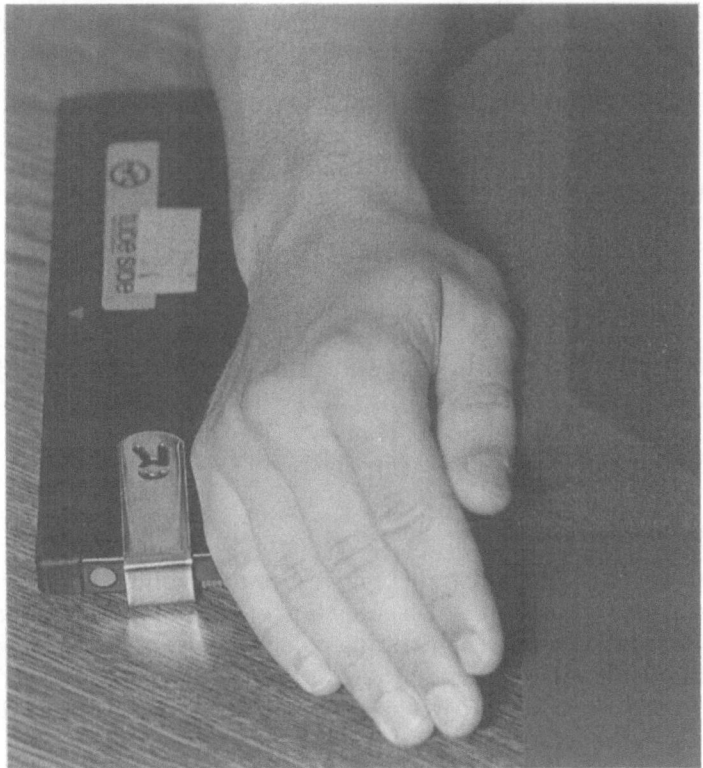

Figure 1.9 Oblique wrist.

Collimate to include proximal third of metacarpals, wrist joint, lower third of radius and ulna and surrounding soft tissues. Apply an AP anatomical marker within the primary beam.

IMAGE EVALUATION

Correct patient identification and anatomical marker included on the radiograph.

Area of interest

Distal third of radius and ulna, proximal third of metacarpals and soft tissue outlines.

Projection

Posteroanterior

- Separation of distal radius and ulna to clearly demonstrate distal radioulnar joint.

- Radial and ulnar styloid processes demonstrated on the lateral and medial aspects of the wrist joint respectively.

Lateral

- Superimposition of distal radius and ulna.
- Superimposition of carpal bones, with lunate demonstrated as a crescent.
- Ulnar styloid process projected in centre of distal surface of ulna.

Posteroanterior oblique

- Slight overlap of distal radius and ulna, obscuring distal radioulnar joint.
- Overlapping of adjacent carpal bones.
- Overlapping of bases of metacarpals.

Exposure factors

- kVp sufficient to demonstrate bony trabeculae within radius, ulna and carpal bones and to enable visualization of each of the carpal bones in areas of bony overlap, maintaining contrast between the bones of the wrist and surrounding soft tissues.
- mAs to provide adequate image density to demonstrate bony detail in contrast to the joint spaces and soft tissue outlines.

No evidence of patient movement.
No artefacts present on the image.

Positional faults

In the LATERAL projection, if the wrist is not sufficiently externally rotated the outline of the distal radius will lie anterior to that of the ulna. If the wrist is externally rotated too far, the outline of the distal radius will lie posterior to that of the ulna.

SCAPHOID

The projections described include all those encountered when examining the scaphoid, and although some imaging departments will utilize all of the five projections, departmental protocols will vary greatly. Indeed, five projections seems a conservative number, since Beamer (1994) discussed as many as 13.

As a scaphoid fracture is rarely demonstrated on X-ray immediately after injury, all patients are treated for fracture of this bone in order to avoid onset of avascular necrosis, and return for further X-ray examination 10–14 days later, when a scaphoid fracture becomes more apparent radiologically owing to demineralization around the fracture site. This presents a scenario where all patients may have up to 10 (or more) X-ray exposures of the area in this short space of time, with additional examinations at regular intervals for those who are found to have this fracture. This should be considered when formulating a departmental routine for scaphoid examination.

The projections demonstrating the scaphoid can be well collimated and therefore accommodated on a 24×30 cm cassette, which is divided into up to four sections by the use of lead–rubber. After each exposure the lead–rubber is repositioned to reveal an unexposed quarter of cassette, and previously exposed areas are covered.

RADIOGRAPHIC TECHNIQUE

Posteroanterior (Fig. 1.10a)

The patient is seated with the affected side next to the table. For radiation protection purposes the legs must not be placed under the table, and a lead–rubber sheet is applied to the lower abdomen and upper thighs. The elbow is flexed to 90° and the anterior aspect of the wrist placed in contact with the first quarter of the cassette, the midpoint between the styloid processes coincident with its centre and the long axis of the forearm parallel to the long axis of the cassette. Slight flexion of the fingers will bring the anterior aspect of the wrist into close contact with the cassette and will ensure that the styloid processes are equidistant from it. The hand is adducted towards the ulna, an action known as 'ulnar deviation', without altering the relationship of the styloid processes to the cassette.

CENTRING: A vertical central ray, at 90° to the cassette, is directed over a point midway between the radial and ulnar styloid processes.

Collimate to include carpal bones, carpometacarpal joints, wrist joint and surrounding soft tissues. Apply an AP anatomical marker within the primary beam.

Ulnar deviation raises the medial aspect of the carpal bones slightly, to bring the scaphoid into a position which is more parallel to the cassette than a conventional PA wrist projection. It will also separate the scaphoid from the other carpal bones and radius.

Posteroanterior oblique/anterior oblique

This projection is similar to the oblique wrist (Fig. 1.9).

From the PA position, the wrist is externally rotated through 45°. The midpoint between the styloid processes is coincident with the centre of the second quarter of the cassette, the long axis of the forearm parallel to

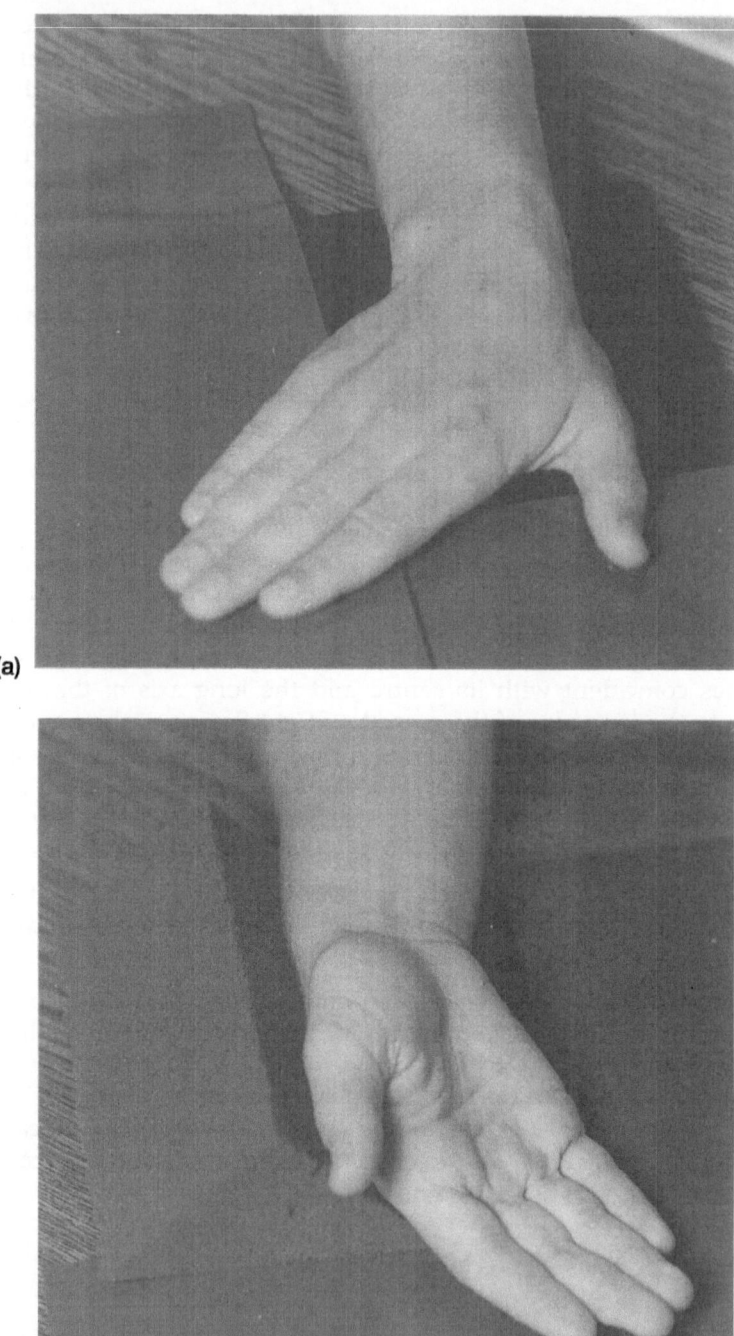

(a)

(b)

Figure 1.10 Scaphoid. (a) PA with ulnar deviation. (b) AP oblique.

the long axis of the cassette. Ulnar deviation is applied to the wrist and a radiolucent pad placed under the anterior aspect of the wrist to aid immobilization.

> CENTRING: A vertical central ray, at 90° to the cassette, is directed over the ulnar styloid process, on the posterior aspect of the wrist.

Collimate to include carpal bones, carpometacarpal joints, wrist joint and surrounding soft tissues.

Lateral

This projection is similar to the lateral wrist (Fig. 1.8b). From the PA oblique position the forearm is externally rotated a further 45° until the radial and ulnar styloid processes are superimposed. The ulnar styloid process is coincident with the centre of the third quarter of the cassette, the long axis of the forearm parallel to the long axis of the cassette. The fingers are extended.

> CENTRING: A vertical central ray, at 90° to the cassette, is directed over the scaphoid bone.

Collimate to include carpal bones, carpometacarpal joints, wrist joint and surrounding soft tissues.

As the area of interest is the scaphoid bone rather than the lower radius and ulna, and as the field size is strictly limited, it is not necessary to straighten the elbow to demonstrate the distal ulna in a lateral projection.

When selecting exposure factors for the lateral projection of the scaphoid, the PA/oblique factors should be altered by doubling the mAs.

Anteroposterior oblique/posterior oblique (Fig. 1.10b)

From the lateral position the arm is extended at the elbow and the hand externally rotated 45° towards supination until the posterior aspect of the ulna is in contact with the cassette. The midpoint of the fourth quarter of the cassette is coincident with the midpoint between styloid processes, the long axis of the forearm parallel to the long axis of the cassette. Ulnar deviation is applied to the wrist and a radiolucent pad placed beneath the posterior aspect of the forearm to aid immobilization.

> CENTRING: A vertical central ray, at 90° to the cassette, is directed over the ulnar styloid process, on the anterior aspect of the wrist.

Collimate to include carpal bones, carpometacarpal joints, wrist joint and surrounding soft tissues.

Posteroanterior 30° with ulnar deviation

This projection may confirm the presence of a fracture and will show better separation of the scaphoid fragments. Its value was highlighted by Groocock (1995) who found it to be the projection in which a definite scaphoid fracture was most likely to be identified.

If carried out in addition to the other four scaphoid projections it may be necessary to use an additional 18×24 cm cassette. However, it can be positioned in the centre of the 24×30 cm cassette if the other four projections are accurately placed.

The patient is positioned as for the PA projection with ulnar deviation (Fig. 1.10a), with the scaphoid bone placed over the centre of the cassette.

> CENTRING: A vertical central ray is directed 30° towards the elbow and over the scaphoid.

The cassette is displaced so that the central X-ray beam, and therefore the image of the scaphoid, is projected on to the centre of the cassette. If the cassette is not displaced at this point, the image of the scaphoid will be projected down over the images in the lower two quarters of the cassette.

Collimate to include the scaphoid bone. Apply an AP anatomical marker within the primary beam if using a separate cassette.

IMAGE EVALUATION

Correct patient identification and anatomical marker included on the radiograph.

Area of interest

All eight carpal bones, distal radius and ulna, bases of metacarpals and soft tissue outlines.

Projection

Posteroanterior with ulnar deviation

- Separation of distal radius and ulna to clearly demonstrate distal radioulnar joint.
- Radial and ulnar styloid processes demonstrated on lateral and medial aspects of wrist joint, respectively.
- Separation of carpal bones with demonstration of the joint spaces around scaphoid through application of ulnar deviation.

- With ulnar deviation the line of first metacarpal should follow that of radius.

Posteroanterior oblique/anterior oblique

- Slight overlapping of bases of metacarpals.
- Overlap of distal radius and ulna, obscuring distal radioulnar joint.
- Separation of scaphoid from adjacent carpal bones with maintenance of ulnar deviation.

Lateral

- Superimposition of distal radius and ulna.
- Superimposition of carpal bones, with lunate projected as a crescent.
- Ulna styloid process demonstrated on posterior aspect of wrist as elbow is flexed.

Anteroposterior oblique/posterior oblique

- Slight overlapping of bases of metacarpals.
- Overlap of distal radius and ulna, obscuring distal radioulnar joint.
- Pisiform projected clear of adjacent carpal bones on anteromedial aspect of wrist.

Posteroanterior 30° with ulnar deviation

- As for PA scaphoid
- Image of scaphoid will be elongated owing to angulation of X-ray beam.

Exposure factors

- kVp sufficient to demonstrate bony trabeculae within the radius, ulna and carpal bones and to enable visualization of each of the carpal bones in areas of bony overlap, maintaining contrast between the carpal bones, joint spaces and surrounding soft tissues.
- mAs to provide adequate image density to demonstrate bony detail in contrast to soft tissue structures.

No evidence of patient movement.
No artefacts present on the image.

RADIOCARPAL JOINT

RADIOGRAPHIC TECHNIQUE

Posteroanterior

The patient position for this projection is similar to that for the PA wrist (Fig. 1.8a).

An 18×24 cm cassette is selected. The patient is seated with the affected side next to the table. For radiation protection purposes the legs must not be placed under the table, and a lead–rubber sheet is applied to the lower abdomen and upper thighs. The elbow is flexed to 90° and forearm pronated with the anterior aspect of the wrist in contact with the cassette. The midpoint between the radial and ulnar styloid processes is coincident with the centre of the cassette, the long axis of the cassette parallel to the long axis of the forearm. The radial and ulnar styloid processes are equidistant from the cassette. The fingers are slightly flexed to bring the anterior aspect of the wrist into close contact with the cassette.

> CENTRING: A vertical central ray is directed 25° towards the elbow, to a point midway between the radial and ulnar styloid processes.

The cassette is displaced so that its centre coincides with the central ray.

Collimate to include proximal third of metacarpals, wrist joint, lower third of radius and ulna and surrounding soft tissues. Apply an AP anatomical marker within the primary beam.

IMAGE EVALUATION

Correct patient identification and anatomical marker included on the radiograph.

Area of interest

Distal third of radius and ulna, proximal third of metacarpals and soft tissue outlines.

Projection

- Separation of distal radius and ulna to demonstrate distal radioulnar joint.
- Radial and ulnar styloid processes demonstrated in profile on lateral and medial aspects of wrist joint, respectively.
- Overlap of metacarpal bases on distal carpal bones and of distal and proximal rows of carpal bones.

● Separation of proximal carpal bones and distal articular surfaces of radius, enabling clear visualization of radiocarpal joint space.

Exposure factors

● kVp sufficient to demonstrate bony trabeculae, maintaining contrast between the bones, adjacent joint spaces and soft tissues outlines.
● mAs to provide adequate image density to demonstrate bony detail in contrast to the surrounding soft tissues.

No evidence of patient movement.
No artefacts present on the image.

CARPAL TUNNEL

RADIOGRAPHIC TECHNIQUE (Fig. 1.11a)

An 18×24 cm cassette is placed on the table top, with its short edge coincident with the edge of the table. A lead–rubber apron is applied to the back of the patient's waist as radiation protection. The patient stands with their back to the table. The affected arm is moved posteriorly and internally rotated until the palm of the hand can be placed in contact with the cassette. The fingers are curled over the edged of the table and cassette, and forced extension of the wrist is carried out by the patient. The forearm should not overlie the area of interest.

> CENTRING: A vertical central ray, at 90° to the cassette, is directed over the anterior aspect of the wrist through the depression formed by the carpal tunnel.

Collimate to include carpal bones, distal radius and ulna, proximal metacarpals and surrounding soft tissues. Apply an AP anatomical marker within the primary beam.

This projection may be too painful for those with carpal tunnel syndrome or degenerative changes in the wrist joint. An alternative method is as follows (Fig. 1.11b):

An 18×24 cm cassette is placed horizontally on a firm support, approximately 15 cm above the table top. The patient is seated, facing the table. For radiation protection purposes the legs must not be placed under the table, and a lead–rubber sheet is applied to the lower abdomen and upper thighs. The affected arm is extended over the table with the forearm pronated and the elbow resting on the table top. The anterior aspect of the forearm rests on the edge of the cassette so that the carpus is coincident with, but does not contact, the centre of the cassette. A bandage is passed around the phalanges and pulled back to extend the

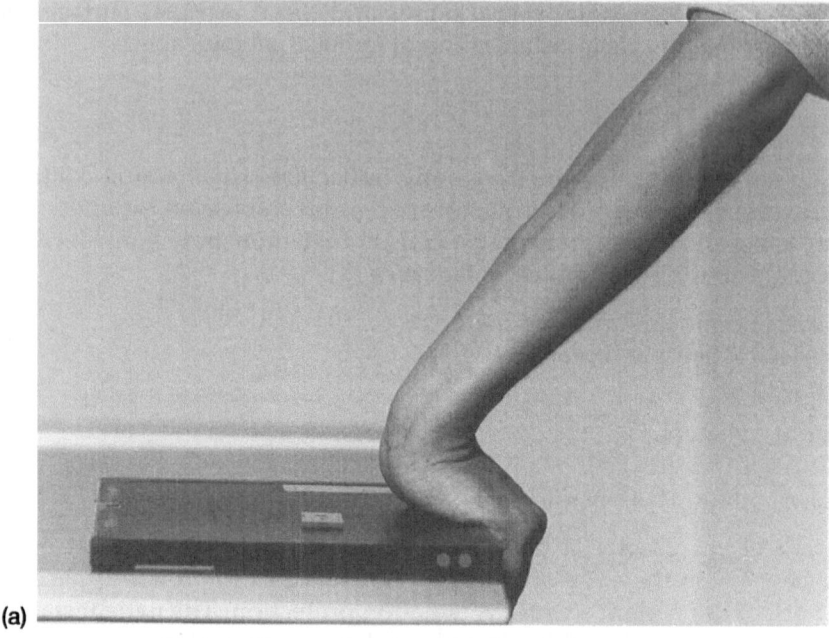

(a)

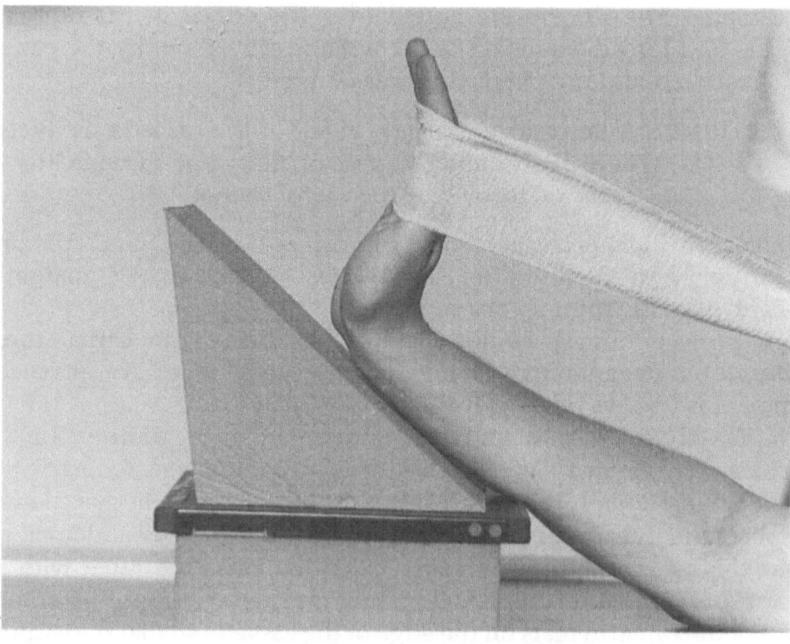

(b)

Figure 1.11 Carpal tunnel. (a) Hand over table edge. (b) Wrist dorsiflexed with crepe bandage.

wrist as far as possible. The patient maintains the position by holding the ends of the bandage with the unaffected hand.

CENTRING: As first method.

Collimation and marker as first method.

Although this method is more easily achieved for some patients, immobilization is more difficult. The increased OFD will result in image magnification and geometric unsharpness, and therefore a compensatory increase in FFD should be considered.

IMAGE EVALUATION

Correct patient identification and anatomical marker included on the radiograph.

Area of interest

Carpal bones, bases of metacarpals, distal radius and ulna and soft tissue outlines.

Projection

- Superimposition of proximal carpal bones on distal carpal bones, and distal radius and ulna on metacarpals.
- Foreshortening along length of metacarpals.
- Hook of hamate and pisiform projected clear of overlying carpal bones on medial aspect of wrist.
- Crest of trapezium and tubercle of scaphoid projected clear of overlying carpal bones on lateral aspect of wrist.
- Carpal tunnel demonstrated as a 'flattened U' anterior to carpal bones.

Exposure factors

- kVp sufficient to demonstrate bony trabeculae within the carpal bones while reducing contrast between the carpal bones and soft tissue area of the carpal tunnel.
- mAs to provide good detail of the soft tissue structures of the carpal tunnel, resulting in slight underexposure of the carpal bones.

No evidence of patient movement.
No artefacts present on the image.

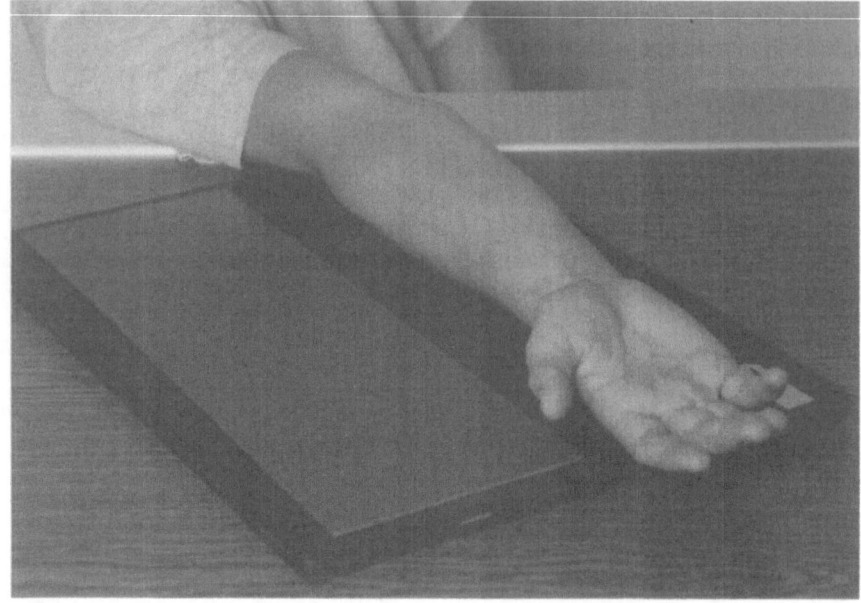

(a)

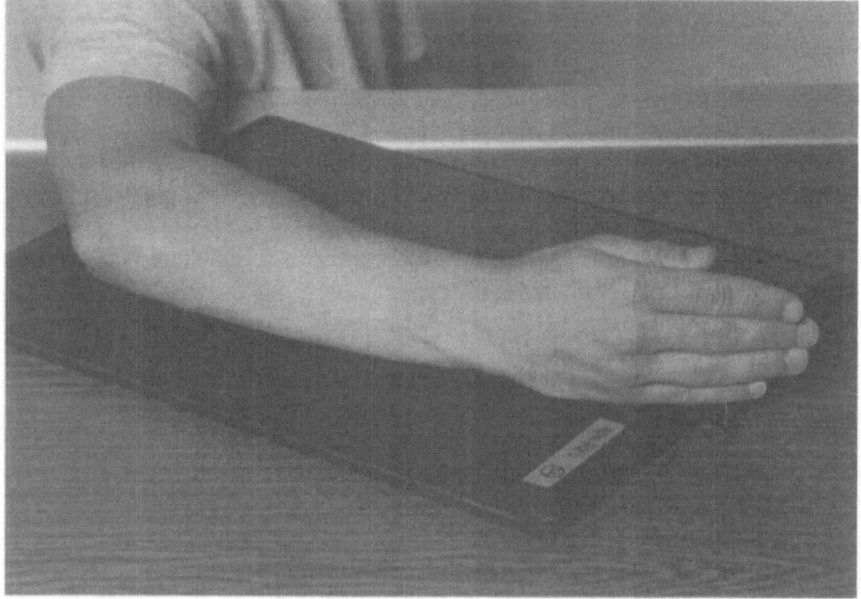

(b)

Figure 1.12 Forearm. (a) AP. (b) Lateral.

FOREARM

RADIOGRAPHIC TECHNIQUE

Anteroposterior (Fig. 1.12a)

An 18×43 cm/24×30 cm cassette is selected. The patient is seated with the affected side next to the table. For radiation protection purposes the legs must not be placed under the table, and a lead–rubber sheet is applied to the lower abdomen and upper thighs. The affected arm is extended at the elbow and supinated. The posterior aspect of the forearm is placed in contact with the cassette, which is positioned to include the wrist and elbow joints in addition to the radius and ulna. The long axis of the cassette is coincident with the long axis of the forearm (the forearm is positioned diagonally across the cassette if a 24×30 cm cassette is used). The radial and ulnar styloid processes are equidistant from the cassette.

> CENTRING: A vertical central ray, at 90° to the cassette, is directed over the middle of the anterior aspect of the forearm and midway between the elbow and wrist joints.

Collimate to include radius and ulna, wrist and elbow joints and surrounding soft tissues. Apply an AP anatomical marker within the primary beam.

Lateral (Fig. 1.12b)

An 18×43 cm/24×30 cm cassette is selected. From the AP position the elbow is flexed through 90° and the arm internally rotated to bring the medial aspect of the forearm in contact with the cassette. The forearm is then adjusted to superimpose the radial and ulnar styloid processes. The long axis of the cassette is coincident with the long axis of the forearm (the forearm is positioned diagonally if a 24×30 cm cassette is used). The cassette is positioned to include the elbow and wrist joints, in addition to the radius and ulna. The shoulder and humerus lie on the same horizontal plane as the forearm in order to superimpose the humeral epicondyles.

> CENTRING: A vertical central ray, at 90° to the cassette, is directed to the middle of the lateral aspect of the forearm, midway between the elbow and wrist joints.

Collimate to include radius and ulna, wrist and elbow joints and surrounding soft tissues. Apply an AP anatomical marker within the primary beam.

IMAGE EVALUATION

Correct patient identification and anatomical marker included on the radiograph.

Ara of intrst

Wrist and elbow joints and soft tissue outlines.

Projection

Anteroposterior

- Separation of radius and ulna, with slight overlap at proximal and distal radioulnar joints.
- Olecranon and coronoid fossae centralized between humeral epicondyles.
- Radial styloid process demonstrated on lateral aspect of wrist joint, with ulnar styloid process demonstrated in centre of distal surface of ulna.

Lateral

- Elbow flexed at 90°.
- Superimposition of distal radius and ulna, with proximal two-thirds of radius projected anterior to shaft of ulna.

Exposure factors

- kVp sufficient to demonstrate bony trabeculae and areas of overlap of the radius, ulna and humerus, maintaining contrast between the bones and soft tissues of the forearm.
- mAs to provide adequate image density to demonstrate bony detail in contrast to the surrounding soft tissues.

No evidence of patient movement.
No artefacts present on the image.

ULNAR GROOVE

RADIOGRAPHIC TECHNIQUE (Fig. 1.13)

An 18×24 cm cassette is selected. The patient is seated with the affected side next to the table. For radiation protection purposes the legs must not be placed under the table, and a lead–rubber sheet is applied to the lower abdomen and upper thighs. The affected arm is fully flexed at the elbow, with the fist clenched and in contact with the shoulder. The posterior

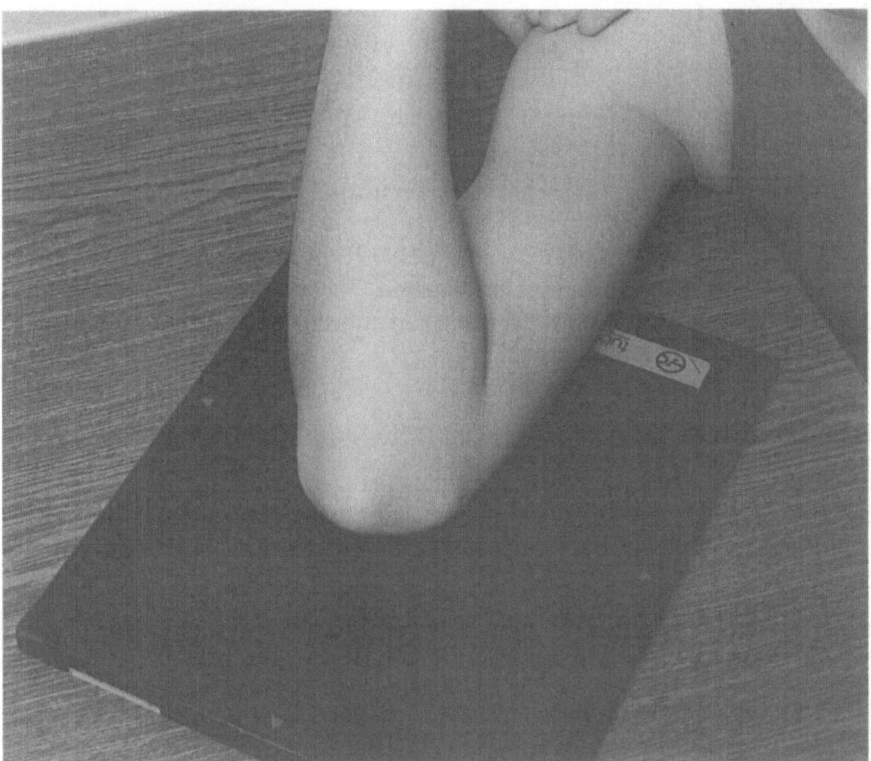

Figure 1.13   Ulnar groove.

aspect of the upper arm is in contact with the cassette, the long axis of the cassette parallel to the long axis of the humerus. The humeral epicondyles are coincident with the middle of the cassette and are initially equidistant from the cassette. The patient leans towards the affected side and externally rotates the arm until the humeral epicondyles are at 45° to the cassette. A 45° radiolucent pad placed under the lateral aspect of the arm will aid immobilization.

CENTRING: A vertical central ray, at 90° to the cassette, is directed
over the medial humeral epicondyle.

Collimate to include distal portion of humerus, olecranon process and surrounding soft tissues. Apply an AP anatomical marker within the primary beam.

IMAGE EVALUATION

Correct patient identification and anatomical marker included on the radiograph.

Area of interest

Humeral epicondyles, olecranon process and soft tissue outlines.

Projection

- Medial epicondyle of humerus demonstrated, with no superimposition of forearm.
- Olecranon process demonstrated distal to humerus, with ulna super-imposed on lateral humeral epicondyle.
- Ulnar groove demonstrated between medial epicondyle and medial aspect of trochlea of humerus.

Exposure factors

kVp sufficient to demonstrate bony trabeculae within the medial epicon-dyle and olecranon process, though not within the distal humerus, maintaining contrast between the ulnar groove and surrounding soft tissues.

mAs to provide adequate image density to demonstrate the ulnar groove in contrast to the humerus and soft tissue structures.

No evidence of patient movement.
No artefacts present on the image.

ELBOW

RADIOGRAPHIC TECHNIQUE

Anteroposterior (Fig. 1.14a)

A 24×30 cm cassette is masked off widthwise with lead–rubber in order to use the film for two projections. The patient is seated with the affected side next to the table. For radiation protection purposes the legs must not be placed under the table, and a lead–rubber sheet is applied to the lower abdomen and upper thighs. The arm is extended at the elbow and the posterior aspect of the elbow is placed in contact with the cassette. The middle of the available area of cassette is coincident with the crease of the elbow, the short axis of the cassette parallel to the long axis of the humerus. The elbow, shoulder and forearm lie in the same horizontal plane. The humeral epicondyles are equidistant from the cassette and the radial and ulnar styloid processes equidistant from the table top.

CENTRING: A vertical central ray, at 90° to the cassette, is directed to a point in the middle of the crease of the elbow.

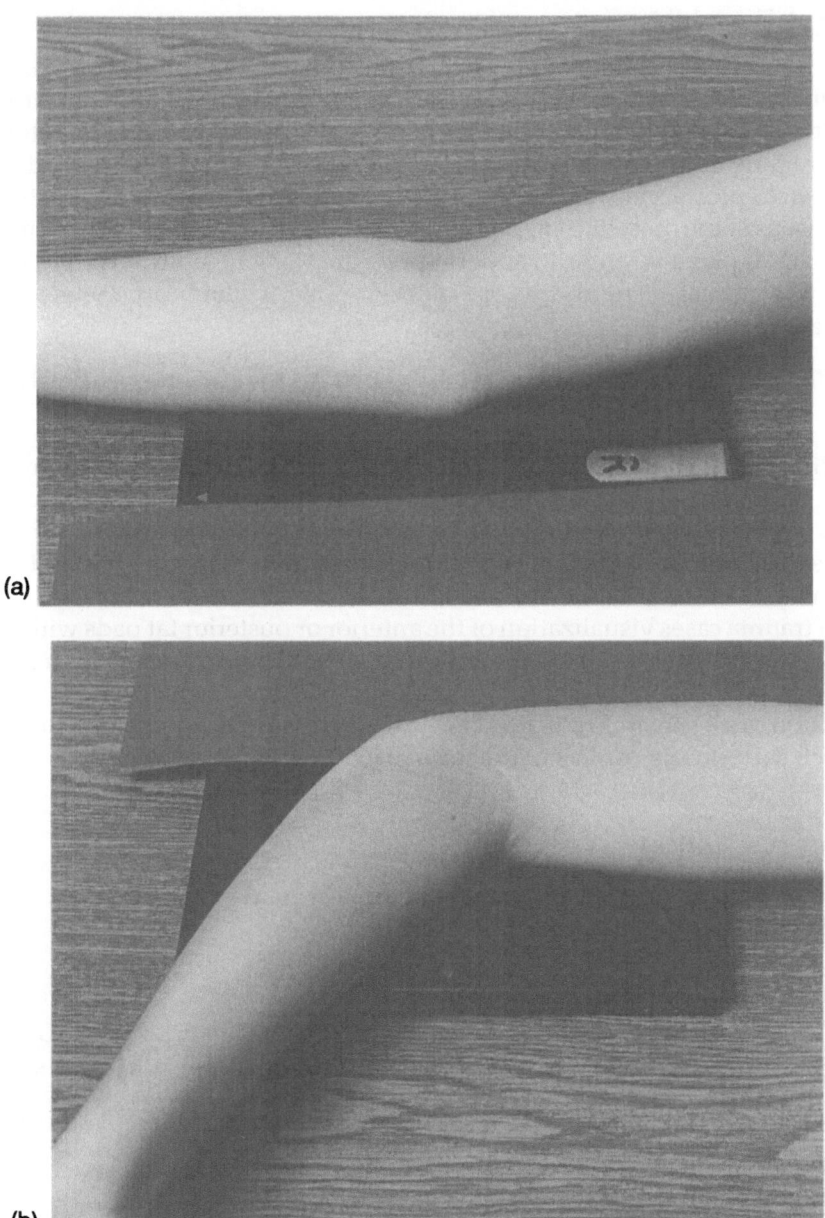

(a)

(b)

Figure 1.14 Elbow. (a) AP. (b) Lateral.

Collimate to include distal third of humerus, proximal third of radius and ulna, and surrounding soft tissues.

Lateral (Fig. 1.14b)

The lead–rubber sheet is moved onto the exposed half of the cassette. From the AP position the elbow is flexed through 90° and the arm internally rotated to bring its medial aspect into contact with the cassette. The middle of the available area of cassette is coincident with the medial humeral epicondyle, the long axis of the humerus coincident with the short axis of the cassette. The shoulder, elbow and forearm lie in the same horizontal plane in order to superimpose the humeral epicondyles. The wrist is adjusted until the radial and ulnar styloid processes are superimposed.

> CENTRING: A vertical central ray, at 90° to the cassette, is directed over the lateral humeral epicondyle.

Collimate to include distal third of humerus, proximal third of radius and ulna, and surrounding soft tissues. Lead–rubber sheets are placed close to the posterior soft tissue outline of the humerus and forearm to absorb the excess primary radiation. Apply an AP anatomical marker within the primary beam.

In trauma cases visualization of the anterior or posterior fat pads within the joint capsule is a significant indication of bony injury, even when the radiographs appear normal. The fat pads will only be seen when an effusion causes them to be raised away from the surfaces of the humerus, which they closely contact in the normal joint.

IMAGE EVALUATION

Correct patient identification and anatomical marker included on the radiograph.

Area of interest

Elbow joint, distal ⅓ humerus, proximal ⅓ radius and ulna and soft tissue outlines.

Projection

Anteroposterior

- Separation of radius and ulna, with slight overlap at proximal radioulnar joint.
- Olecranon and coronoid fossae centralized between humeral epicondyles.

Lateral

- Elbow flexed at 90°.
- Superimposition of trochlea and capitulum of humerus, demonstrating a clear joint space.

Exposure factors

- kVp sufficient to demonstrate bony trabeculae and areas of overlap of the radius, ulna and humerus, maintaining contrast between the bones and soft tissues.
- mAs to provide adequate image density to demonstrate bony detail in contrast to the surrounding soft tissues.

No evidence of patient movement.
No artefacts present on the image.

Positional faults

Epicondyles not equidistant from the cassette in the AP projection:

- Excessive external rotation of the arm will lead to opening of the proximal radioulnar joint and separation of the radius and ulna.
- Internal rotation of the arm will lead to overlap of the shafts of the radius and ulna.

Shoulder, elbow and wrist joints not on the same horizontal plane in the lateral projection:

- With the wrist raised/lowered in relation to the elbow and shoulder the capitulum will be projected posterior/anterior to the trochlea, respectively.
- With the shoulder raised/lowered in relation to the elbow and wrist the capitulum will be projected inferior/superior to the trochlea, respectively.

In cases of trauma the radiographer often encounters patients who cannot extend their elbow. The routine AP projection, thrfor, cannot carried out and modification of technique is required in order that a diagnostic image be produced.

Some imaging departments employ an '**equal angles**' technique for elbows in slight partial flexion, but as this requires the patient to place the olecranon process in contact with the cassette it is not possible in cases of severe trauma. With the forearm and humerus supported on pads, the arm is positioned so that the angles between forearm/humerus and cassette are equal. The advantage of this method is that an AP projection of the complete joint is produced on a single image. However, there will be some distortion of all aspects of the image, and therefore the projection should not be utilized if flexion of the joint is through more than 30°.

If the patient arrives from the trauma unit wearing a collar and cuff sling, it is important **not** to remove the sling or extend the elbow. Similarly, if the patient cannot fully extend the joint, even when not wearing a sling, forced extension is to be avoided. The commonest reason for the use of a collar and cuff sling is for suspected supracondylar fracture of the humerus (mostly found in children), and it is vital that there be no movement at the elbow joint in order to avoid brachial vascular injury or damage to radial, median or ulnar nerves. In these instances, in addition to the lateral, an AP projection of the elbow in partial or full flexion is undertaken; both methods are described below.

Elbow flexed through less than 90°

Following the lateral projection, the lead–rubber sheet is moved on to the exposed half of the cassette.

(a) To demonstrate proximal radius and ulna in an AP projection (Fig. 1.15a)
The affected arm is abducted and extended at the elbow, as far as is comfortable. The posterior aspect of the forearm is placed in contact with the cassette. The crease of the elbow is coincident with the centre of the cassette, the short axis of the cassette parallel to the long axis of the forearm. The humeral epicondyles are equidistant from the cassette. A large pad placed under the axilla will help to immobilize in this position.

CENTRING: A vertical central ray, at 90° to the cassette, is directed 2.5 cm distal to the midpoint of the crease of the elbow.

Collimate to include distal third of humerus, proximal third of radius and ulna and surrounding soft tissues. Apply an AP anatomical marker within the primary beam.

(b) To demonstrate distal humerus in an AP projection (Fig. 1.15b)
The affected arm is abducted and extended at the elbow, as far as is comfortable. The posterior aspect of the upper arm is placed in contact with the cassette. The crease of the elbow is coincident with the centre of the cassette, the short axis of the cassette parallel to the long axis of the humerus. The humeral epicondyles are equidistant from the cassette. A large pad placed under the forearm will help to immobilize in this position.

CENTRING: A vertical central ray, at 90° to the cassette, is directed midway between the humeral epicondyles.

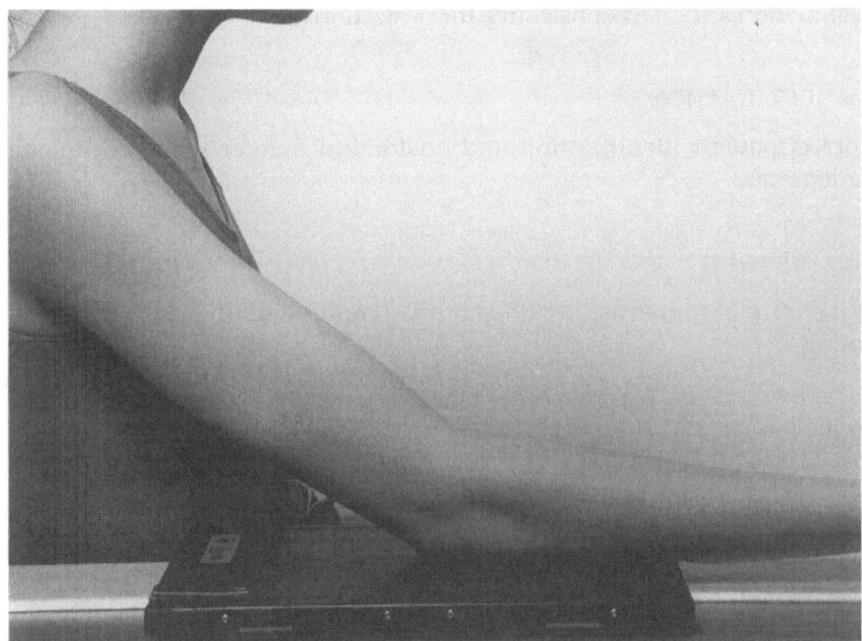

(a)

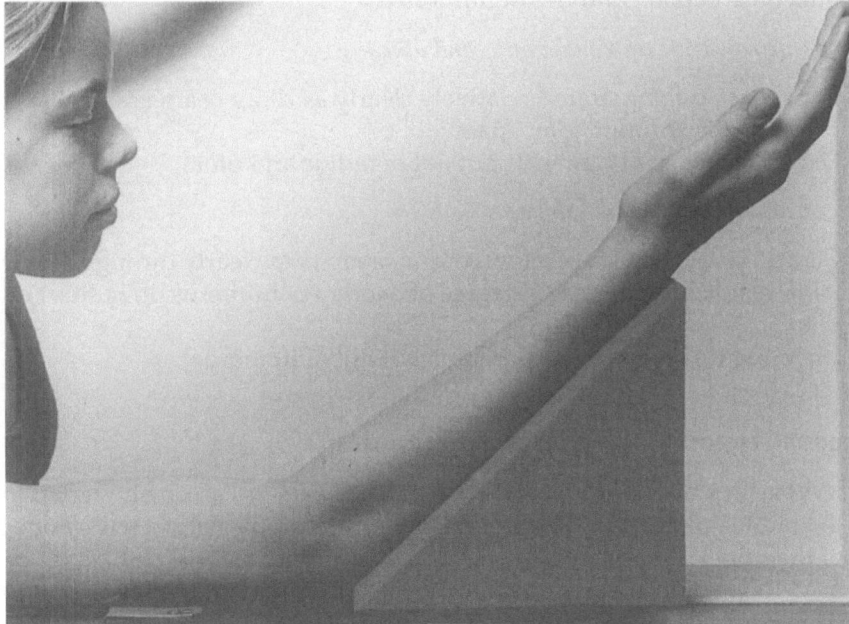

(b)

Figure 1.15 Partial flexion of elbow. (a) Proximal radius and ulna. (b) Distal humerus.

Collimation and marker as above for projection (a).

IMAGE EVALUATION

Correct patient identification and anatomical marker included on the radiograph.

Area of interest

Distal third of humerus, proximal third of radius and ulna and soft tissue outlines.

Projection

Elbow flexed through less than 90°

- Separation of shafts of radius and ulna, with slight overlap at proximal radioulnar joint.
- Olecranon and coronoid fossae centralized between humeral epicondyles.
- Joint space obscured by partial superimposition of proximal radius and ulna on articular condyles of humerus.

(a) To demonstrate proximal radius and ulna

- Joint space demonstrated relatively clearly as X-ray beam is still able to pass directly through joint space.
- Distorted image of humerus but not of radius and ulna.

(b) To demonstrate distal humerus

- Centring point does not allow central ray to pass clearly through elbow joint, resulting in a greater degree of overlap of humerus on radius and ulna.
- Distorted image of radius and ulna but not of humerus.

Exposure factors

- kVp sufficient to demonstrate bony trabeculae and areas of overlap of the radius, ulna and humerus, maintaining contrast between the bones of the upper and lower arm and the surrounding soft tissues.
- mAs to provide adequate image density to demonstrate bony detail in contrast to the surrounding soft tissues.

No evidence of patient movement.
No artefacts present on the image.

Elbow flexed through more than 90°

When a patient presents with the elbow in full flexion, often in a collar and cuff sling, the elbow must not be extended. Axial projections in full flexion can be undertaken as follows.

(c) To demonstrate distal humerus and olecranon process in an AP projection (Fig. 1.16a)
An 18×24 cm cassette is placed near the edge of the table. The patient is seated with the affected side next to the table. For radiation protection purposes the legs must not be placed under the table, and a lead–rubber sheet is applied to the lower abdomen and upper thighs. The affected arm is abducted and the posterior aspect of the upper arm is placed in contact with the cassette, the long axis of the cassette parallel to the long axis of the humerus. The humeral epicondyles are coincident with and equidistant from the centre of the cassette. The head is turned towards the unaffected side.

> CENTRING: A vertical central ray, at 90° to the long axis of the humerus, is directed over the posterior aspect of the forearm, midway between the humeral epicondyles.

Collimate to include olecranon process, proximal third of radius and ulna, distal third of humerus and surrounding soft tissues. Apply an AP anatomical marker within the primary beam.

(d) To demonstrate proximal radius and ulna in an AP projection (Fig 1.16b)
An 18×24 cm cassette is placed near the edge of the table. A lead-rubber apron is applied behind the patient's lower abdomen as radiation protection. The patient is seated with their back to the table. The affected arm is moved posteriorly and the posterior aspect of the forearm placed in contact with the cassette, the long axis of the forearm parallel to the long axis of the cassette. The humeral epicondyles are coincident with and equidistant from the middle of the cassette.

> CENTRING: A vertical central ray, at 90° to the long axis of the forearm, is directed over the posterior aspect of the upper arm, midway between the humeral epicondyles.

Collimate to include olecranon process, proximal third of radius and ulna, distal third of humerus and surrounding soft tissues. Apply an AP anatomical marker within the primary beam.

If the soft tissues on the aspect of the arm which should make contact with the cassette are injured severely enough to prevent such contact, both techniques should be adapted thus:

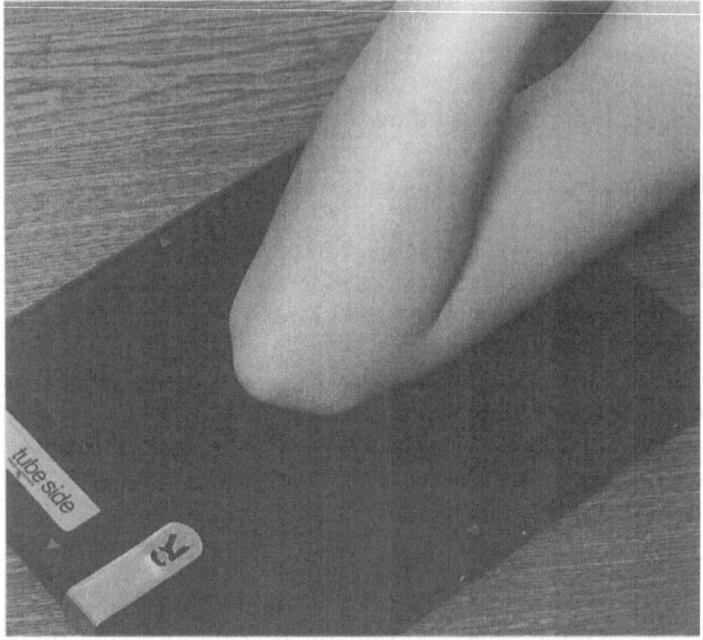

(a)

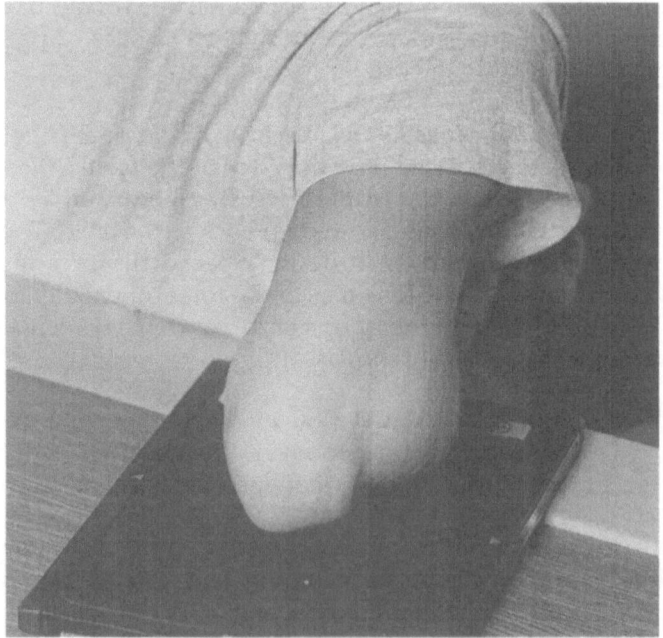

(b)

Figure 1.16 Fully flexed elbow. (a) Distal humerus. (b) Proximal radius and ulna.

To demonstrate distal humerus and olecranon process
The patient is positioned as for the proximal radius and ulna, projection (d), and the central ray is angled to 90° to the long axis of the humerus and centred midway between the humeral epicondyles.

To demonstrate proximal radius and ulna
The patient is positioned as for the humerus and olecranon process, projection (c), and the central ray is angled to 90° to the long axis of the forearm and centred midway between the humeral epicondyles.

IMAGE EVALUATION

Correct patient identification and anatomical marker included on the radiograph.

Area of interest

Distal third of humerus, proximal third of radius and ulna and soft tissue outlines.

Projection

Elbow flexed through more than 90°

- Separation of shafts of radius and ulna.
- Superimposition of humerus on the radius and ulna.

Central ray at 90° to the humerus

- Olecranon process projected clear of distal humerus.
- Radiohumeral joint obscured, with superior aspect of head of radius demonstrated elliptically.
- No distortion of image of humerus.

Central ray at 90° to the forearm

- Olecranon process superimposed on distal humerus.
- Radiohumeral joint clearly demonstrated.
- No distortion of images of radius and ulna.

Exposure factors

- kVp sufficient to demonstrate bony trabeculae in the humerus and radius and ulna, maintaining contrast between the bones of the upper and lower arm and the surrounding soft tissues.
- mAs to provide adequate image density to demonstrate bony detail of

the radius, ulna, humerus and olecranon process in contrast to the surrounding soft tissues.

No evidence of patient movement.
No artefacts present on the image.

HEAD OF RADIUS

RADIOGRAPHIC TECHNIQUE

The head of the radius is inadequately demonstrated on routine projections of the elbow, being significantly superimposed over the ulna on the lateral. In addition to the routine AP and lateral projections of the elbow, one or more of the following may be undertaken.

Lateral

An 18×24 cm cassette is selected. The patient is seated and positioned as for the routine lateral elbow projection (Fig. 1.14b) and the forearm and wrist are rotated to demonstrate different aspects of the radial head as follows.

Position of hand and wrist	To demonstrate
Lateral: medial aspect of hand in contact with table	Anterior aspect of radial head
Pronated: palm of hand in contact with table	Lateral aspect of radial head
Internally rotated: dorsum of thumb in contact with table	Posterior aspect of radial head

CENTRING: A vertical central ray, at 90° to the cassette, is directed over the lateral humeral epicondyle.

Collimation and marker as for lateral elbow.

Anteroposterior oblique (Fig. 1.17)

An 18×24 cm cassette is selected. The patient is seated and positioned as for the AP projection of the elbow. The patient leans towards the affected side and the arm is externally rotated through 20°.

CENTRING: A vertical central ray, at 90° to the cassette, is directed over a point in the middle of the crease of the elbow.

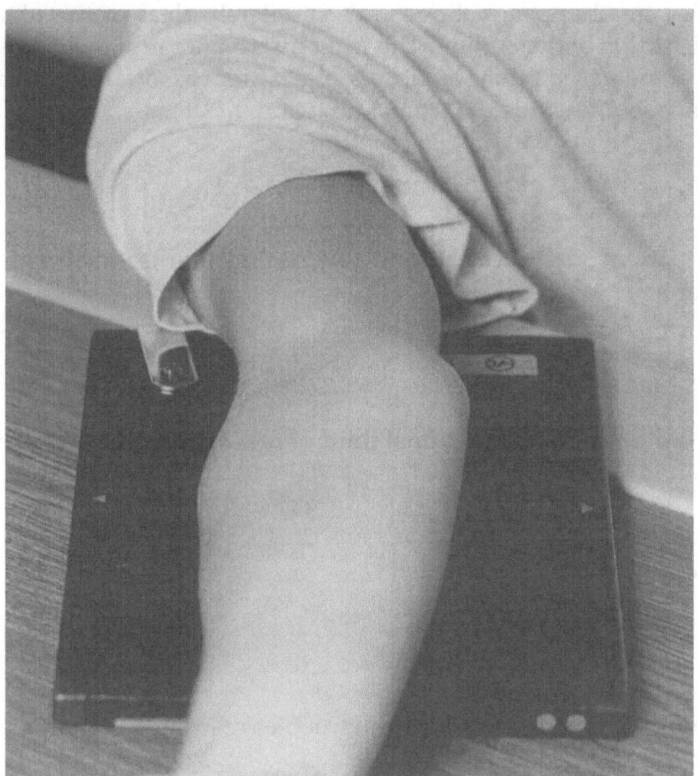

Figure 1.17   Head of radius.

Collimation and marker as for AP elbow projection.

The anteroposterior oblique projection described above is also under-taken to demonstrate the **superior radioulnar joint**.

Lateral with 45° angulation

Bearing in mind that rotation of the forearm is often very difficult for the injured patient, a suitable alternative is suggested by Greenspan and Norman (1982).

The patient wears a full-length lead–rubber apron as radiation protec-tion and is positioned as for the routine lateral elbow projection (Fig. 1.14b), with their head turned away from the primary beam. The cassette is displaced until the forearm runs along its lower edge, to ensure that the resultant image is projected on to the centre of the film.

CENTRING: A vertical central ray is angled 45° along the humerus, towards the shoulder, and directed over the radial head.

The radial head appears above and completely clear of the ulna, with slight distortion of the outline. The main disadvantage of this projection is the risk of increased radiation dose to the patient associated with angling the X-ray beam towards the trunk and head.

IMAGE EVALUATION

Correct patient identification and anatomical marker included on the radiograph.

Area of interest

Distal third of humerus, proximal third of radius and ulna and soft tissue outlines.

Projection

Lateral

- Elbow flexed to 90°.
- Superimposition of capitulum and trochlea of humerus, demonstrating a clear joint space.
- Head of radius overlying coronoid process of ulna.
- Different aspects of radial head and radial tuberosity demonstrated, depending on degree of rotation of forearm.

Anteroposterior oblique

- Separation of proximal radius and ulna with visualization of proximal radioulnar joint.

Exposure factors

- kVp sufficient to demonstrate bony trabeculae and areas of overlap of the radius, ulna and humerus, maintaining contrast between the bones of the upper limb and surrounding soft tissues.
- mAs to provide adequate image density to demonstrate bony detail in contrast to the surrounding soft tissues and elbow joint.

No evidence of patient movement.
No artefacts present on the image.

HUMERUS

RADIOGRAPHIC TECHNIQUE

Anteroposterior (Fig. 1.18)

A 30×40 cm cassette is placed longitudinally in the vertical cassette holder. The patient is erect, facing the X-ray tube, with their back towards the cassette. A lead–rubber apron is applied to the patient's lower abdomen as radiation protection. The affected arm is extended at the elbow and abducted slightly, with the palmar aspect of the hand facing the X-ray tube. The posterior aspect of the upper arm is placed in contact with the cassette, which is positioned to include the shoulder and elbow joints. The humeral epicondyles are equidistant from the cassette. The head is turned away from the affected side.

> CENTRING: A horizontal central ray, at 90° to the cassette, is directed to a point in the middle of the anterior aspect of the upper arm, midway between the shoulder and elbow joints.

Collimate to include humerus, shoulder and elbow joints and surrounding soft tissues. Apply an AP anatomical marker within the primary beam.

It is important to separate the upper arm adequately from the trunk, otherwise there may be partial superimposition of the soft tissues of the trunk over the humerus.

Lateral (Fig. 1.19)

A 30×40 cm cassette is placed longitudinally in the vertical cassette holder. The patient is erect, facing the cassette, with their back to the X-ray tube. A lead–rubber waist apron is applied behind the patient's lower abdomen as radiation protection. The affected limb is abducted and flexed at the elbow, the palmar aspect of the hand resting on the hip. The patient leans forward slightly, to bring the lateral aspect of the upper arm into contact with the cassette, which is positioned to include the shoulder and elbow joints. The humeral epicondyles are superimposed, perpendicular to the cassette. The head is turned away from the affected side.

> CENTRING: A horizontal central ray, at 90° to the cassette, is directed over a point on the medial aspect of the upper arm, midway between the shoulder and elbow joints.

Collimate to include humerus, shoulder and elbow joints and surrounding soft tissues. Apply a PA anatomical marker within the primary beam.

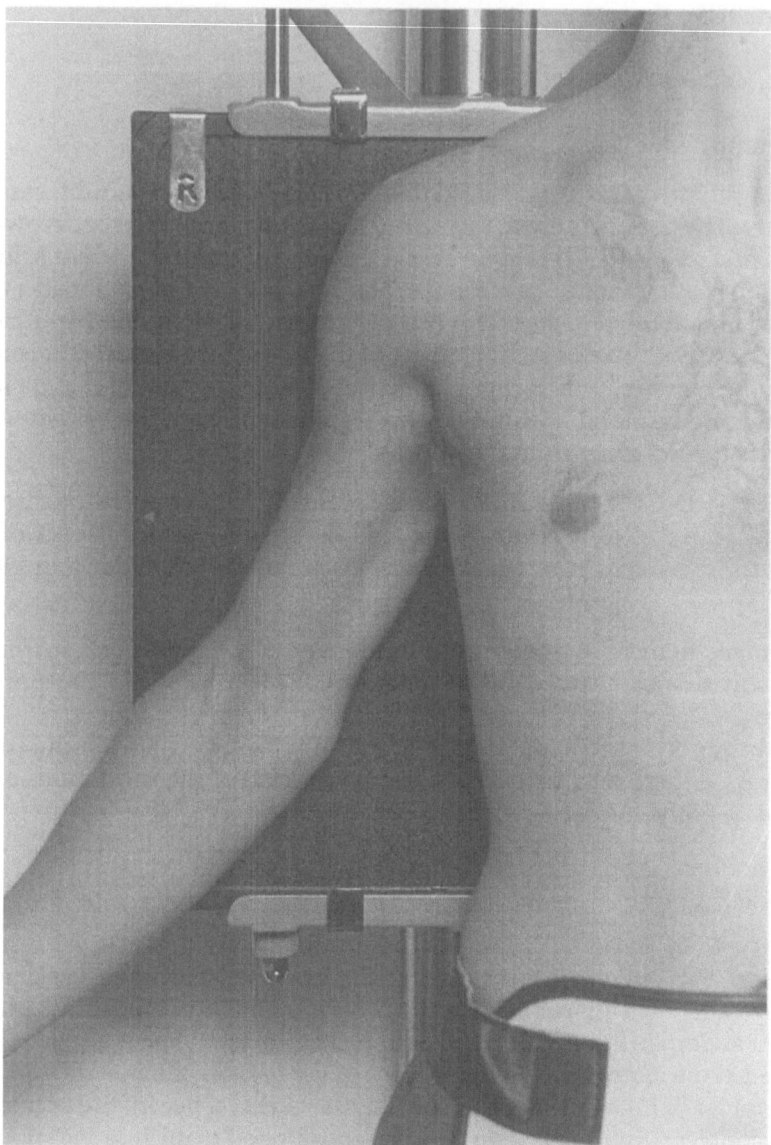

Figure 1.18 AP humerus.

In the severely injured patient the AP humerus can be adequately carried out in the supine position. The lateral projection is more awkward, but not impossible if the patient can flex the elbow and place the dorsum of the hand under the buttock.

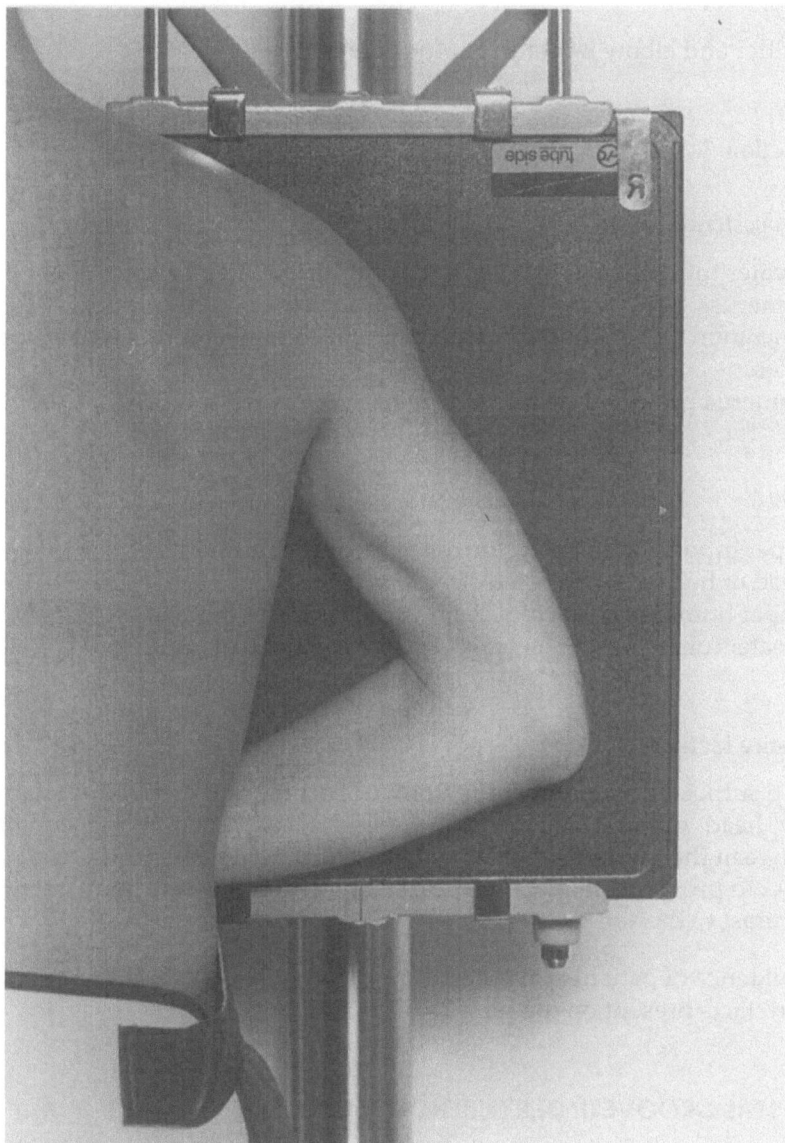

Figure 1.19   Lateral humerus.

IMAGE EVALUATION

Correct patient identification and anatomical marker included on the radiograph.

Area of interest

Shoulder and elbow joints and soft tissue outlines.

Projection

Anteroposterior

- Greater tuberosity demonstrated in profile on lateral aspect of head of humerus.
- Olecranon and coronoid fossae centralized between humeral epicondyles.
- Humerus projected clear of overlying soft tissues of thorax.

Lateral

- Superimposition of capitulum and trochlea of humerus.
- Head of humerus projected clear of scapula.
- Upper humerus projected clear of soft tissues of thorax.
- Greater tuberosity projected over centre of head of humerus.

Exposure factors

- kVp sufficient to demonstrate bony trabeculae and areas of overlap of the head of humerus on the glenoid fossa, maintaining contrast between the humerus and surrounding soft tissue structures.
- mAs to provide adequate image density to demonstrate bony detail in contrast to the soft tissues.

No evidence of patient movement.
No artefacts present on the image.

BICIPITAL GROOVE (INTERTUBEROUS SULCUS)

RADIOGRAPHIC TECHNIQUE (Fig. 1.20)

An 18×24 cm cassette is selected. The patient lies supine on the table. A lead–rubber sheet is applied to the thorax and abdomen as radiation protection. The cassette is placed in contact with the superior aspect of the affected shoulder, vertical to the table top, and is supported in this position with pads and sandbags. The middle of the cassette is coincident with the head of humerus. The arm is slightly abducted and in partial

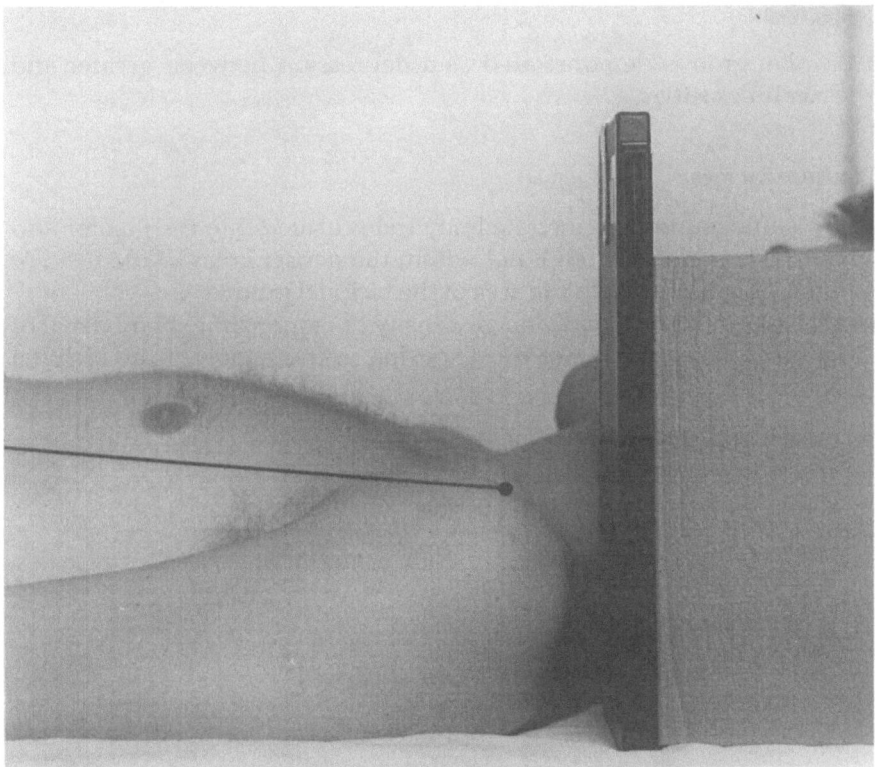

Figure 1.20 Bicipital groove.

supination, the line joining the humeral epicondyles at 45° to the table top. The head is turned towards the unaffected side.

    CENTRING: A horizontal central ray is angled down 5° and directed over the middle of the anterior aspect of the head of the humerus.

Collimate to include head of humerus and surrounding soft tissues. Apply an AP anatomical marker within the primary beam.

IMAGE EVALUATION

Correct patient identification and anatomical marker included on the radiograph.

Area of interest

Anterior aspect of head of humerus, including greater and lesser tuberosities and soft tissue outlines.

Projection

- Bicipital groove demonstrated as a depression between greater and lesser tuberosities.

Exposure factors

- kVp sufficient to demonstrate bony trabeculae within the greater and lesser tuberosities, though not within the denser areas of the head of humerus, in contrast to the area of the bicipital groove.
- mAs to provide adequate image density to demonstrate bony detail of the tuberosities while not overexposing in the region of the bicipital groove.

No evidence of patient movement.
No artefacts present on the image.

Shoulder girdle 2

SHOULDER

RADIOGRAPHIC TECHNIQUE

Anteroposterior (Fig. 2.1)

A 24×30 cm cassette is placed transversely in the erect cassette holder. A lead–rubber apron is applied to the patient's lower abdomen as radiation protection. The patient is erect, with the posterior aspect of the affected shoulder in contact with the cassette, which is positioned with its upper border 5 cm above the level of the acromion process. The lateral soft tissue outline of the upper humerus should lie within the lateral border of the cassette. The affected arm is extended and slightly abducted, with the humeral epicondyles equidistant from the cassette. The patient is rotated approximately 20° towards the affected side until the blade of the scapula is parallel to the cassette. The patient's head is turned away from the affected side.

CENTRING: A horizontal central ray, at 90° to the cassette, is directed to the centre of the cassette.

Collimate to include head and upper third of humerus, scapula, clavicle and surrounding soft tissues. Apply an AP anatomical marker within the primary beam.

Superoinferior shoulder (Fig. 2.2)

An 18×24 cm cassette is selected. The patient sits with the affected side next to the table. For radiation protection purposes the legs must not be placed under the table, and a lead–rubber sheet is applied to the lower abdomen and upper thighs. The cassette is placed on the table. The arm is

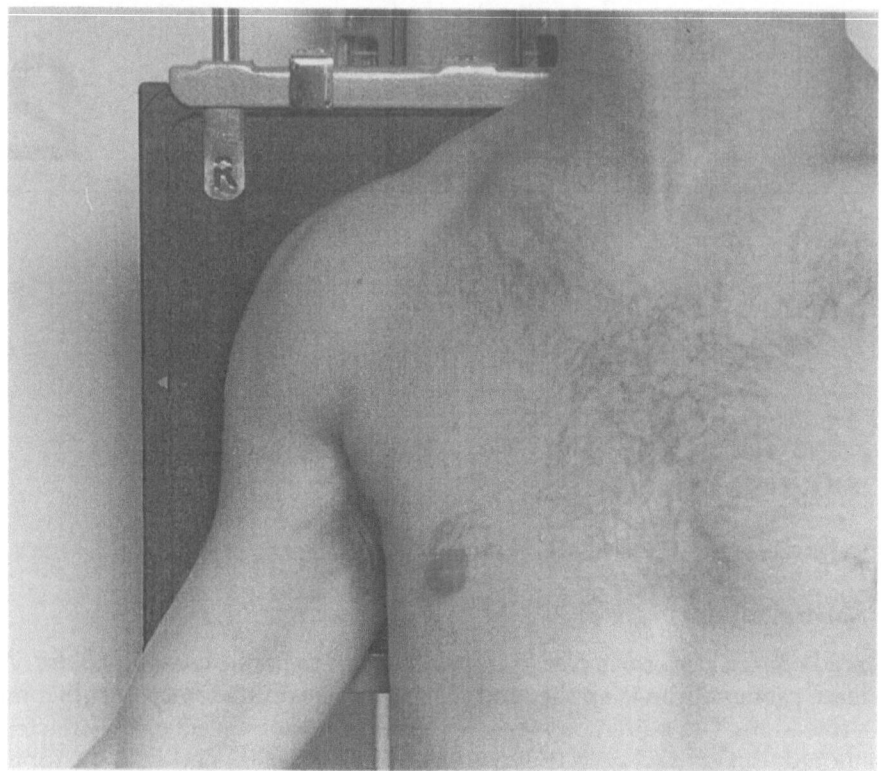

Figure 2.1 AP shoulder.

fully abducted and the patient leans across the cassette to place their axilla over its centre. The long axis of the cassette is parallel to the long axis of the humerus. The patient lowers the axilla as close to the cassette as possible. The elbow is flexed to 90° and the humeral epicondyles superimposed vertically. The neck is flexed to clear the head from the area of interest.

> CENTRING: A vertical central ray, at 90° to the cassette, is directed over the superior aspect of the head of humerus.

Collimate to include the head and proximal third of humerus, glenoid cavity, acromion, coracoid process and surrounding soft tissues. Apply an AP anatomical marker within the primary beam.

Owing to the extreme abduction of the arm, the supero-inferior projection is frequently inappropriate for trauma cases. In these cases the 45° modified superoinferior projection will demonstrate the presence and direction of dislocation. With reference to one of the basic rules of radiography, images of objects that are further away from the cassette are

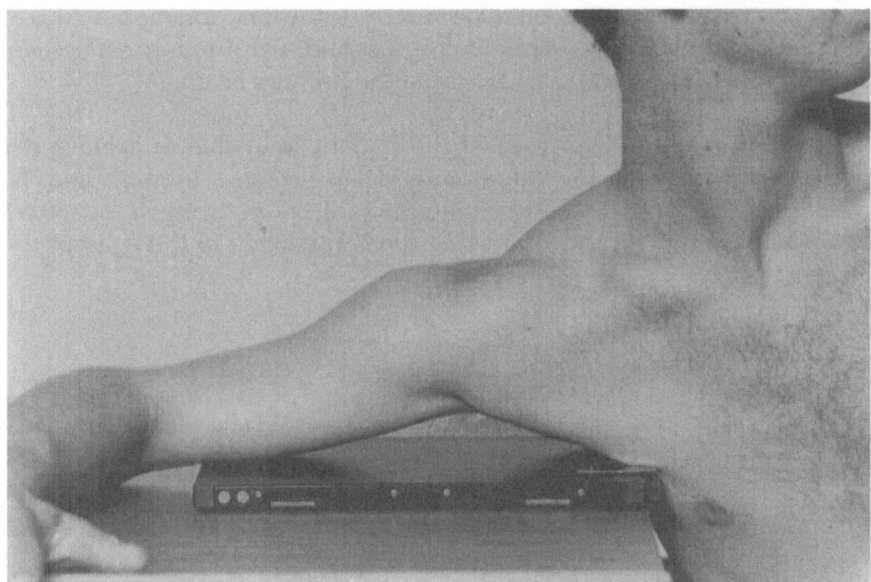

Figure 2.2 Superoinferior shoulder.

projected to a greater extent in the same direction as the angle applied; images of objects closer to the cassette are projected to a much lesser degree in the direction of angulation. Therefore, with 45° caudal angulation, the head of the humerus will be projected inferior to the glenoid in the case of an anterior dislocation and superior to the glenoid in the case of a posterior dislocation.

45° Modified superoinferior shoulder

This is an adaptation of the technique described by Wallace and Hellier (1983). The positions of patient and cassette are similar to those of the AP shoulder (Fig. 2.1).

A 24×30 cm cassette is placed longitudinally in the vertical cassette holder. A lead–rubber apron is applied to the patient's lower abdomen as radiation protection. The patient is seated with the posterior aspect of the shoulder in contact with the cassette. The upper edge of the cassette is level with the superior aspect of the shoulder. The trunk is rotated towards the affected side, to bring the blade of scapula parallel to the cassette. The humeral epicondyles are equidistant from the cassette.

CENTRING: A horizontal central ray is directed 45° caudally and over the head of humerus.

The cassette is displaced to ensure that the central ray is coincident with the centre of the cassette. Collimate to include the head and upper third of humerus, glenoid cavity, acromion process and surrounding soft tissues. Apply an AP anatomical marker within the primary beam.

This projection does not provide a view of the shoulder at 90° to the AP in cases of suspected fracture. If the patient is unable to achieve the position for the routine superoinferior projection, they should be positioned as for the lateral humerus projection, using a 24×30 cm cassette longitudinally and directing the X-ray beam to the head of the humerus.

IMAGE EVALUATION

Correct patient identification and anatomical marker included on the radiograph.

Area of interest

Anteroposterior

Head and proximal third of humerus, medial end of clavicle, inferior angle of scapula and acromioclavicular joint.

Superoinferior

Head and proximal third of humerus, glenoid fossa, lateral end of clavicle, coracoid process and acromion.

Modified superoinferior

Head and proximal shaft of humerus, glenoid fossa, lateral end of clavicle and acromion.

Projection

Anteroposterior

- Greater tuberosity demonstrated in profile on lateral aspect of head of humerus.
- No foreshortening of image of clavicle.

- Glenohumeral joint obscured by head of humerus overlying glenoid fossa.
- Acromion demonstrated clear of superior aspect of head of humerus.

Superoinferior

- Lesser tuberosity demonstrated in profile on anterior aspect of head of humerus.
- Acromion and lateral end of clavicle superimposed on superoposterior aspect of head of humerus.
- No distortion along length of humerus.
- Coracoid process demonstrated on anteromedial aspect of head of humerus.

45° modified superoinferior

- Greater tuberosity demonstrated on lateral aspect of head of humerus.
- Elongation of head of humerus.
- Partial superimposition of acromion on superolateral aspect of head of humerus.
- Partial superimposition of coracoid process on inferomedial aspect of head of humerus.
- Glenoid fossa and head of humerus projected clear of lateral margin of rib cage.

Exposure factors

- kVp sufficient to demonstrate bony trabeculae within the bones of the shoulder girdle and the head of humerus through the overlying structures of the scapula, maintaining contrast between the bony structures and surrounding soft tissues.
- mAs to provide adequate image density to demonstrate bony detail in contrast to the shoulder joint and surrounding soft tissues.

No evidence of patient movement.
No artefacts present on the image.

SCAPULA

RADIOGRAPHIC TECHNIQUE

Anteroposterior (Fig. 2.3)

A 24×30 cm cassette is placed in the erect cassette holder. A lead–rubber apron is applied to the patient's lower abdomen as radiation protection.

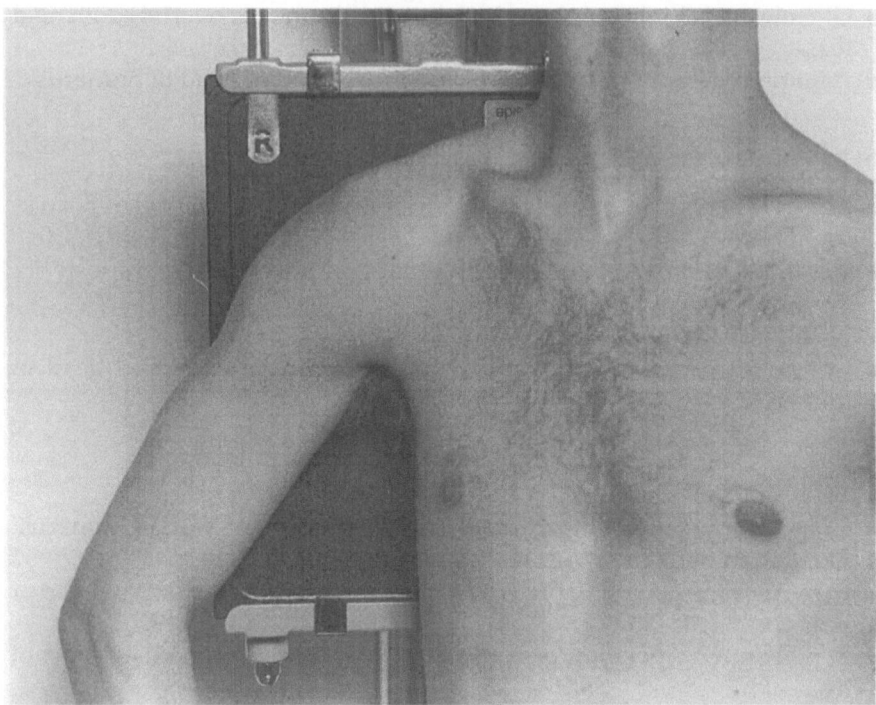

Figure 2.3 AP shoulder with medial rotation for scapula, calcified tendons and glenohumeral joint.

The patient is erect with their back in contact with the cassette, the centre of which should be coincident with a point 5 cm below the midpoint of the clavicle. The trunk is rotated approximately 20° towards the affected side to bring the blade of the scapula parallel to the cassette. The elbow of the affected limb is flexed and the dorsum of the hand rests on the hip. The arm is internally rotated to move the scapula laterally away from the rib cage. The head is turned towards the unaffected side.

CENTRING: A horizontal central ray, at 90° to the cassette, is directed over a point 5 cm below the midpoint of the clavicle.

Collimate to include scapula, head and upper third of humerus and surrounding soft tissues. Apply an AP anatomical marker within the primary beam.

A long exposure time, in conjunction with a low mA, with the patient breathing gently, will blur out the images of the overlying ribs.

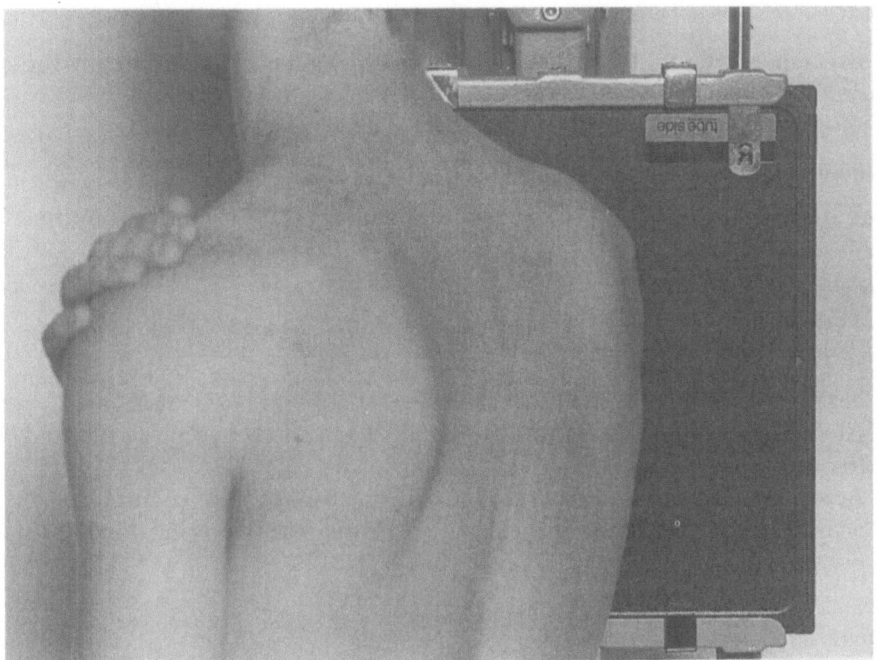

Figure 2.4 Lateral scapula.

Lateral (Fig. 2.4)

A 24×30 cm cassette is placed longitudinally in the vertical cassette holder. A lead–rubber apron is applied behind the patient's lower abdomen as radiation protection. The patient is erect, with the affected side next to the cassette and the MSP parallel to it. The centre of the cassette should be at the level of T4. The affected arm is either flexed at the elbow and adducted across the trunk, with the palm of the hand resting on the unaffected shoulder, or flexed at the elbow and abducted from the trunk, with the dorsum of the hand resting on the hip. Either position will avoid superimposition of the shaft of the humerus over the body of the scapula. Keeping the affected shoulder in contact with the cassette, the trunk is rotated approximately 20° towards the affected side, until the body of the scapula is perpendicular to the cassette. This is checked by palpating the lateral and medial borders of the scapula.

> CENTRING: A horizontal central ray, at 90° to the cassette, is directed over the centre of the palpable medial border of the scapula at the level of T4.

Collimate to include scapula, upper third of humerus and surrounding soft tissues. Apply a PA anatomical marker within the primary beam.

IMAGE EVALUATION

Correct patient identification and anatomical marker included on the radiograph.

Area of interest

Superior and inferior angles of scapula, head of humerus and acromion.

Projection

Anteroposterior

- No foreshortening of image of clavicle.
- Glenohumeral joint obscured by head of humerus overlying glenoid fossa.
- Acromion demonstrated clear of superior aspect of head of humerus.
- Scapula projected laterally, clearing as much of overlying thorax as possible.

Lateral

- Superimposition of medial and lateral borders of scapula.
- Shaft of humerus not overlying body of scapula.
- Body of scapula projected clear of thorax.

Exposure factors

Anteroposterior

- kVp sufficient to demonstrate bony trabeculae within the scapula through the overlying bony thorax, head of humerus and clavicle, maintaining contrast between the scapula, air-filled lungs and surrounding soft tissues.

Lateral

- kVp sufficient to reduce the subject contrast inherent along the length of scapula and demonstrate bony trabeculae, maintaining contrast between the scapula, ribcage and surrounding soft tissues.

Anteroposterior and lateral

- mAs to provide adequate image density to demonstrate bony detail of the scapula in contrast to the lungs, mediastinum and surrounding soft tissue structures.

No evidence of patient movement other than blurring due to the breathing technique.

No artefacts present on the image.

CLAVICLE

RADIOGRAPHIC TECHNIQUE

Anteroposterior

A 24×30 cm cassette is placed transversely in the erect cassette holder. A lead–rubber apron is applied to the patient's lower abdomen as radiation protection. The patient is erect, facing the X-ray tube, with the posterior aspect of the affected shoulder in contact with the cassette. The general plane of the clavicle lies parallel to the cassette (rather than the scapula lying parallel, as in Figure 2.1 for AP shoulder). The affected arm is made comfortable, either remaining in a sling or supported by the unaffected arm.

CENTRING: A horizontal central ray, at 90° to the cassette, is directed over the midpoint of the clavicle.

Collimate to include clavicle, acromioclavicular and sternoclavicular joints. Apply an AP anatomical marker within the primary beam.

Posteroanterior (Fig. 2.5)

This is the preferred projection, as the clavicle lies closer to the film, but can only be attempted if the patient's condition permits.

A 24×30 cm cassette is placed transversely in the erect cassette holder. A lead–rubber apron is applied behind the patient's lower abdomen as radiation protection. The patient faces the cassette to bring the anterior aspect of the shoulder in contact with it. The clavicle is coincident with the central long axis of the cassette. The general plane of the clavicle is parallel to the cassette. The affected arm is made comfortable.

CENTRING: A horizontal central ray, at 90° to the cassette, is directed to the superior angle of the scapula.

Collimation as for AP clavicle. Apply a PA anatomical marker within the primary beam.

Inferosuperior (Fig. 2.6)

A 24×30 cm cassette is selected. The patient lies supine, with the arms resting at their sides. The cassette, resting on its long axis, is placed in

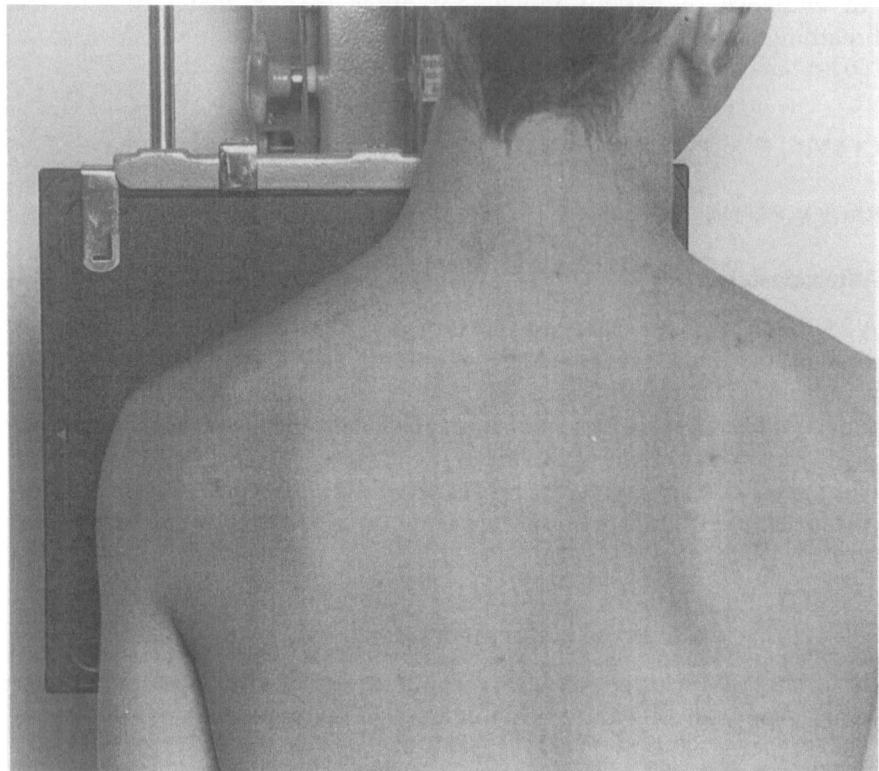

Figure 2.5 PA clavicle.

contact with the posterosuperior aspect of the shoulder, at an angle of 20°
from the vertical. It is parallel to the long axis of the clavicle and supported
in position by a sandbag. The head is turned away from the affected side.

CENTRING: A vertical central ray is angled 45° cranially and 15°
laterally, over the midpoint of the clavicle.

Collimate to include clavicle, acromioclavicular and sternoclavicular
joints. Apply an AP anatomical marker within the primary beam.

IMAGE EVALUATION

Correct patient identification and anatomical marker included on the
radiograph.

Area of interest

Full length of clavicle, including sternoclavicular and acromioclavicular
joints.

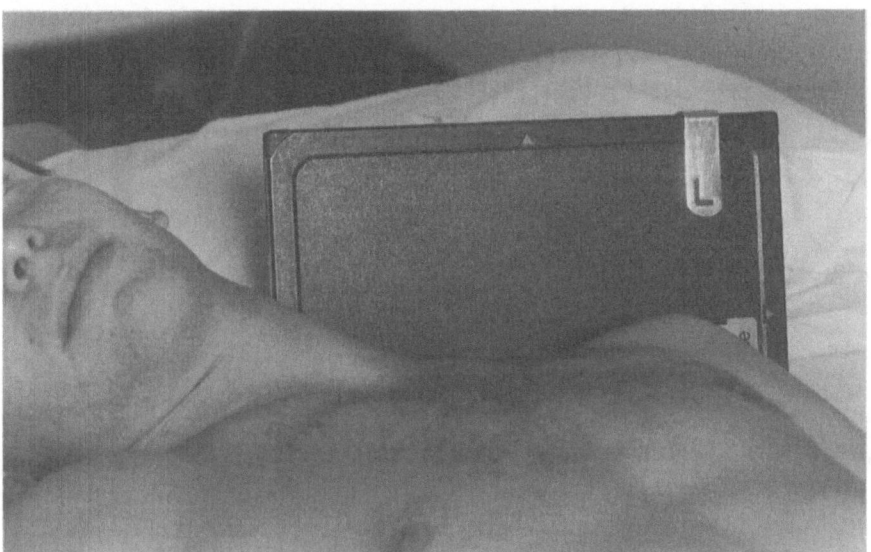

Figure 2.6 Inferosuperior calvicle.

Projection

Anteroposterior and posteroanterior

- No distortion along length of clavicle.
- Medial end of clavicle slightly inferior to lateral end.
- Visualization of acromioclavicular joint.

Inferosuperior

- Clavicle projected above apices of chest.
- Anterior and posterior portions of ribs are almost on same horizontal level.
- Tubercle of clavicle visible on its undersurface, at junction of middle and lateral portions.
- Medial end of clavicle slightly superior to lateral end.

Exposure factors

- kVp sufficient to demonstrate bony trabeculae within the clavicle, including areas of overlap of the clavicle on the adjacent bony structures, and to reduce the subject contrast along the length of the clavicle, maintaining contrast between the bony structures, air-filled lungs and surrounding soft tissues.

- mAs to provide adequate image density to demonstrate bony detail within the medial portion of the clavicle, without overexposing the lateral, superficial portion.

No evidence of patient movement.
No artefacts on the image.

ACROMIOCLAVICULAR JOINTS

RADIOGRAPHIC TECHNIQUE

Anteroposterior

An 18×24 cm cassette is placed transversely in the erect cassette holder. This may be used for both acromioclavicular joints by using one half of the cassette for each side. A lead–rubber apron is applied to the patient's lower abdomen as radiation protection. The patient is erect, with the posterior aspect of the relevant shoulder in contact with the cassette. The middle of the available area of film is coincident with the acromioclavicular joint under examination. The arm remains at the side of the trunk and the patient is turned 10° towards the side under examination, to bring the acromioclavicular joint at 90° to the cassette, similar to Figure 2.1. The head is turned away from the side under examination.

>   CENTRING: A horizontal central ray, at 90° to the cassette, is directed over the acromioclavicular joint.

Collimate to include acromioclavicular joint, acromion process and surrounding soft tissues. Apply an AP anatomical marker within the primary beam. Both sides are examined for comparison.

In cases of suspected subluxation of the acromioclavicular joints these projections are repeated with the patient holding a weight in each hand. The patient is instructed to relax the arm so that the weight is borne in the shoulder. This should not be attempted before the initial radiographs have been examined and possible fractures excluded. Subluxation will be demonstrated as a widening of the affected joint compared to the normal joint, the difference being more apparent on the 'weight-bearing' radiographs.

IMAGE EVALUATION

Correct patient identification and anatomical marker included on the radiograph.

Area of interest

Acromion process, lateral end of clavicle and soft tissue outlines.

Projection

- Acromioclavicular joint spaces clearly demonstrated.
- Comparable images of left and right sides.
- 'Neutral' and 'weight-bearing' legends included as appropriate.

Exposure factors

A reduction in objective contrast is necessary to provide bony detail, for the identification of a possible fracture, together with soft tissue information of the acromioclavicular joint space.

- kVp sufficient to demonstrate bony trabeculae within the acromion and clavicle, reducing the subjective contrast between the bony structures and soft tissues of the joint space.
- mAs to provide adequate image density to demonstrate bone detail while not overexposing in the region of the acromioclavicular joint.

No evidence of patient movement.
No artefacts present on the image.

DEMONSTRATION OF CALCIFICATION OF THE SHOULDER TENDONS

Although MRI will provide high-quality images of the tendons without exposure to radiation, the resource implications for its use should be considered against those of plain radiography. Plain radiography will often adequately demonstrate the presence of calcification, but images which fail to exclude pathology should be followed with MRI examination whenever possible.

Plain radiography to demonstrate calcified tendons is infrequently requested and thus seen to be 'complicated', since the projections vary according to the tendons to be demonstrated. However, these projections are simply variations on the basic AP and superoinferior shoulder projections.

Using cassette size and initial patient positioning as for the routine AP and superoinferior projections of the shoulder, modifications are made to demonstrate tendons as follows:

Projection	Demonstrates
Anteroposterior shoulder Patient position as in Fig. 2.1.	Insertion of supraspinatus tendon into higher impression of greater tuberosity.
Anteroposterior shoulder with 25° caudal angulation Patient position as in Fig. 2.1.	1. Acromial portion of supraspinatus tendon. 2. Insertion of infraspinatus tendon into middle impression of greater tuberosity.
AP shoulder with internal rotation of humerus Elbow flexed with internal rotation of the humerus to superimpose the epicondyles. The lateral epicondyle faces the X-ray tube. (Patient position as in Fig. 2.3).	1. Insertion of teres minor tendon into the lower impression of greater tuberosity. 2. Insertion of subscapularis tendon into lesser tuberosity.
AP shoulder with external rotation of humerus Elbow flexed with external rotation of the humerus to superimpose the epicondyles. The medial epicondyle faces the X-ray tube (Fig. 2.7).	Movement of any calcification demonstrated in any of the tendons shown in the projections described above.
Superoinferior shoulder (Fig. 2.2)	1. Insertion of teres minor into the lower impression of greater tuberosity. 2. Insertion of subscapularis into lesser tuberosity. 3. Passage of shoulder tendons on the anterior and posterior aspects of the shoulder joint.

CENTRING: For all projections listed above, the central ray is directed over the head of humerus.

Collimate to include head of humerus, acromion, lateral half of scapula and surrounding soft tissues. Apply an AP anatomical marker within the primary beam.

A reduction in the values of mAs and kVp selected for routine examination of the shoulder will be necessary, as soft tissue information is required rather than bony detail. Excess mAs will cause overblackening

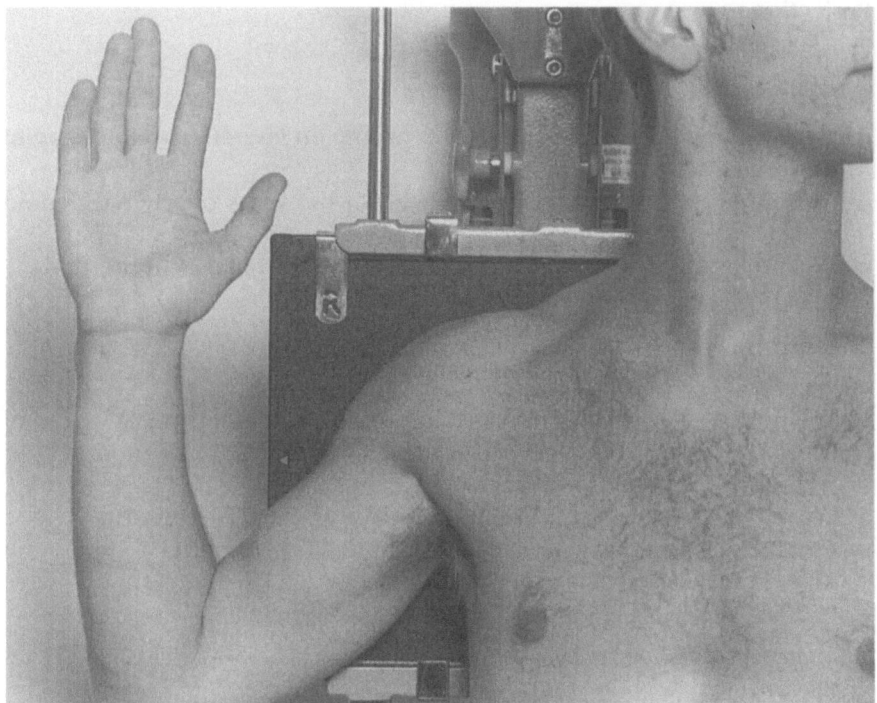

Figure 2.7   Humerus in external rotation.

and excess kVp will reduce the subject contrast in the areas of interest. Both will lead to calcifications within the shoulder tendons not being demonstrated.

IMAGE EVALUATION

Correct patient identification and anatomical marker included on the radiograph.

Area of interest

Anteroposterior

- Head and proximal shaft of humerus, lateral half of scapula, acromion process and lateral third of clavicle.

Superoinferior

- Head and proximal shaft of humerus, glenoid cavity, acromion and coracoid process.

Projection

Anteroposterior

- Greater tuberosity demonstrated in profile on lateral aspect of head of humerus.
- Glenohumeral joint obscured by head of humerus overlying glenoid fossa.
- Slight overlap of acromion on superior aspect of head of humerus.

Anteroposterior with 25° caudal angulation

- Greater tuberosity demonstrated in profile on lateral aspect of head of humerus.
- Elongation of head of humerus.
- Acromion projected superior to, and clear of, head of humerus.
- Superimposition of coracoid process on head of humerus.

Anteroposterior with internal rotation

- Greater tuberosity demonstrated *'en face'*, superimposed on head of humerus and acromion.
- Lesser tuberosity demonstrated in profile on medial aspect of head of humerus, superimposed on glenoid cavity.
- Slight overlap of acromion on head of humerus.

Anteroposterior with external rotation

- Greater tuberosity demonstrated *'en face'*, superimposed on head of humerus.
- Lesser tuberosity demonstrated in profile on lateral aspect of head of humerus.
- Slight overlap of acromion on superior aspect of head of humerus.

Superoinferior

- Lesser tuberosity demonstrated in profile on anterior aspect of head of humerus.
- Acromion and lateral end of clavicle superimposed on superoposterior aspect of head of humerus.
- No evidence of elongation or foreshortening along shaft of humerus.

- Coracoid process demonstrated on anteromedial aspect of head of humerus.

Exposure factors

kVp is selected in order to enhance subject contrast, enabling the detection of tiny areas of calcification within the shoulder tendons.

- kVp sufficient to demonstrate bony trabeculae within the acromion, though not within the dense head of humerus, maintaining contrast between the bones and soft tissues of the shoulder girdle.

mAs is selected so as not to overexpose the soft tissues around the head of humerus and acromion.

- mAs to provide adequate image density to demonstrate detail of the shoulder tendons, in contrast to the head of humerus and acromion.

No evidence of patient movement.
No artefacts present on the image.

GLENOHUMERAL JOINT AND DEMONSTRATION OF THE EFFECTS OF RECURRENT DISLOCATION OF THE SHOULDER

The glenohumeral joint and the effects of recurrent dislocation of the shoulder are demonstrated on the anteroposterior shoulder with internal rotation of the humerus, described on page 66, and the routine superoinferior shoulder projections. Exposure factors are selected to demonstrate bony detail.

In cases of recurrent anterior dislocation an area of bony erosion will be demonstrated on the posterolateral aspect of the head of the humerus. In cases of posterior dislocation the defect will be seen on the anterior aspect of the humeral head.

Lower limb
3

RADIOGRAPHIC TECHNIQUE

Dorsiplantar – all toes

The toes are positioned as for the DP foot (see Fig. 3.2a), but differing in centring point and position of cassette.

An 18×24 cm cassette is placed on the table top and masked off widthways with lead–rubber in order to use the cassette for two projections. The patient is seated on the table with the unaffected limb extended and abducted, leaning back on their hands for support. A lead–rubber apron is applied to the lower abdomen as radiation protection. The affected limb is flexed at the knee and the plantar aspect of the forefoot placed in contact with the cassette, the middle of which is coincident with the metatarsophalangeal joint of the toe under examination. The short axis of the cassette is parallel to the long axis of the foot.

> CENTRING: A vertical central ray, at 90° to the cassette, is directed over the metatarsophalangeal joint of the toe under examination.

Collimate to include phalanges and metatarsal of relevant toe and surrounding soft tissues. Apply an AP anatomical marker within the primary beam.

Dorsiplantar oblique – toes 2–5

The toes are positioned as for the DPO foot (Fig. 3.2b), differing in centring point and position over the cassette.

The lead–rubber sheet is moved on to the exposed half of the cassette. The plantar aspect of the forefoot is placed in contact with the unexposed area of the cassette and the foot internally rotated until the dorsum is parallel to the table top. The metatarsophalangeal joint of the toe under examination is coincident with the midpoint of the unexposed area of the cassette, the short axis of which is parallel to the long axis of the foot. The plantar aspect of the foot is supported with a radiolucent pad.

> CENTRING: A vertical central ray, at 90° to the cassette, is directed over the metatarsophalangeal joint of the toe under examination.

Collimate to include phalanges and metatarsal of relevant toe and surrounding soft tissues.

Lateral hallux (Fig. 3.1)

The lead–rubber sheet is moved on to the exposed half of the cassette. The affected limb is internally rotated until the medial aspect of the hallux is in contact with the unexposed area of the cassette, the interphalangeal joint coincident with its midpoint. The short axis of the cassette is parallel to the long axis of the hallux. To clear the other toes from the hallux, a

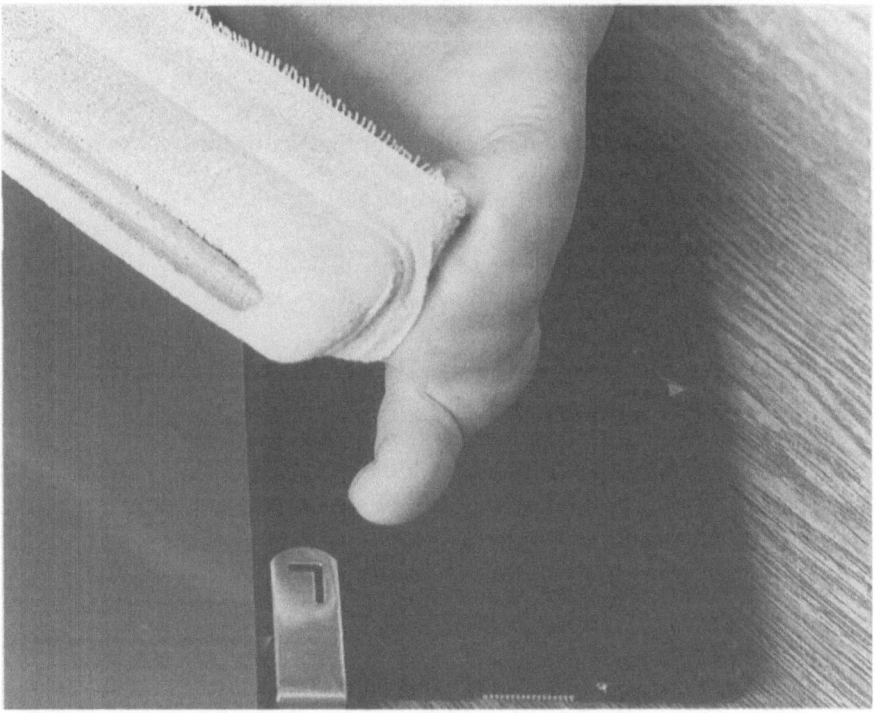

Figure 3.1 Lateral hallux.

radiolucent bandage is placed around toes 2–5, and pulled towards either the dorsal or plantar aspect of the foot and held in place by the patient.

> CENTRING: A vertical central ray, at 90° to the cassette, is directed over the interphalangeal joint.

Collimate to include phalanges and head of first metatarsal and surrounding soft tissues.

IMAGE EVALUATION

Correct patient identification and anatomical marker included on the radiograph.

Area of interest

Dorsiplantar and dorsiplantar oblique

Distal phalanx, base of metatarsal and soft tissue outlines of the toe.

Lateral

Distal phalanx, head of metatarsal and soft tissue outlines of the toe.

Projection

Dorsiplantar

- Separation of adjacent phalanges and metatarsals.
- Separation of bases of first and second metatarsals.
- Slight overlap at bases of metatarsals 2–5.
- Metatarsophalangeal joints clearly demonstrated.
- Interphalangeal joints may/may not be demonstrated, depending on degree of flexion of the toes.

Dorsiplantar oblique

- Separation of adjacent phalanges and metatarsals.
- Overlap of bases of first and second metatarsals.
- Separation of bases of metatarsals 2–5.

- Sesamoid bones below head of first metatarsal projected over head of second metatarsal.

Lateral hallux

- Superimposition of medial and lateral borders of phalanges and head of metatarsal.
- Image of hallux not obscured by other toes.

Exposure factors

- kVp sufficient to demonstrate bony trabeculae and any sesamoid bones below the heads of metatarsals, maintaining contrast between the bones and surrounding soft tissues.
- mAs to provide adequate image density to demonstrate bony detail in contrast to the joint spaces and soft tissues outlines.

No evidence of patient movement.
No artefacts present on the image.

DEMONSTRATION OF HALLUX VALGUS

The term hallux valgus (bunions) describes malalignment of the toes with displacement of the phalanges away from the midline. Both sides are examined for comparison, with the patient taking the full body weight on the feet in order to demonstrate the full extent of the condition.

RADIOGRAPHIC TECHNIQUE

A 24×30 cm cassette is placed on a lead–rubber sheet on the floor. A lead–rubber apron is applied to the patient's lower abdomen as radiation protection. The patient stands on the cassette with their back to the table, feet slightly separated and positioned to include distal phalanges and distal tarsal bones. The long axis of the cassette is parallel to the long axis of the feet. The patient leans back slightly, supporting him/herself against the table in order to clear the upper thighs from the area of interest, and is instructed to maintain the full body weight equally on both feet.

CENTRING: A vertical central ray is directed midway between the first metatarsophalangeal joints. Owing to the size of the X-ray tube head it is often necessary to angle the beam towards the calcanei to achieve the correct centring point. This angle should be kept to a minimum to reduce image distortion.

Collimate to include phalanges of toes 1–5, distal tarsal bones and surrounding soft tissues. Apply Right and Left AP anatomical markers within the primary beam.

IMAGE EVALUATION

Correct patient identification and anatomical marker included on the radiograph.

Area of interest

Distal phalanges, distal tarsal bones and soft tissue outlines of the foot.

Projection

- Feet slightly separated, with first metatarsophalangeal joints level.
- Separation of bases of first and second metatarsals, with slight overlap at bases 2–5.
- Inclusion of a 'weight bearing' legend.

Exposure factors

- kVp sufficient to demonstrate bony trabeculae within phalanges and metatarsals, maintaining contrast between the bones and soft tissue outlines.
- mAs to provide adequate image density to demonstrate bony detail in contrast to the surrounding soft tissues.

No evidence of patient movement.
No artefacts present on the image.

FOOT

RADIOGRAPHIC TECHNIQUE

Dorsiplantar (Fig. 3.2a)

A 24×30 cm cassette is masked off lengthways with a sheet of lead–rubber in order to use it for two projections. The patient is seated on the table with their legs extended, leaning back on the hands for support. A lead–rubber sheet is placed over the lower abdomen as radiation protection. The knee of the affected side is flexed and the plantar aspect of

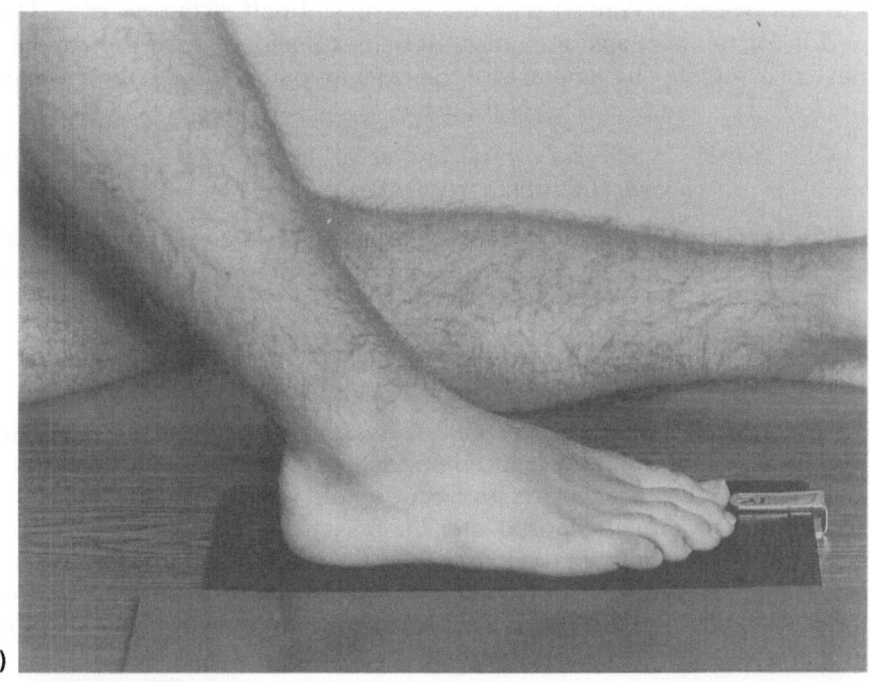

(a)

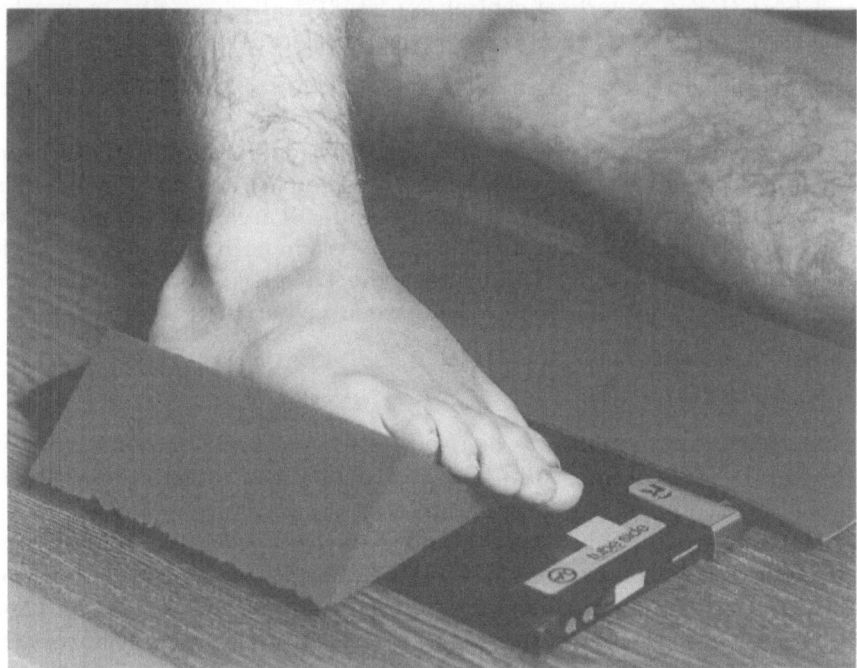

(b)

Figure 3.2 Foot and toes. (a) Dorsiplantar. (b) Dorsiplantar oblique.

the foot placed in contact with the unexposed half of the cassette. The middle of the available area of cassette is coincident with the cuboid–navicular region, the long axis of the cassette parallel to the long axis of the foot. The unaffected leg is abducted.

> CENTRING: A vertical central ray, at 90° to the cassette, is directed over the cuboid–navicular region.

Collimate to include phalanges, metatarsals, tarsal bones and surrounding soft tissues. Apply an AP anatomical marker within the primary beam.

Dorsiplantar oblique (Fig. 3.2b)

The lead–rubber sheet is moved on to the exposed half of the cassette. The plantar aspect of the foot is placed on the unexposed half of the cassette and the foot internally rotated until the dorsum is parallel to the table top. The centre of the unexposed area of cassette is coincident with the cuboid–navicular region, the long axis of the cassette parallel to the long axis of the foot. A radiolucent pad is placed below the plantar aspect of the foot, or the knee of the affected side rested against the opposite leg, for immobilization.

> CENTRING: A vertical central ray, at 90° to the cassette, is directed over the cuboid–navicular region.

Collimate to include phalanges, metatarsals, tarsal bones and surrounding soft tissues.

The kVp selected for the DP and DPO projections should be sufficient to reduce the subject contrast inherent between the toes and tarsal bones, producing a suitable density to demonstrate all areas on a single image. For adequate demonstration of the tarsal area in both projections a slight increase in mAs will be required for the DP projection, owing to the increased density of this region compared to when the foot is obliqued.

Lateral (Fig. 3.3)

This projection must always be used for foreign-body demonstration in the foot, in place of the routine DPO projection, and for demonstration of dorsal/plantar bone displacement in cases of fracture.

The lead–rubber sheet is moved on to the exposed half of the cassette, or a separate 24×30 cm cassette is selected. From the dorsiplantar position the affected leg is externally rotated until the lateral aspect of the foot and little toe is in contact with the cassette. The centre of the available area of cassette is coincident with the navicular–cuneiform joint, the long axis of the cassette parallel to the long axis of the foot. The plantar aspect of the

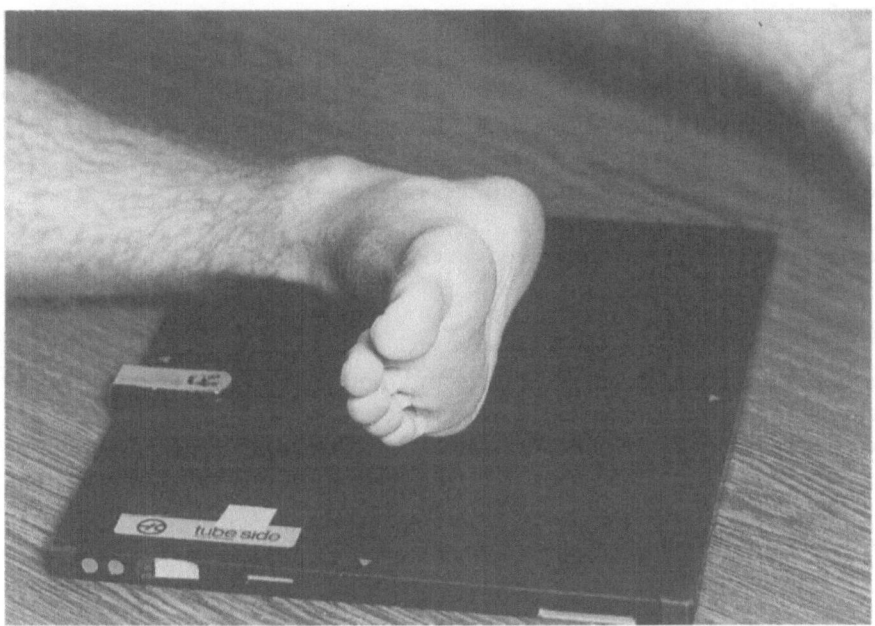

Figure 3.3 Lateral foot.

foot is at 90° to the cassette and this is maintained by supporting the leg with radiolucent pads under its lateral aspect.

CENTRING: A vertical central ray, at 90° to the cassette, is directed over the medial aspect of the foot to the navicular–cuneiform joint.

Collimate to include phalanges, metatarsals, tarsal bones, ankle joint and surrounding soft tissues. Apply an AP anatomical marker within the primary beam.

When selecting exposure factors for the lateral projection, the DP/DPO factors should be altered by doubling the mAs and adding approximately 5 kVp.

IMAGE EVALUATION

Correct patient identification and anatomical marker included on the radiograph.

Area of interest

Distal phalanges, calcaneum and soft tissue outlines of the foot.

Projection

Dorsiplantar

- Separation of adjacent phalanges and metatarsals.
- Slight overlap of bases of metatarsals 2–5.
- Separation of bases of first and second metatarsals.
- Overlapping of tarsal bones.
- Tibia and fibula superimposed on calcaneum and talus.

Dorsiplantar oblique

- Separation of adjacent phalanges and metatarsals.
- Overlap of bases of first and second metatarsals.
- Separation of bases of metatarsals 2–5.
- Separation of tarsal bones, with the exception of medial and middle cuneiforms.
- Posterior aspect of calcaneum and talus demonstrated clear of overlying tibia and fibula.

Lateral

- Superimposition of phalanges.
- Superimposition of metatarsals.
- Cuboid and tubercle of fifth metatarsal demonstrated on plantar aspect of foot.

Exposure factors

kVp selected to reduce the subject contrast inherent in the foot from the phalanges to the much denser tarsus.

- kVp sufficient to demonstrate bony trabeculae, individual outlines in areas of bony overlap and any sesamoid bones below the heads of metatarsals, maintaining contrast between the bones and soft tissues of the foot.
- mAs to provide adequate image density to demonstrate bony detail in contrast to the surrounding soft tissues.

No evidence of patient movement.
No artefacts present on the image.

LATERAL WEIGHT-BEARING FEET FOR PES PLANUS

Both feet are examined for comparison, and it is essential that certain criteria are fulfilled for accuracy of assessment:

1. Weight bearing should be equal on both feet during exposure. This must be explained to the patient.
2. To assist with this an immobilization aid should be available for patients to hold on to in order to stand steadily with even weight distribution.
3. Special equipment should be available for film support. This usually consists of an elevated platform upon which the patient stands. The platform contains a groove for cassette insertion so that it remains vertical, with its lower border below the soft tissue on the plantar aspect of the foot. There should also be a rectangle of lead–rubber, slightly larger than the cassette, placed vertically behind the cassette so that the foot not currently under examination is shielded from the primary beam.

A 24×30 cm cassette is selected. A lead–rubber apron is applied to the patient's lower abdomen as radiation protection. The patient stands with both feet on the platform and the medial aspect of the foot under examination in contact with the cassette, which is placed in the groove of the platform described above.

The long axis of the foot is parallel to the long axis of the cassette, the centre of which is coincident with the tubercle of the fifth metatarsal. The patient stands with the weight distributed evenly on both feet and holds on to the immobilization device as described above.

CENTRING: A horizontal central ray, at 90° to the cassette, is directed over the tubercule of the fifth metatarsal.

Collimate to include phalanges, metatarsals, tarsal bones and surrounding soft tissues. Apply an AP anatomical marker within the primary beam.

IMAGE EVALUATION

Correct patient identification and anatomical marker included on the radiograph.

Area of interest

Distal phalanges, calcaneum, ankle joint and soft tissue outlines of the foot.

Projection

- Superimposition of phalanges.
- Superimposition of metatarsals.

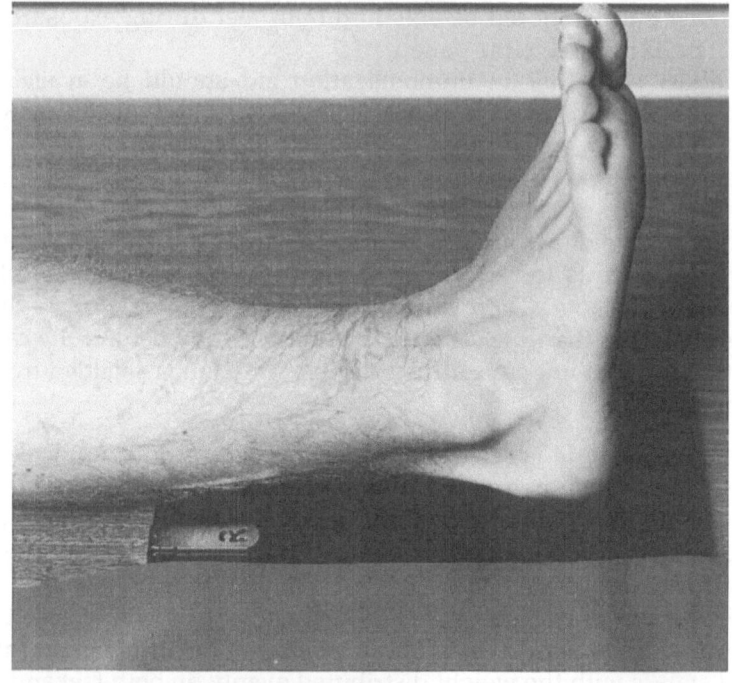

(a)

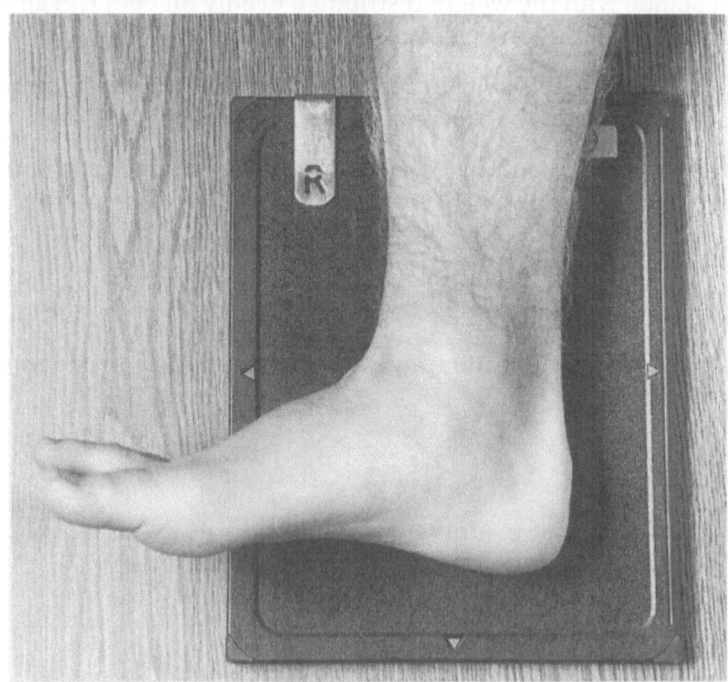

(b)

Figure 3.4 Ankle. (a) AP. (b) Lateral.

- Superimposition of medial and lateral articular surfaces of talus.
- Inclusion of a 'weight-bearing' legend.

Exposure factors

- kVp sufficient to demonstrate the individual outlines of the five sets of phalanges and metatarsals and the bony trabeculae within the calcaneum, maintaining contrast between the bones and soft tissues of the foot.
- mAs to provide adequate image density to demonstrate bony detail within all bones of the foot in contrast to the surrounding soft tissues.

No evidence of patient movement.
No artefacts present on the image.

ANKLE

RADIOGRAPHIC TECHNIQUE

Anteroposterior (Fig. 3.4a)

A 24×30 cm cassette is masked off widthways with lead–rubber to include two projections on one film. The patient is seated on the X-ray table with legs extended, leaning back on their hands for support. A lead–rubber sheet is applied to their lower abdomen as radiation protection. The posterior aspect of the ankle is placed in contact with the unmasked area of the cassette, the plantar aspect of the heel 1 cm above its lower border. The long axis of the tibia is parallel to the short axis of the cassette. The patient flexes the ankle to 90°, maintaining this position with the aid of a pad and sandbag placed below the plantar aspect of the foot. The foot is slightly internally rotated so that the malleoli are equidistant from the cassette.

CENTRING: A vertical central ray, at 90° to the cassette, is directed to a point midway between the malleoli.

Collimate to include ankle joint, talus, lower thirds of tibia and fibula, both malleoli and surrounding soft tissues. Apply an AP anatomical marker within the primary beam.

Lateral (Fig. 3.4b)

The lead–rubber sheet is moved on to the exposed half of the cassette. The patient turns onto the affected side and leans on the elbow for support. The affected leg is extended and externally rotated until the lateral aspect of the foot is in contact with the cassette, the plantar aspect of the heel 1 cm above its lower border. The long axis of the tibia is parallel to the short axis of the cassette. The ankle is flexed to 90° and the malleoli are superimposed. The ankle is immobilized in position with a pad and sandbag below the plantar surface of the foot.

CENTRING: A vertical central ray, at 90° to the cassette, is directed over the medial malleolus.

Collimate to include ankle joint, lower thirds of tibia and fibula, talus, calcaneum, navicular and surrounding soft tissues.

Generally, a perfect lateral projection can be produced if the patient is instructed to keep the knee straight and turn fully on to their side, rather than sitting on the table and externally rotating the leg at the hip. The lateral aspect of the foot is placed in contact with the cassette with the ankle dorsiflexed to 90°.

In the case of severely injured patients a horizontal beam lateral projection should be undertaken. The cassette is supported vertically in contact with the lateral or medial aspect of the ankle, and the X-ray beam directed from the opposite side to pass parallel to the line adjoining the malleoli.

Anteroposterior oblique (Fig. 3.5)

An 18×24 cm cassette is selected. From the AP position the ankle is internally rotated through 30° and dorsiflexed to 90°. The plantar aspect of the heel is 1 cm above the lower border of the cassette, its long axis parallel to the long axis of the tibia. Position is maintained with a pad and sandbag below the plantar aspect of the foot and a radiolucent pad under the medial aspect of the foot.

CENTRING: A vertical central ray, at 90° to the cassette, is directed to a point midway between the malleoli.

Collimate to include ankle joint, lower thirds tibia and fibula, talus, calcaneum and surrounding soft tissues. Apply an AP anatomical marker within the primary beam.

The oblique projection is used to separate the lower ends of tibia and fibula.

In all three projections, because of the low centring point and in order to include the lower thirds of tibia and fibula on the image, there is considerable excess primary radiation below the plantar aspect of the foot. A piece of lead–rubber placed at the lower border of the cassette will absorb this, reducing patient dose and improving image quality.

Inversion/eversion injuries of the ankle can cause rupture or stretching of the ligaments, leading to subluxation. Following routine AP and lateral

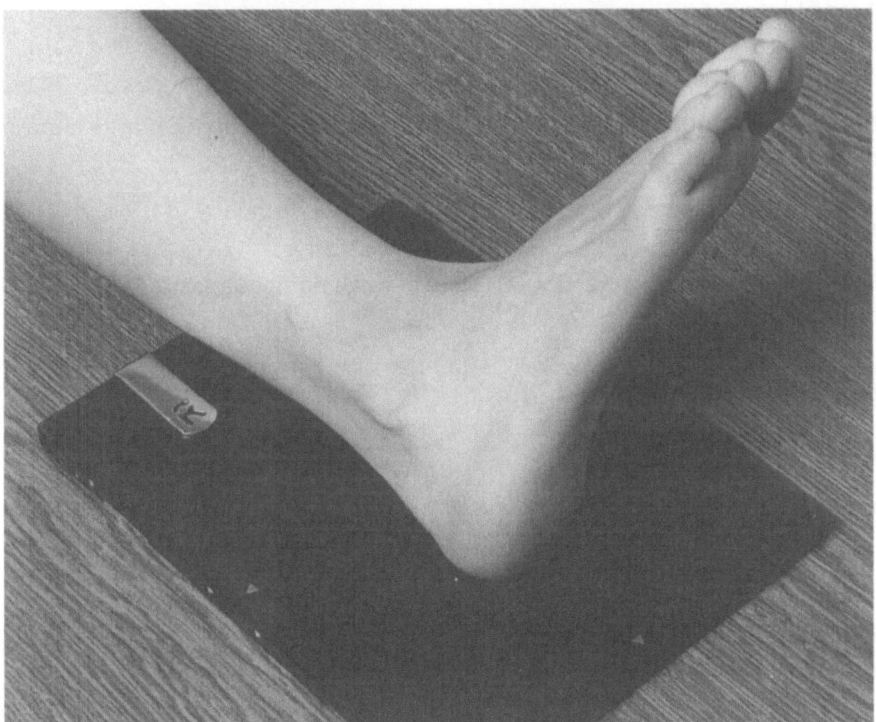

Figure 3.5   Medial oblique ankle.

projections a further AP projection may be taken, with a medical officer placing and maintaining stress (internal or external) on the joint during the exposure. The medical officer must be provided with a full-length lead–rubber apron and lead–rubber gloves to avoid irradiation of the hands. The limb must be carefully position as for the routine AP projection, ensuring that the malleoli are equidistant from the cassette immediately the stress is applied by the medical officer. Widening of the joint space between the malleolus and talus, in comparison to the neutral AP projection, indicates damage to the ligament and may be associated with a flake fracture of the malleolus.

IMAGE EVALUATION

Correct patient identification and anatomical marker included on the radiograph.

Area of interest

Anteroposterior and anteroposterior oblique

Lower thirds tibia and fibula, plantar aspect of foot, medial and lateral malleoli and soft tissue outlines.

Lateral

Lower thirds tibia and fibula, calcaneum, navicular and soft tissue outlines.

Projection

Anteroposterior

- Demonstration of clear joint spaces between inferior articular surface of tibia and superior aspect of talus, lateral aspect of medial malleolus and medial border of talus, medial aspect of lateral malleolus and lateral border of talus.
- Distal tibiofibular joint obscured.
- Superimposition of phalanges, metatarsals and tarsal bones.

Lateral

- Superimposition of medial and lateral malleoli.
- Superimposition of medial and lateral borders of talus, demonstrating a clear joint space between inferior articular surface of tibia and superior aspect of talus.
- Shaft of fibula projected slightly posteriorly in relation to shaft of tibia.

Anteroposterior oblique

- Demonstration of a clear joint space between inferior articular surface of tibia and superior aspect of talus.
- Clear demonstration of distal tibiofibular joint.

Exposure factors

Anteroposterior and anteroposterior oblique

- kVp sufficient to penetrate tibia and fibula, demonstrating bony trabeculae, and reduce subject contrast between areas of greater soft tissue volume (lower calf) and those where there is virtually none (around the malleoli).

- mAs to provide adequate image density to demonstrate bony detail while not overexposing in the area of the malleoli.

Lateral

- kVp sufficient to demonstrate fibula through tibia and the malleoli through talus, enabling visualization of bony trabeculae.
- mAs to provide adequate image density to demonstrate bony detail along the shafts of tibia and fibula and within the malleoli, talus and calcaneum in contrast to the surrounding soft tissues.

No evidence of patient movement.
No artefacts present on the image.

Positional faults

AP projection:

- Insufficient dorsiflexion at the ankle joint will lead to superimposition of the calcaneum over the lateral malleolus, with visualization of the medial malleotalar joint space. The joint space between the superior aspect of the talus and inferior aspect of the tibia will be obscured.
- With insufficient internal rotation the fibiotalar joint space will not be demonstrated.
- Excessive internal rotation will lead to demonstration of the distal tibiofibular joint space.
- If the foot is externally rotated the joint spaces between the malleoli and talus will not be demonstrated, and the distal fibula will be superimposed on the tibia.

Lateral projection:

- Insufficient rotation of the foot will lead to the shaft of the fibula being superimposed over the midshaft of the tibia.
- Excessive rotation of the foot will lead to the shaft of the fibula being projected too far posteriorly in relation to the tibia.
- In both of the above there will be horizontal separation of the medial and lateral articular surfaces of the talus.
- With insufficient dorsiflexion, or if the tibia is not parallel to the film, there will be vertical separation of the medial and lateral articular surfaces of the talus.

CALCANEUM (OS CALCIS)

RADIOGRAPHIC TECHNIQUE

Lateral

For this projection the patient's ankle is turned externally as for the lateral ankle position (see Fig. 3.4b). An 18×24 cm cassette is masked off widthways with a sheet of lead–rubber in order to include two projections on one film. The patient is seated upon the table with their legs extended. A lead–rubber sheet is applied to the lower abdomen as radiation protection. The patient is turned on to the affected side until the lateral aspect of the foot is in contact with the cassette. The middle of the calcaneum is coincident with the centre of the available area of the cassette, long axis of tibia parallel to short axis of cassette. The ankle is dorsiflexed to 90° and the malleoli superimposed.

> CENTRING: A vertical central ray, at 90° to the cassette, is directed to a point 2.5 cm below the medial malleolus, in the middle of the calcaneum.

Collimate to include calcaneum, ankle joint, adjacent tarsal bones and surrounding soft tissues. Apply an AP anatomical marker within the primary beam.

If both calcanei are to be examined in the lateral projection it may be possible to expose them simultaneously, so reducing radiation dose to the patient. The patient does, however, need to be reasonably supple to achieve the required position: sitting on the table with both knees flexed and the plantar aspects of the feet in contact with each other. The legs are relaxed laterally and supported on pads.

> CENTRING: A vertical central ray is directed between the heels, at the level of the medial malleoli.

Axial (Fig. 3.6)

The lead–rubber sheet is moved on to the exposed half of the cassette. The patient is seated with legs extended. The posterior aspect of the affected heel is placed in contact with the unmasked area of cassette, the inferior border of the heel coincident with its lower edge and the long axis of the tibia parallel to the short axis of the cassette. The foot is dorsiflexed and this position maintained by the patient holding a radiolucent bandage looped around the forefoot and pulled towards the knee. The malleoli are equidistant from the cassette.

> CENTRING: A vertical central ray is directed 40° cranially to a point in the middle of the plantar aspect of the foot, at the level of the tubercule of the fifth metatarsal.

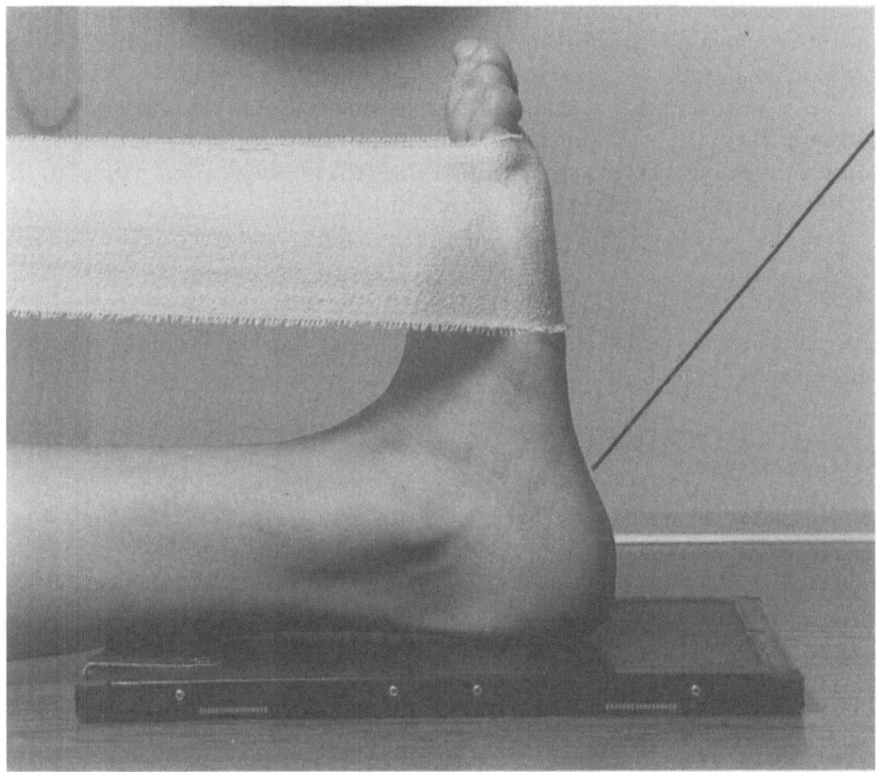

Figure 3.6   Axial calcaneum with central ray angled cranially 40° from vertical.

Collimate to include the calcaneum, adjacent tarsal bones and surrounding soft tissues.

In cases of serious injury the axial projection described above should be carried out. One disadvantage of this projection is that the X-ray beam is directed towards the patient's gonads, potentially increasing the dose to this radiosensitive area. If the patient is mobile, without serious injury to the foot, an alternative is as follows. Stand the patient on the cassette with 2.5 cm of the cassette projecting beyond the back of the heel. The patient bends the knees slightly, holding on to a chair or the table for support.

CENTRING: With the X-ray tube behind the patient's legs, a vertical central ray is directed 30° towards the toes over a point on the posterior aspect of the heel, level with the lateral malleolus.

This projection is only possible if the X-ray tube can be lowered sufficiently to achieve a suitable FFD (100 cm) from the floor.

Either axial technique can be adapted to examine both calcanei simultaneously. The cassette is positioned to include both calcanei and the X-ray beam directed midway between the two, at the levels previously stated.

kVp selection for the axial projection is vital in order to demonstrate the full length of the calcaneum on the image. kVp must be sufficient to reduce the subject contrast, demonstrating the cubocalcaneal articulation on the same image as the distal calcaneum.

IMAGE EVALUATION

Correct patient identification and anatomical marker included on the radiograph.

Area of interest

Lateral

Calcaneum, talocalcaneal and cubocalcaneal joints and soft tissue outlines.

Superoinferior

Calcaneum, cubocalcaneal articulation and soft tissue outlines.

Projection

Lateral

● Superimposition of medial and lateral malleoli.

Superoinferior

● Cubocalcaneal joint space clearly visualized, with no superimposition of metatarsals.
● Lateral malleolus demonstrated on lateral aspect of calcaneum.

Exposure factors

Lateral

● kVp sufficient to demonstrate bony trabeculae within the calcaneum, maintaining contrast with the surrounding soft tissues.

- mAs to provide adequate image density to demonstrate bony detail in contrast to the surrounding soft tissues.

Superoinferior

- kVp sufficient to penetrate calcaneum, demonstrating bony trabeculae, and demonstrate the cubocalcaneal joint.
- mAs to provide adequate image density to demonstrate bony detail throughout calcaneum, providing information in the region of the cubocalcaneal joint while not overexposing the distal portion.

No evidence of patient movement.
No artefacts present on the image.

TIBIA AND FIBULA

RADIOGRAPHIC TECHNIQUE

Anteroposterior (Fig. 3.7a)

An 18×43 cm cassette (or 35×43 cm used diagonally) is selected in order to include ankle and knee joints on one image. The patient is seated on the table, leaning back on their hands for support, with both legs extended and the unaffected leg abducted. A lead–rubber apron is applied to the lower abdomen as radiation protection. The posterior aspect of the lower leg is placed in contact with the cassette, which is positioned to include the knee and ankle joints, long axis of cassette parallel to long axis of tibia. The malleoli at the ankle joint are equidistant from the cassette. The ankle is flexed through 90° and the position maintained with a radiolucent pad and sandbag below the plantar aspect of the foot.

> CENTRING: A vertical central ray, at 90° to the long axis of the tibia, is directed to a point midway between the ankle and knee joints, on the anterior aspect of the lower leg.

Collimate to include tibia and fibula, ankle and knee joints and surrounding soft tissues. Apply an AP anatomical marker within the primary beam.

Lateral (Fig. 3.7b)

An 18×43 cm cassette (or 35×43 cm used diagonally) is selected. The patient turns on to the affected side and leans on their forearm and elbow for stability. The lateral aspect of the lower leg is in contact with the cassette, which is positioned to include ankle and knee joints, long axis of

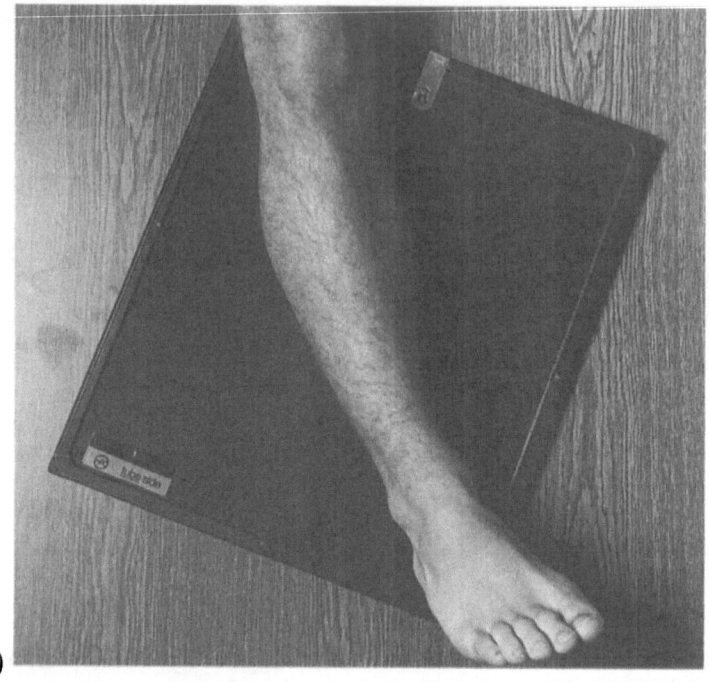

(a)

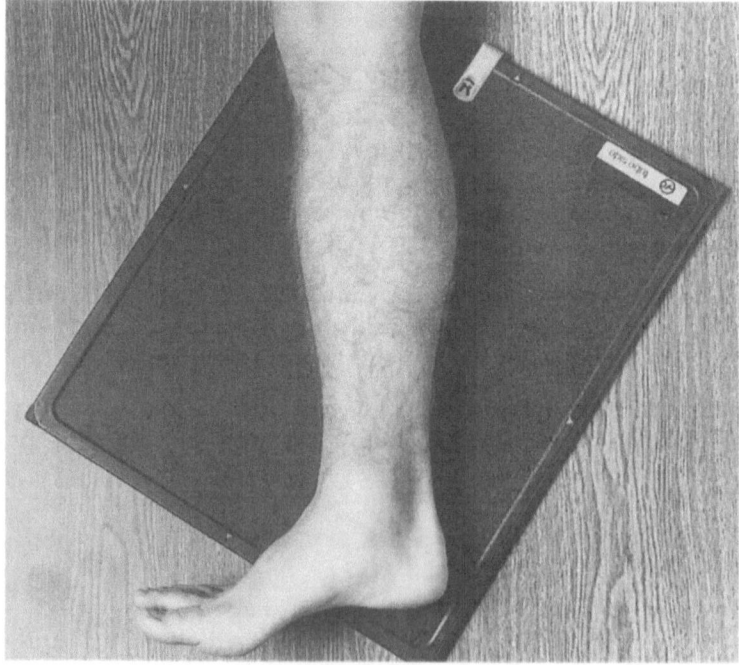

(b)

Figure 3.7 Tibia and fibula. (a) AP. (b) Lateral.

cassette parallel to long axis of tibia. The plantar aspect of the heel is level with the lower edge of the cassette. The ankle is flexed at 90° and the position maintained with a radiolucent pad and sandbag. The malleoli are superimposed vertically.

> CENTRING: A vertical central ray, at 90° to the long axis of the tibia, is directed over the medial aspect of the lower leg midway between the knee and ankle joints.

Collimate to include tibia and fibula, ankle and knee joints and surrounding soft tissues. Apply an AP anatomical marker within the primary beam.

The fibula acts as a stay for the tibia, and therefore a fracture at one end of the tibia or fibula is often associated with a fracture at the opposite end of the other bone. For this reason, when examining the tibia and fibula for a possible fracture it is imperative that both the ankle and knee joints are demonstrated.

IMAGE EVALUATION

Correct patient identification and anatomical marker included on the radiograph.

Area of interest

Ankle and knee joints and soft tissue outlines of the lower leg.

Projection

Anteroposterior

- Separation of shafts of tibia and fibula.
- Superimposition of tibia and fibula at proximal and distal tibiofibular joints.
- Demonstration of joint spaces between medial and lateral borders of the talus and medial and lateral malleoli respectively.

Lateral

- Superimposition of medial and lateral malleoli;
- Superimposition of proximal and distal shafts of tibia and fibula, with midshaft of fibula projected slightly posteriorly in relation to tibia.

Exposure factors

- kVp sufficient to demonstrate bony trabeculae and areas of overlap of tibia, fibula and talus, maintaining contrast between the bones of the lower limb and surrounding soft tissues.
- mAs to provide adequate image density to demonstrate bony detail in contrast to the joint spaces and soft tissue outlines.

No evidence of patient movement.
No artefacts present on the image.

KNEE

RADIOGRAPHIC TECHNIQUE

Anteroposterior (Fig. 3.8a)

An 18×24 cm cassette is selected. The patient sits upon the table, leaning back on their hands for support, with their legs extended and the unaffected leg abducted. A lead–rubber apron is applied to the lower abdomen as radiation protection. The posterior aspect of the affected knee is in contact with the cassette. The centre of the cassette is coincident with a point 2.5 cm below the apex of the patella, long axis of cassette parallel to long axis of tibia. The patella is centralized between the femoral condyles.

CENTRING: A vertical central ray, at 90° to the long axis of the tibia, is directed over a point 2.5 cm below the apex of the patella.

Collimate to include distal third of femur, knee joint, proximal third of tibia, head of fibula and surrounding soft tissues. Apply an AP anatomical marker within the primary beam.

Lateral (Fig. 3.8b)

An 18×24 cm cassette is selected. The patient turns on to the affected side and leans on the forearm for support. The knee is flexed through 60° and the lateral aspect of the leg is in contact with the cassette. The cassette is positioned so that the soft tissue outlines of the patella and tibia are 2.5 cm within the edge of the cassette, its centre level with a point 2.5 cm below the apex of the patella. The femoral condyles are superimposed and a small pad is placed under the lateral aspect of the ankle, to bring the long axis of the tibia parallel to the cassette.

CENTRING: A vertical central ray, at 90° to the long axis of the tibia, is directed to a point 2.5 cm behind and below the apex of the patella.

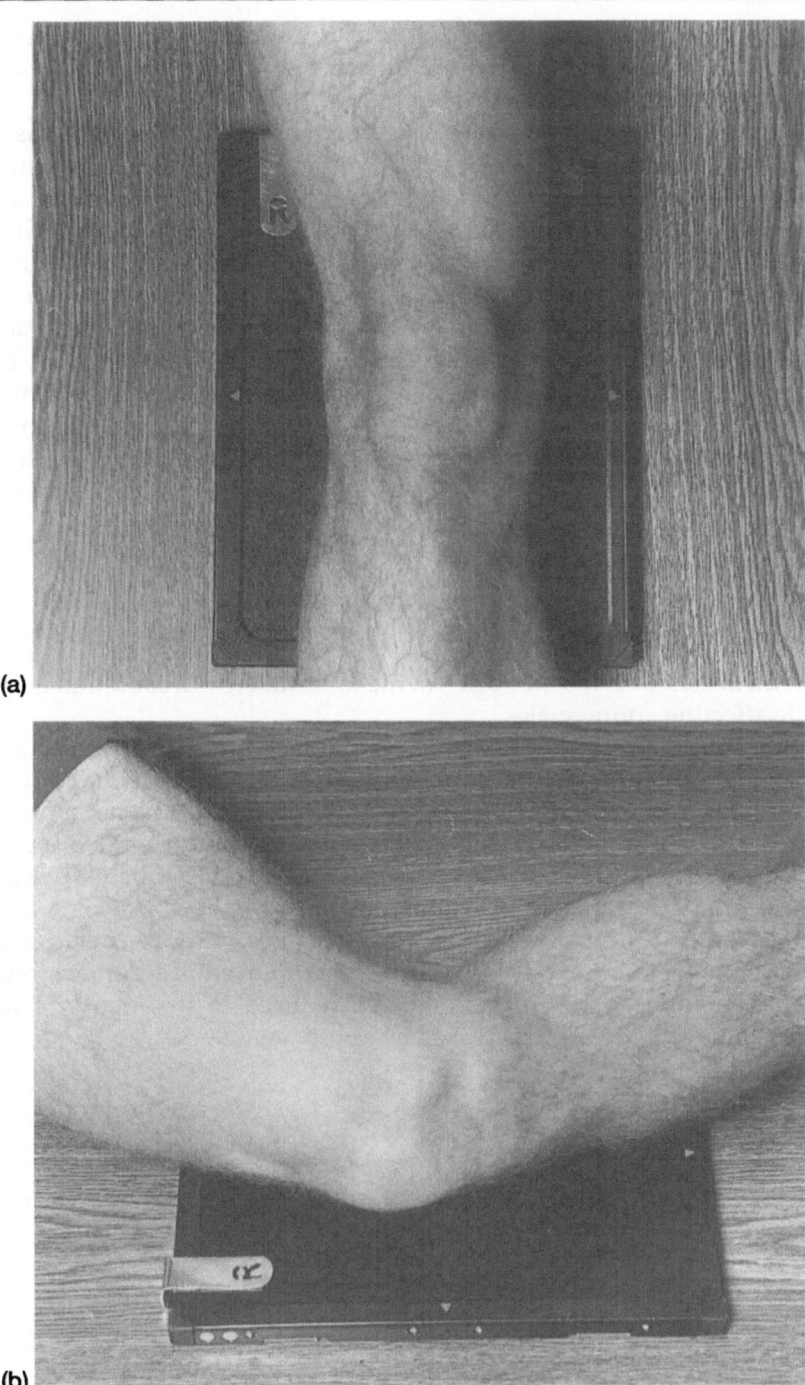

(a)

(b)

Figure 3.8   Knee. (a) AP. (b) Lateral.

Collimate to include distal third of femur, knee joint, patella, proximal third of tibia, head of fibula and surrounding soft tissues. Apply an AP anatomical marker within the primary beam.

A horizontal beam lateral projection should be undertaken in all cases of trauma (Swallow *et al.*, 1986). The cassette should be supported vertically against the lateral or medial aspect of the limb, with the horizontal X-ray beam directed from the opposite side. This may confirm the presence of an intracapsular fracture through demonstration of a fluid level indicating lipohaemarthrosis (Swallow *et al.*, 1986), caused when fat released from the bone marrow at the fracture site enters the joint space and floats on top of the associated effusion. Exposure factors must be selected to demonstrate soft tissue detail, particularly in the region of the suprapatellar bursa, if a fluid level is to be detected as well as bony information. Selection of a relatively high kVp, so as to demonstrate a wider range of densities on the one image, in conjunction with a reduced mAs, will help to achieve this.

Osgood–Schlatter's disease

This term describes osteochondritis of the tibial tubercle, a condition most usually affecting young males.

In order to confirm the disease lateral projections of both knees are taken for comparison. Commonly, the positioning and centring for the routine lateral knee projection is used, but some departments may require an adaptation of this technique so that the central X-ray beam is directed over the tibial tubercle itself. In this case the tibial tubercle will be demonstrated in profile, with slight obliquity of the knee joint and femoral condyles. In either technique small changes will not be detected if the routine knee joint exposure factors are employed. To demonstrate this area adequately the mAs should be reduced to two-thirds of its original value and the kVp decreased by approximately 5.

IMAGE EVALUATION

Correct patient identification and anatomical marker included on the radiograph.

Area of interest

Distal third of femur, proximal third of tibia, head of fibula, patella and soft tissue outlines.

Projection

Anteroposterior

- Patella centralized between femoral condyles.
- Proximal tibiofibular joint obscured owing to slight overlap of head of fibula on tibia.
- Separation of shafts of tibia and fibula.

Lateral

- Superimposition of medial and lateral femoral condyles.
- Patellofemoral joint space clearly demonstrated.
- Proximal tibiofibular joint obscured owing to slight overlap of head of fibula on tibia.
- Shaft of fibula projected posteriorly in relation to shaft of tibia.

Exposure factors

- kVp sufficient to demonstrate bony trabeculae, areas of overlap of tibia, fibula, femur and patella, and the fabella if present, maintaining contrast between the bones and adjacent soft tissue structures.
- mAs to provide adequate image density to demonstrate bony detail in contrast to the surrounding soft tissues.

No evidence of patient movement.
No artefacts present on the image.

Positional faults

Anteroposterior:

- If the central ray is not directed at right-angles to the long axis of the tibia, the superior aspect of the tibial plateau will be projected elliptically and it will not be possible to demonstrate the true width of the joint space.
- Excessive internal rotation of the limb will cause the patella to be projected medially. The head of fibula will be projected clear of the lateral margin of the tibia, demonstrating the proximal tibiofibular joint.
- Excessive external rotation of the limb will cause the patella to be

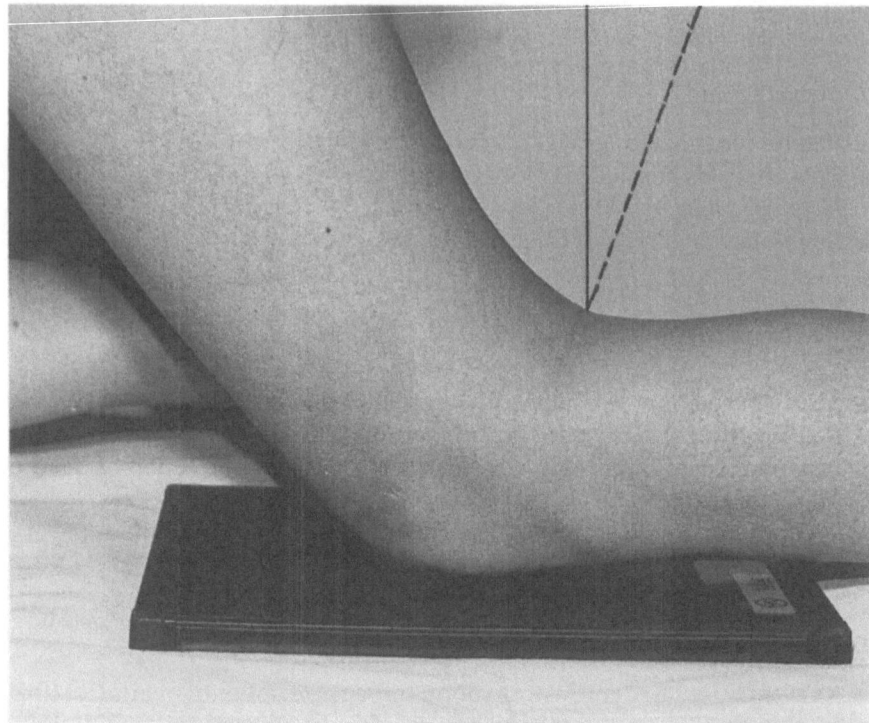

Figure 3.9 Intercondylar notch – patient prone. _____ central ray at 90° to tibia; _ _ _ _ central ray at 70° to tibia.

projected laterally. The head of the fibula will be totally obscured by the proximal tibia.

Lateral:

- Insufficient external rotation will cause a horizontal separation of the femoral condyles, with the head of the fibula superimposed on the proximal tibia.
- Excessive external rotation will cause a horizontal separation of the femoral condyles, with the head of the fibula projected clear of the posterior aspect of the tibia, demonstrating the proximal tibiofibular joint.
- In either of the above, the patellofemoral joint space will not be visible.
- An accurate way of assessing incorrect patient position in the lateral projection is through identification of the adductor tubercule, if apparent, on the superoposterior aspect of the medial condyle of the femur. It should then be obvious whether the medial condyle is anterior to the lateral condyle, indicating over-rotation, or posterior to

it, indicating under-rotation. If the adductor tubercle is not obvious, position can be assessed by comparing the relative position of the head of the fibula to the proximal tibia.

• If the central ray is not directed at right-angles to the long axis of the tibia, the femoral condyles will be separated vertically.

INTERCONDYLAR NOTCH

RADIOGRAPHIC TECHNIQUE

Loose bodies within the knee joint, commonly indicated through 'locking' of the joint, can be seen on routine AP and lateral projections, but demonstration of the intercondylar notch of the femur will show loose bodies clear of other structures. Frequently called 'tunnel' projections, the radiographic appearances of the intercondylar notch resemble the shape of a railway tunnel.

Method 1 (Fig. 3.9)

An 18×24 cm cassette is selected. A lead–rubber apron is applied to the back of the patient's waist as radiation protection. The patient kneels on the X-ray table, with the apex of the patella of the affected knee over the centre of the cassette and leaning forward on to their arms for support. The angle between the femur and tibia is 120° and the patella is centralized between the femoral condyles.

> CENTRING: *To demonstrate the posterior aspect of the notch and full space within the 'tunnel':*
> A vertical central ray, at 90° to the long axis of the tibia, is directed to a point in the middle of the crease at the back of the knee.
> *To demonstrate the anterior aspect of the notch:*
> A vertical central ray, angled cranially until 70° to the long axis of the tibia, is directed to a point in the middle of the crease at the back of the knee.

Collimate to include the femoral and tibial condyles and surrounding soft tissues. Apply a PA anatomical marker within the primary beam.

This is the method of choice as it does not require a special curved cassette and the X-ray beam is not directed at the gonads. However, it is difficult for some patients to achieve or maintain the kneeling position, and in these cases the following method may be used.

Method 2 (Fig. 3.10)

An 18×24 cm (curved or straight) cassette is selected. The patient is seated on the X-ray table and a lead–rubber apron applied to their lower

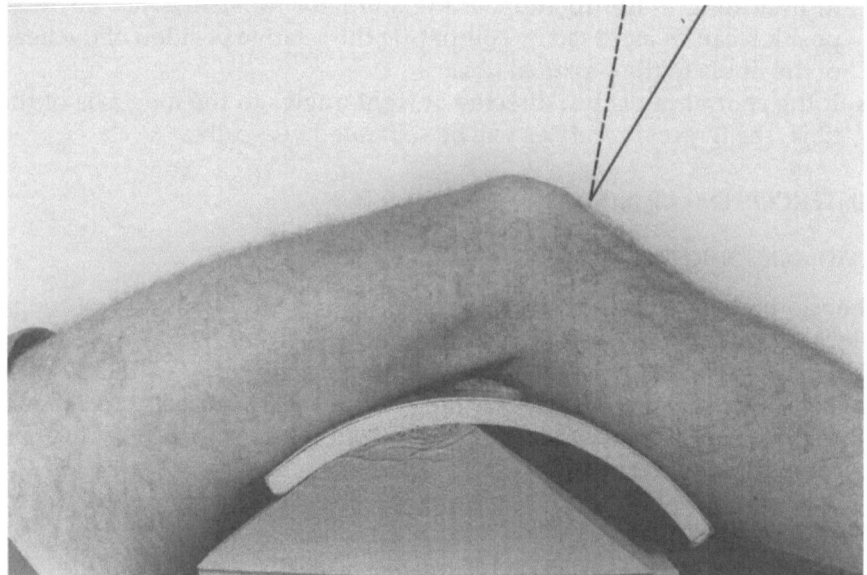

Figure 3.10 Intercondylar notch – patient seated. _____ central ray at 90° to tibia; _ _ _ _ central ray at 110° to tibia. ·

abdomen as radiation protection. The affected knee is flexed through 60° so that the angle between femur and tibia is 120°. The cassette is placed under the flexed knee on top of pads, which help maintain close contact with the leg. The centre of the cassette is coincident with the apex of the patella. The patella is centralized between the femoral condyles.

CENTRING: *To demonstrate the posterior aspect of the notch and full space within the 'tunnel':*
A vertical central ray, angled cranially until at 90° to the long axis of the tibia, is directed immediately below the apex of the patella.
To demonstrate the anterior aspect of the notch:
A vertical central ray is angled 20° caudally from the previous projection until at 110° to the long axis of the tibia, and directed immediately below the apex of the patella.

The cassette is displaced until the central ray is coincident with its centre. Collimate to include femoral and tibial condyles and surrounding soft tissues. Apply an AP anatomical marker within the primary beam.

It is very difficult to change the cassette between projections without some movement of the leg. To ensure that the leg is re-positioned precisely as it was for the 90° projection, do not move the X-ray tube or alter the angle. After exchanging the cassettes, use the light beam and flex the patient's knee until the central ray is directed to the same point over the apex of the patella as for the 90° projection. Once the leg is correctly positioned the angle of the X-ray beam is altered for the 110° projection and the beam recentred to the apex of the patella.

In Method 2, owing to the direction of the X-ray beam in the 90° projection, a lead–rubber sheet **must** be placed between the thighs to provide radiation protection to the gonad region.

IMAGE EVALUATION

Correct patient identification and anatomical marker included on the radiograph.

Area of interest

Femoral and tibial condyles and soft tissues outlines.

Projection

- Patella projected over femoral condyles and clear of intercondylar notch.
- Patella centralized between femoral condyles.

Central ray at 90° to tibia

- Intercondylar notch demonstrated as an inverted 'U'.
- Joint space obscured laterally and medially by partial superimposition of femoral and tibial condyles.

Central ray at 70°/110° to tibia

- Intercondylar notch demonstrated as an inverted, flattened 'U'.
- Joint space clearly visible between femoral and tibial condyles.

Exposure factors

- kVp sufficient to demonstrate bony trabeculae within femoral and tibial condyles, maintaining contrast between the bony structures and soft tissues of the knee joint.
- mAs to provide adequate image density to demonstrate bony detail and

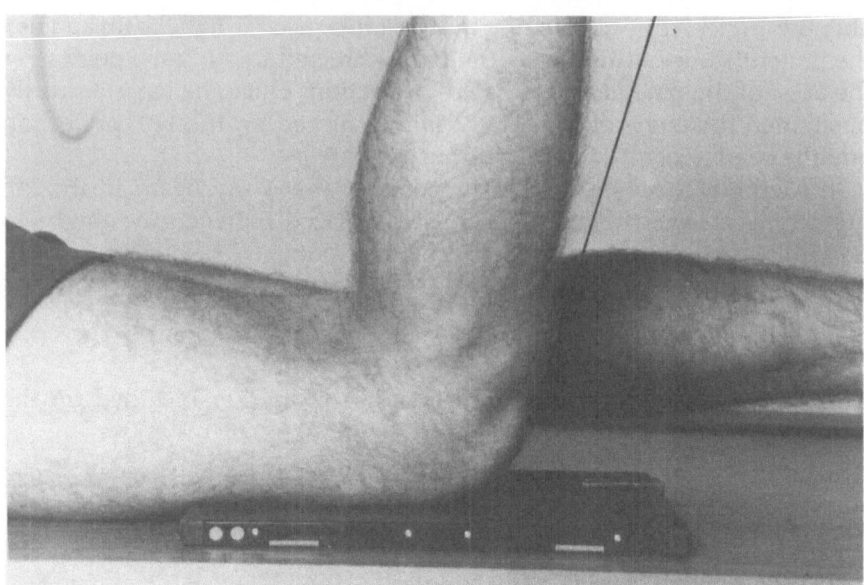

Figure 3.11 Inferosuperior patella – patient prone.

the presence of any loose bodies within the joint space in contrast to the surrounding soft tissues.

No evidence of patient movement.
No artefacts present on the image.

PATELLA

RADIOGRAPHIC TECHNIQUE

Inferosuperior: method 1 (Fig. 3.11)

An 18×24 cm cassette is selected. The patient lies prone with the anterior aspect of the affected limb in contact with the cassette. A lead–rubber apron is applied behind their pelvis as radiation protection. The centre of the cassette is coincident with the upper border of the patella. The knee is flexed through 60° and the limb is immobilized with a bandage placed around the ankle and held by the patient. The patella is centralized between the femoral condyles.

CENTRING: A vertical central ray is directed approximately 15° cranially, to coincide with the long axis of the patella, to a point immediately behind the apex of the patella.

Collimate to include the patellofemoral joint space, articular surfaces of femur, anterior surface of patella and surrounding soft tissues. Apply an AP anatomical marker within the primary beam.

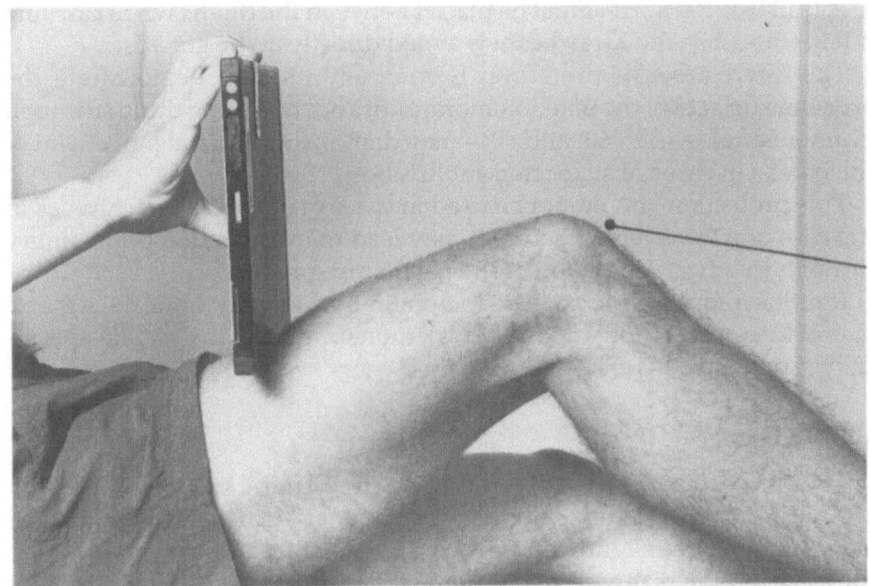

Figure 3.12 Inferosuperior patella – patient seated.

With regard to radiation protection, this is the method of choice as the X-ray beam is not directed towards the gonads. Also, the risk of movement unsharpness on the image is reduced as the cassette is placed on the table top. Many patients, however, will have difficulty in lying prone and an alternative method is as follows.

Inferosuperior: method 2 (Fig. 3.12)

An 18×24 cm cassette is selected. The patient is seated with the affected knee flexed through 60°. For radiation protection purposes a full-length lead–rubber apron is applied to the trunk and abdomen and a sheet of lead–rubber is placed vertically between the thighs. The cassette is placed vertically, with its long edge in contact with the anterior aspect of the thigh, at 90° to the long axis of the patella. The centre of the cassette is coincident with the patella, which is centralized between the femoral condyles. The patient supports the cassette, which is immobilized by placing a radiolucent pad between the distal femur and the cassette.

CENTRING: A horizontal central ray is directed cranially, to coincide with the long axis of the patella, to a point immediately behind the apex of the patella.

Collimate to include the patellofemoral joint space, articular surfaces of the femur, anterior surface of the patella and surrounding soft tissues. Apply an AP anatomical marker within the primary beam.

A lead–rubber apron **must** be placed between the thighs when carrying out Method 2 as the X-ray beam is aimed directly at the gonads.

The inferosuperior projection is routinely used to demonstrate the articular surfaces of the patellofemoral joint and, by flexing the leg through different angles – 30°, 60° and 90° – may demonstrate lateral movement of the patella in cases of suspected subluxation.

This projection should not be used in cases of suspected fracture, as in the case of a transverse fracture it may lead to exacerbation of the injury through (further) separation of the patellar fragments.

Routine requests for patella demonstration usually indicate AP and lateral knee projections. However, demonstration of the patella specifically can be carried out as follows.

Lateral

For this projection the patient position is as for a lateral knee (see Fig. 3.8b).

An 18×24 cm cassette is selected. The patient is turned on to the affected side with the knee slightly flexed. A lead–rubber waist apron is applied to the lower abdomen as radiation protection. The patella is coincident with the centre of the cassette, the transverse axis of the patella perpendicular to it. A radiolucent pad under the ankle will aid immobilization.

CENTRING: A vertical central ray, at 90° to the cassette, is directed to the midpoint of the medial aspect of the patella.

Collimate to include patella, the patellofemoral joint space and surrounding soft tissues. Apply an AP anatomical marker within the primary beam.

Posteroanterior

An 18×24 cm cassette is selected. The patient lies prone with their legs extended and the unaffected leg abducted. A lead–rubber apron is applied to the pelvis as radiation protection. The patella is placed in contact with the centre of the cassette, long axis of the leg coincident with long axis of the cassette. A small pad is placed below the anterior aspect of the lower tibia to prevent rotation of the limb.

CENTRING: A vertical central ray, at 90° to the cassette, is directed to a point in the middle of the crease at the back of the knee.

Collimate to include patella, femoral condyles, knee joint and surrounding soft tissues. Apply a PA anatomical marker within the primary beam.

Posteroanterior obliques (Fig. 3.13)

As the patella is superimposed over the femur on the AP/PA projection, obliques will assist in demonstrating each half of the patella in turn, clear of the femoral condyles.

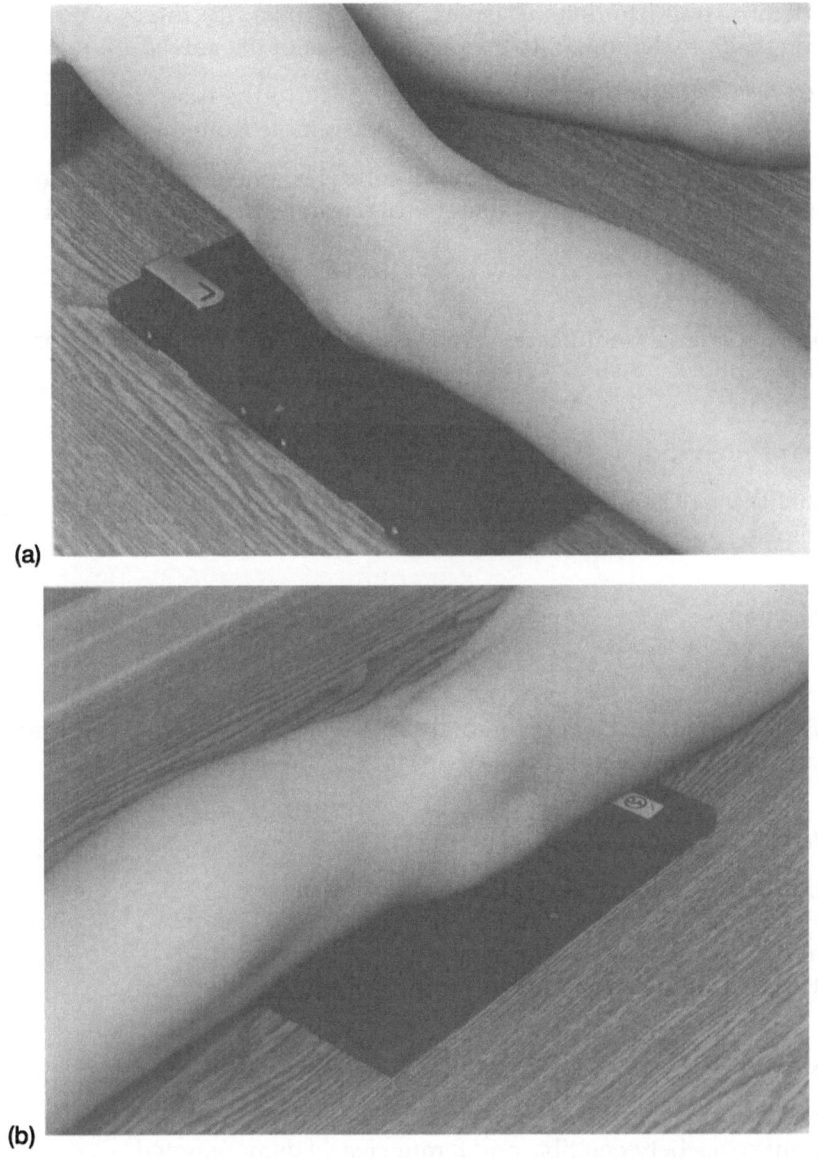

(a)

(b)

Figure 3.13 Oblique left patella. (a) External rotation. (b) Internal rotation.

An 18×24 cm cassette is selected. The patient lies prone with their legs extended and the unaffected leg abducted. A lead–rubber apron is applied to the pelvis as radiation protection. The patella is placed in contact with the centre of the cassette, long axis of the leg coincident with long axis of the cassette. The leg is then (1) externally rotated through 45°

to demonstrate the lateral aspect of the patella; (2) internally rotated through 45° to demonstrate the medial aspect of the patella.

> CENTRING: A vertical central ray, at 90° to the cassette, is directed over the femoral condyle remote from the cassette.

Collimate to include patella, femoral condyles, knee joint and surrounding soft tissues. Apply a PA anatomical marker within the primary beam.

IMAGE EVALUATION

Correct patient identification and anatomical marker included on the radiograph.

Area of interest

Distal third of femur, proximal third of tibia and fibula and soft tissue outlines.

Projection

Inferosuperior

- Patella projected clear of femoral condyles, enabling clear visualization of patellofemoral joint space.

Lateral

- Superimposition of posterior borders of patella.
- Patella demonstrated anterior to femoral condyles, with clear visualization of patellofemoral joint space.
- Femoral condyles will not be perfectly superimposed.

Posteroanterior

- Patella centralized between femoral condyles.
- Joint space between tibia and femur clearly demonstrated.

Posteroanterior oblique

- Half of patella remote from cassette demonstrated clear of femoral condyles.
- Internal rotation: Head of fibula projected posterior to tibia, with clear demonstration of proximal tibiofibular joint.
- External rotation: Head and proximal shaft of fibula superimposed down centre of tibia.

Exposure factors

Inferosuperior

- kVp sufficient to demonstrate bony trabeculae within patella, though not within condyles of femur, maintaining contrast between patella and the surrounding soft tissues.

Lateral

- kVp sufficient to demonstrate bony trabeculae within patella and femoral condyles, maintaining contrast between patella and the surrounding soft tissues.

Posteroanterior and posteroanterior oblique

- kVp sufficient to demonstrate bony trabeculae within patella through overlying femur, maintaining contrast between the bones of the lower limb and the surrounding soft tissues.

All projections

- mAs to provide adequate image density to demonstrate bony detail of patella in contrast to the joint space and surrounding soft tissues.

No evidence of patient movement.
No artefacts present on the image.

HEAD OF FIBULA AND PROXIMAL TIBIOFIBULAR JOINT

RADIOGRAPHIC TECHNIQUE

An 18×24 cm cassette is selected. The patient lies on the affected side on the table. The unaffected leg rests on the table in front of the affected one. The affected knee is flexed through 20°, its lateral aspect in contact with the cassette. The long axis of the cassette is parallel to the long axis of the tibia. The patient rolls forward slightly to externally rotate the leg through 30° until the head of the fibula can be felt in profile behind the tibia. The centre of the cassette is coincident with the lateral femoral condyle.

CENTRING: A vertical central ray, at 90° to the cassette, is directed over the head of the fibula.

Collimate to include head of fibula, proximal tibia and surrounding soft tissues. Apply a PA anatomical marker within the primary beam.

IMAGE EVALUATION

Correct patient identification and anatomical marker included on the radiograph.

Area of interest

Condyles of femur, proximal third of tibia and fibula and soft tissue outlines.

Projection

- Fibula projected posterior to tibia, enabling clear visualization of tibiofibular joint space.
- Patella projected medially and partially superimposed on medial condyle of femur.

Exposure factors

- kVp sufficient to demonstrate bony trabeculae within head of fibula and proximal tibia, and to demonstrate the outline of the patella through the overlying femur, maintaining contrast between the bones and surrounding soft tissues.
- mAs to provide adequate image density to demonstrate detail of the proximal tibiofibular joint in contrast to the adjacent bones and surrounding soft tissues.

No evidence of patient movement.
No artefacts present on the image.

FEMUR

RADIOGRAPHIC TECHNIQUE

Anteroposterior (Fig. 3.14a)

An 18×24 cm cassette is selected (or a 35×43 cm cassette used diagonally) in order to include knee and hip joints on one image. The patient lies supine on the table with their legs extended and the unaffected leg abducted. A lead–rubber apron is applied to the lower abdomen as radiation protection. The posterior aspect of the thigh is placed in contact with the cassette, which is positioned to include the knee and hip joints. The lower edge of the cassette is at the level of the tibial tuberosity, in order to include the knee joint on the radiograph. The patella is centralized between the femoral condyles.

>   CENTRING: A vertical central ray, at 90° to the long axis of the femur, is directed to a point on the anterior aspect of the thigh, to coincide with the centre of the cassette.

Collimate to include knee and hip joints and surrounding soft tissues. Apply an AP anatomical marker within the primary beam.

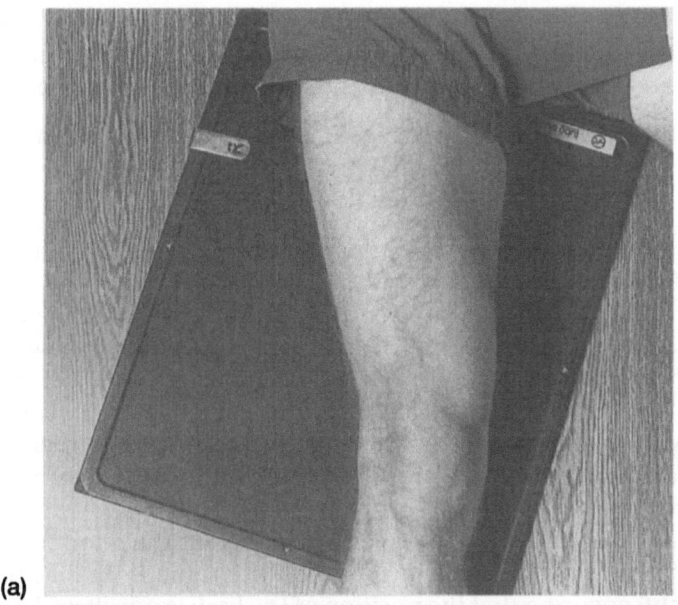

(a)

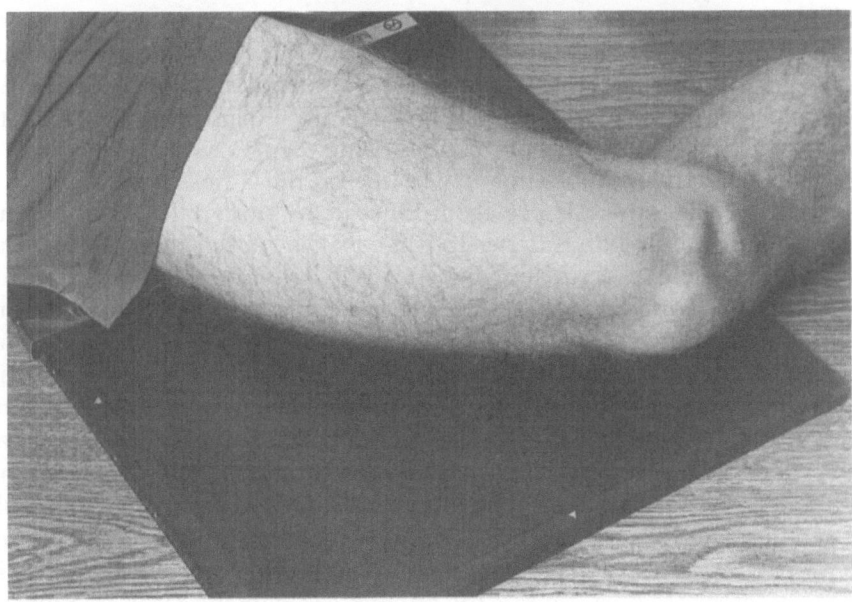

(b)

Figure 3.14 Femur. (a) AP. (b) Lateral.

Lateral (Fig. 3.14b)

An 18×43 cm cassette is selected (or 35×43 cm used diagonally). The patient turns on to the affected side. The knee is slightly flexed and the lateral aspect of the thigh placed in contact with the cassette, which is positioned to include the hip and knee joints. The lower edge of the cassette is coincident with the tibial tuberosity. The femoral condyles are superimposed and pads placed under the lower leg to aid immobilization.

> CENTRING: A vertical central ray, at 90° to the cassette, is directed to a point on the medial aspect of the thigh, midway between knee and hip joints.

Collimate to include knee and hip joints and surrounding soft tissues. Apply an AP anatomical marker within the primary beam.

Owing to the variation in subject contrast between the knee and hip joints, selection of a relatively high kVp, in conjunction with a lower mAs, is necessary to produce an exposure which demonstrates the full length of the femur on one image. Alternatively, the patient may positiond on the table with the knee at the anode end of the X-ray tube, utilizing the 'anode–heel effect' in order to produce a more uniform density along the image of the femur.

When undertaking radiographic examinations of the femur, both the hip and knee joints should be included on the same image if possible. Alternatively, ensuring that the position of the limb is not altered, so as to allow assessment for rotation of the limb at a fracture site, two films for each projection should be taken to include the knee joint and lower femur and the hip joint and upper femur, with the midshaft area included on each. In either case, the full length of the femur must be demonstrated, to reduce the possibility of abnormalities being overlooked.

With severely injured patients who attend the X-ray department on a casualty trolley, the AP projection should be undertaken placing the cassette in the cassette tray beneath the trolley, rather than moving the limb to place the cassette directly beneath it. A horizontal beam lateral of the knee joint and lower two-thirds of the femur may be taken, with the cassette supported vertically on either the medial or lateral aspects of the limb, bearing in mind that a mediolateral projection will require the patient to raise the opposite leg clear of the primary beam. The hip joint and upper femur may be demonstrated using the same technique as that described for a horizontal beam lateral projection of the hip, but again the patient must be able to raise the unaffected limb, with the thigh vertical. Together, these two images will provide a lateral projection of the full length of the femur. For follow-up examinations of a fractured femur it is only necessary to demonstrate the fracture site plus the associated joint.

Radiation protection to the gonads is an important consideration when examining the femur. Protection in the form of a lead–rubber sheet should be used, ensuring that it is accurately positioned so as not to obscure any part of the femur. It should always be used for the full AP projection and the lateral projection of the lower femur, but may be excluded from the lateral projection of the upper femur, where placement is more difficult and its use may lead to a need for repeat exposure.

IMAGE EVALUATION

Correct patient identification and anatomical marker included on the radiograph.

Area of interest

Hip and knee joints, patella and soft tissue outlines.

Projection

Anteroposterior

- Patella centralized between femoral condyles.
- Greater trochanter demonstrated in profile on lateral aspect of femur.
- Lesser trochanter demonstrated on medial aspect of shaft of femur.

Lateral

- Superimposition of femoral condyles.
- Patellofemoral joint space clearly demonstrated.
- Greater trochanter superimposed on shaft of femur.
- Lesser trochanter demonstrated in profile on posterior aspect of femur.

Exposure factors

Particularly in the AP projection, kVp needs to be selected to reduce the subject contrast inherent along the length of the femur.

- kVp sufficient to demonstrate bony trabeculae within femur and areas of overlap of patella on femoral condyles (AP projection) and head of femur on acetabulum, maintaining contrast between the bony structures and surrounding soft tissues.
- mAs to provide adequate image density to demonstrate bony detail in contrast to the surrounding soft tissues.

No evidence of patient movement.
No artefacts present on the image.

MEASUREMENT OF LEG LENGTH (BONE MENSURATION)

Certain childhood problems, e.g. Perthes' disease or trauma involving the epiphyses, may lead to a foreshortening of the long bones in the lower limb. Treatment to reduce the difference in leg length may involve osteotomy and traction of the shorter limb, rendering it the same length as the normal leg.

Alternatively, the epiphyseal plate of the normal limb may be stapled, restricting its growth, and so allowing the shorter limb to 'catch up'. Prior to either method of intervention radiographic examination is necessary to accurately demonstrate the relative lengths of the lower limbs.

CT is the technique of choice, mainly because of its low patient dose, being estimated at 50–100 times lower than conventional scanography (Webb *et al.*, 1991), which was previously the most common method of leg length measurement. The CT scanogram facilitates the production of a series of accurately comparable images of the growing limbs. Following the scanogram, callipers are applied to the extreme ends of the femora, tibial plateaux and distal tibiae, the computer providing an instant readout of leg length.

RADIOGRAPHIC TECHNIQUE

In the absence of CT, the most commonly used conventional X-ray method is also one of the more accurate, because the X-ray beam is always centred vertically over the joint under examination.

The patient lies on an orthopaedic rule placed on the X-ray table or a special cassette tunnel. The orthopaedic rule incorporates a radio-opaque scale marked at 1 cm intervals, which allows the distance between the ankle, knee and hip joints of each limb to be calculated directly. Placing 30×40 cm or 35×43 cm cassettes transversely in the table bucky or underneath the cassette tunnel, three separate exposures are made with the vertical X-ray beam centred midway between the limbs, at the level of each of the three joints in turn. If the difference in leg length is greater than 5 cm, six separate exposures will be necessary, with the vertical X-ray beam centred accurately to each joint on each limb in turn. This avoids the use of a divergent X-ray beam, which would lead to inaccurate measurements. Through simple arithmetic subtraction the radio-opaque ruler enables the orthopaedic surgeon to accurately compare the leg lengths.

As these patients may require a series of radiographs to monitor leg length during their treatment, radiation protection is essential and must include lead–rubber gonad protectors, accurate technique and beam collimation and the recording of exposure factors used. This will serve as a record of patient dose as well as indicating suitable exposure factors to the radiographers undertaking subsequent examinations of the same patient.

Pelvic girdle

4

PELVIS AND HIPS

RADIOGRAPHIC TECHNIQUE

Anteroposterior pelvis

For this projection the patient is initially positioned as for the supine abdomen (see Chapter 9, Fig. 9.1).

A 35×43 cm cassette is placed transversely in the table bucky. The patient lies supine on the table with their legs extended. The MSP is coincident with, and perpendicular to, the midline of the table. The ASISs are equidistant from the table top. The arms are abducted, resting by the patient's sides. With the FFD set at 100 cm and the bucky tray fully out, the vertical X-ray beam is centred to the middle of the cassette and collimated to its longitudinal and transverse limits. The bucky tray is pushed under the table and the X-ray tube centred to it transversely. The X-ray tube or patient is moved until the iliac crests lie just within the upper border of collimation. The legs are placed in slight internal rotation to bring the necks of the femora parallel to the cassette.

> CENTRING: The vertical X-ray beam, at 90° to the cassette, will be directed over the midline, approximately midway between the ASISs and the upper border of the symphysis pubis.

The cassette is aligned with the X-ray beam. Collimate to include iliac crests and greater and lesser trochanters. Apply an AP anatomical marker within the primary beam.

Anteroposterior, both hips

The technique is exactly as described above for the pelvis, with the ASISs included within the upper border of collimation and the centring point

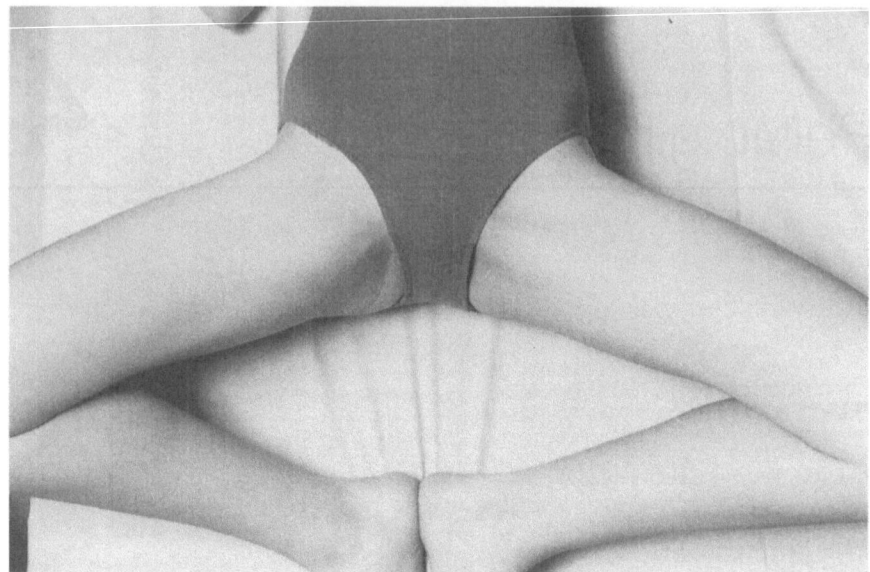

Figure 4.1 'Frog' laterals, demonstrating both hips.

approximately 2.5 cm above the upper border of the symphysis pubis. Areas for inclusion are ASISs, greater and lesser trochanters and upper third of femur.

Collimating to the cassette in this way is good practice in terms of radiation protection, as the area of the primary beam will not exceed the available area of film. Restriction of the primary beam will result in less secondary radiation being produced, reducing the dose received by the patient and improving image quality. Some units incorporate a scale in the light beam diaphragm housing which relates field size to FFD, enabling the radiographer to manually collimate to the limits of the cassette. Others may incorporate a device which automatically sets the maximum field size according to the size of cassette locked into the bucky tray.

Gonad protection should not be used in preliminary examinations of the pelvis and hips, but should be used in subsequent examinations in a series.

It is sometimes difficult to include both greater trochanters on the image, particularly in a female with a wide pelvis. This problem can be overcome by increasing the FFD, so reducing the divergence of the X-ray beam. In order to produce a correctly exposed radiograph, the mAs should be increased according to the inverse square law.

Overexposure in the region of the greater trochanters can be a problem, particularly when X-raying thin patients with minimal soft tissue in this area. This can be avoided by selecting a relatively low value of mAs, to reduce the degree of film blackening, in conjunction with a kVp of at least 70, in order to reduce the level of subject contrast. kVp alone should **not** be reduced, as this will have the effect of increasing subject contrast, compounding the exposure problem as well as increasing skin dose.

Lateral oblique, both hips (Fig. 4.1)

A lateral projection of both hips is required when comparison of both sides is necessary, for example in Perthes' disease. This project is **not** to be used in cases of trauma.

A 30×40 cm cassette is placed transversely in the table bucky and the vertical X-ray beam centred and collimated to it as in the AP projections above. From the position used for AP pelvis/hips, both knees and hips are flexed. The plantar aspects of the feet are placed together, the knees are separated and both legs externally rotated through 60°. The legs are supported with radiolucent pads under their lateral aspects. The X-ray tube or patient is moved until the ASISs lie just within the upper border of collimation.

> CENTRING: The vertical X-ray beam, at 90° to the cassette, will be directed over a point in the midline, approximately 2.5 cm above the upper border of the symphysis pubis.

The cassette is aligned with the X-ray beam. Collimate to include ASISs and greater and lesser trochanters. Apply an AP anatomical marker within the primary beam.

Anteroposterior, single hip

For this projection the patient is positioned initially as for AP pelvis.

A 24×30 cm cassette is placed longitudinally in the table bucky and the vertical X-ray beam centred and collimated to it as above. The patient lies supine with the legs extended, MSP perpendicular to the table top, ASISs equidistant from it. The hip joint under examination is over the centre of the cassette. The affected leg is slightly internally rotated and the unaffected leg abducted. The X-ray tube or patient is moved until the ASIS lies just within the upper border of collimation and the greater trochanter within the lateral border.

> CENTRING: The vertical beam, at 90° to the cassette, will be directed approximately over the femoral pulse. (See p. 114.)

The cassette is aligned with the X-ray beam. Collimate to include ASIS, greater and lesser trochanters and upper third of femur. Apply an AP anatomical marker within the primary beam.

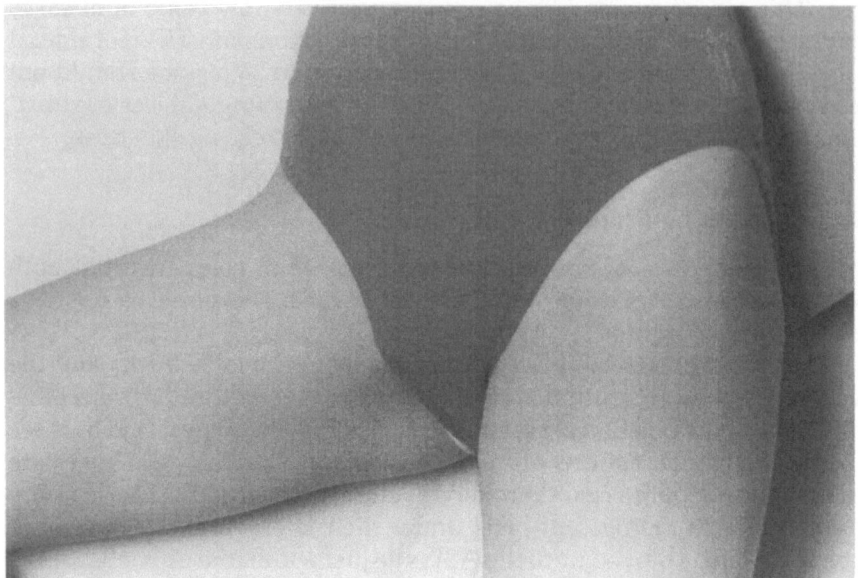

Figure 4.2 Lateral oblique single hip.

To locate the **femoral pulse** draw an imaginary line between the ASIS on the side under examination and the upper border of the symphysis pubis. Bisect this line with another at 90° to it. The femoral pulse is found 2.5 cm inferiorly along the line of bisection.

Lateral-oblique, single hip (Fig. 4.2)

This is *not* to be used in cases of trauma.

A 24×30 cm cassette is placed longitudinally in the table bucky and the X-ray beam centred and collimated to it as before. The patient lies supine on the table, MSP coincident with its long axis, and is rotated 45° towards the affected side. Radiolucent pads are placed under the raised trunk and leg to support in this position. The affected leg is flexed at the knee and externally rotated until the lateral aspect of the thigh is in contact with the table. The hip joint is over the centre of the cassette. The X-ray tube or patient is moved until the ASIS lies just within the upper border of collimation.

CENTRING: The vertical beam, at 90° to the cassette, will be directed approximately over the femoral pulse.

The cassette is aligned with the X-ray beam. Collimate to include ASIS, greater and lesser trochanters and anterior and posterior soft tissues of femur. Apply an AP anatomical marker within the primary beam.

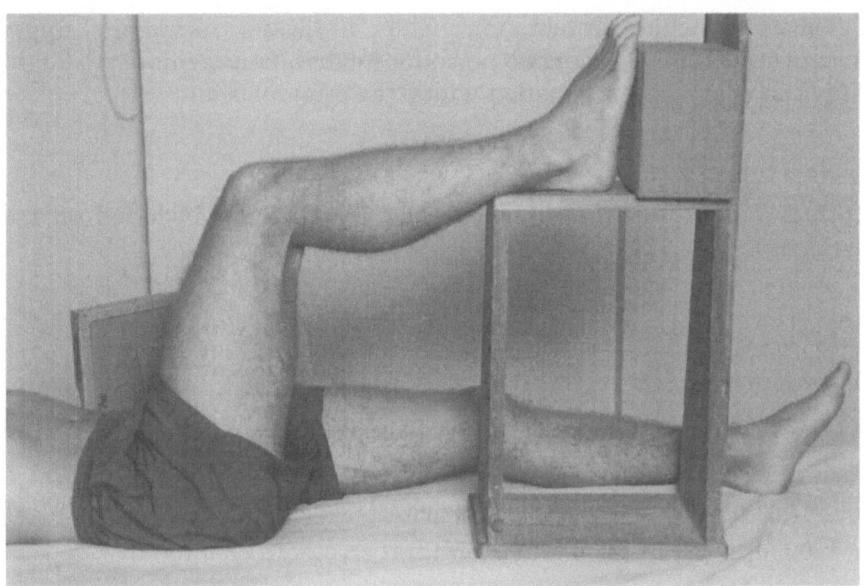

Figure 4.3   Horizontal beam lateral hip.

Horizontal beam lateral for neck of femur (Fig. 4.3)

Must be used in cases of trauma.

The patient lies supine on the trolley with both legs extended, MSP perpendicular to the trolley. A 24×30 cm gridded cassette, placed transversely in a vertical cassette holder, is placed against the lateral aspect of the affected hip at approximately 45° to the MSP. The long axis of the cassette is parallel to the neck of the femur (a 45° radiolucent pad between cassette and patient will assist in gauging the angle). The upper border of the cassette is tucked well into the waist and the cassette wedged down on to the trolley mattress, so as to include the ischial tuberosity on the image. The unaffected leg is flexed to 90° at the knee and hip joints and raised to bring the thigh as near vertical as possible. External rotation of the uninjured limb will assist in clearing the soft tissue of the raised thigh from the area of interest. A leg support is used to maintain this position.

> CENTRING: A horizontal central ray, at 90° to the neck of femur and gridded cassette, is directed through the crease of the groin to the centre of the long axis of the cassette and midway between the anterior and posterior soft tissue margins of the thigh.

Collimate to include acetabulum, greater and lesser trochanters, upper third of femur and anterior and posterior soft tissues margins of the thigh. Apply an AP anatomical marker within the primary beam.

IMAGE EVALUATION

Correct patient identification and anatomical marker included on the radiograph.

Area of interest

Anteroposterior pelvis

Iliac crests and greater and lesser trochanters.

Anteroposterior and lateral-oblique, single and both hips

ASIS(s), upper third(s) of femur(ora) and greater trochanter(s).

Horizontal beam lateral for neck of femur

Acetabulum, upper third of femur, ischial tuberosity and ASIS.

Projection

Anteroposterior pelvis and both hips

- MSP coincident with midline of film.
- Symmetry of right and left iliac bones and obturator foramina.
- Symmetry of right and left necks of femora and comparable visualization of greater and lesser trochanters.

Lateral-oblique, both hips

- MSP coincident with midline of film.
- Greater trochanters superimposed over necks of femora, with the lesser trochanters demonstrated in profile on medial aspects of shafts of femora.
- No superimposition of superior pubic rami over acetabula and heads of femora.

Anteroposterior, single hip

- Greater trochanter seen in profile on lateral aspect of head of femur, with lesser trochanter just visible on medial margin of upper shaft of femur.

- Obturator foramen 'open', with no superimposition of ischium on pubis.

Lateral-oblique, single hip

- Greater trochanter superimposed over neck of femur, with lesser trochanter demonstrated in profile on medial aspect of shaft of femur.
- Ischium superimposed on superior pubic ramus.
- No superimposition of superior pubic ramus over acetabulum and head of femur.

Horizontal beam lateral for neck of femur

- Greater trochanter superimposed on neck of femur, with lesser trochanter superimposed on greater trochanter.
- Proximal two-thirds of neck of femur visible, with no superimposition of other structures.
- ASIS demonstrated in profile on anterior aspect of pelvis, with ischial tuberosity demonstrated posteriorly.

Exposure factors

Anteroposterior projections

- kVp selected to reduce the inherent subject contrast between the greater trochanters and pelvis.
- mAs to provide adequate overall image density, avoiding overexposure in the region of the greater trochanters.

Anteroposterior and lateral-oblique projections

- kVp sufficient to demonstrate bony trabeculae within the pelvic bones and to demonstrate the acetabulum(a) through the head(s) of femur(ora), maintaining contrast between the bony structures and pelvic viscera.
- mAs to provide adequate image density to demonstrate bony detail in contrast to the soft tissue organs within the pelvic cavity.

Horizontal beam lateral for neck of femur

kVp selected to reduce the subject contrast inherent in the area from the dense hip joint down the shaft of femur.

- kVp sufficient to demonstrate the head of femur within the acetabulum and bony trabeculae within the head, neck and proximal shaft of femur.

- mAs to provide adequate image density to demonstrate bony detail within the acetabulum and head of femur and along the shaft of femur in contrast to the surrounding soft tissues.

No evidence of patient movement.
No artefacts present on the image.

LATERAL PELVIMETRY

Pelvimetry is the radiographic examination of the maternal pelvis for the purpose of obtaining measurements of the pelvic inlet and outlet. By comparing these figures with the biparietal diameter of the baby's skull, ascertained during ultrasound, cases of cephalopelvic disproportion may be identified. This would indicate the need for caesarian section rather than natural delivery. Pelvimetry may be carried out towards the end of pregnancy, where there is concern over the size of the baby's head in relation to the pelvic outlet, or following caesarian section to provide measurements in anticipation of future pregnancies.

CT will provide images for accurate pelvimetry with a radiation dose approximately 30 times lower than conventional radiographic pelvimetry, using AP and lateral scanograms and a single axial CT slice at the level of the fovea of the heads of the femora (Webb *et al.*, 1991). Badr *et al.* (1995), however, recommend the use of a single lateral scanogram only, with accurate positioning to ensure that the scan field commences at the iliac crests and the scan length limited to 250 mm whenever possible. This will further reduce the radiation dose to the mother, and in particular to the foetus. In the absence of CT, they state that the method of choice should be that of erect lateral pelvimetry using an air-gap technique. This will obviate the need for a secondary radiation grid, reducing the amount of scatter/back-scatter reaching the film or patient, maintaining image quality and reducing radiation dose to both mother and foetus.

Special adaptation of the equipment is required, in the form of a frame which allows the cassette to be supported 25 cm behind a perspex screen, against which the patient stands. An FFD of 180 cm will compensate for image magnification caused by the increased OFD.

It must be remembered, however, that there will still be some degree of image magnification, and this should be accounted for when taking measurements of the pelvic inlet and outlet. To ensure accuracy, one of two methods can be employed.

1. A radio-opaque ruler, marked at 1 cm intervals, is placed between the buttocks to coincide with the midline, as all landmarks used for pelvic measurement are midline structures. The markings on the ruler will therefore be magnified proportionally to these structures, allowing actual measurements to be obtained.

2. The distance from the gluteal cleft to the perspex on the air-gap frame is measured and added to the 25 cm air-gap to give an actual OFD. This measurement is written on the resulting image and used in conjunction with a pelvimetry chart which converts the image measurements into actual size.

RADIOGRAPHIC TECHNIQUE

A 35×35 cm cassette is placed in the back of the vertical air-gap frame and the appropriate AP anatomical marker applied. With a horizontal FFD of 180 cm, the X-ray beam is centred to the middle of the cassette, turning the light box through 45° to produce a diamond shape. The beam is collimated so that the points of the diamond just reach the edges of the cassette, enabling the bony landmarks required for pelvic measurement to be included without excessive irradiation of the lower abdomen. The patient stands with their side against the perspex front of the frame. The vertical height of the X-ray tube is altered and the patient moved backwards/forwards until the central ray is coincident with a point 2.5 cm above the greater trochanters. The feet are slightly separated for stability and positioned so that the backs of the heels are level. The patient is instructed to look forward, taking the body weight equally on both legs. The arms are folded on to the chest away from the primary beam. The MSP is parallel to the cassette and the greater trochanters are superimposed horizontally and vertically. If the patient has one leg shorter than the other, a small wooden block is placed under the shorter leg to bring the trochanters level. The cassette is positioned to coincide with the X-ray beam.

Collimate to include iliac crest, upper femora, symphysis pubis and sacrum/coccyx.

IMAGE EVALUATION

Correct patient identification and anatomical marker included on the radiograph.

Area of interest

Sacral promontory, greater trochanters, symphysis pubis and sacrococcygeal junction (plus the radio-opaque ruler if used).

Projection

• Perfect superimposition of heads of femora.

Exposure factors

- kVp sufficient to penetrate the dense pelvis, demonstrating the outlines of both femoral heads and bony trabeculae within.
- mAs to provide adequate image density to demonstrate the posterior border of the symphysis pubis, without overexposing the region of the coccyx.

ILIUM AND ACETABULUM

RADIOGRAPHIC TECHNIQUE

The ilium and acetabulum are demonstrated on routine projections of the hips and pelvis, but the anterior and posterior aspects of the acetabular rim are superimposed over the ischium and head of femur, whereas the ilium is seen at an angle. To demonstrate these areas adequately, the following projections are undertaken:

Acetabulum 'en face' and lateral ilium (Fig. 4.4)

A 24×30 cm cassette is placed longitudinally in the table bucky. The patient lies supine on the X-ray table, MSP coincident with its central long axis, and is rotated 45° away from the side under examination. Radiolucent pads are placed under the raised trunk and leg for support in this position.

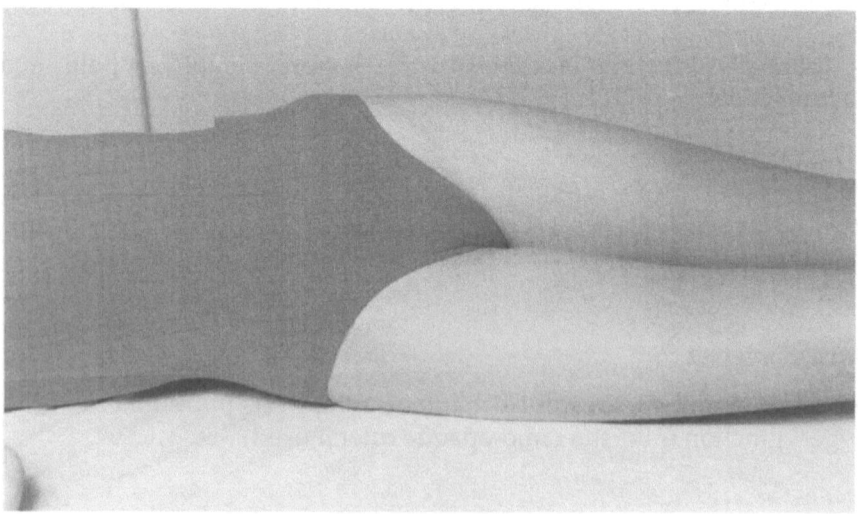

Figure 4.4 45° posterior oblique to show lateral ilium and acetabulum *en face* (left side), with centring altered according to area required.

For the acetabulum the hip joint is coincident with the centre of the cassette; *for the ilium* the long axis of the ilium is coincident with the central long axis of the cassette, the upper border of which is 5 cm above the iliac crest.

CENTRING: *Acetabulum*
A vertical central ray, at 90° to the cassette, is directed over the femoral pulse. (See page 114.)
Ilium
A vertical central ray, at 90° to the cassette, is directed over the ASIS on the raised side.

For acetabulum collimate to include ASIS, ischium and pubic ramus.
For ilium collimate to include iliac crest, ischium and sacroiliac joint.
Apply an AP anatomical marker within the primary beam.

Lateral acetabulum and anteroposterior ilium

A 24×30 cm cassette is placed longitudinally in the table bucky. The patient lies supine on the X-ray table, MSP coincident with its central long axis, and is rotated 45° towards the side under examination. Radiolucent pads are placed under the raised trunk and leg for support in this position.
For the acetabulum the hip joint is coincident with the centre of the cassette; *for the ilium* the upper border of the cassette is placed 5 cm above the iliac crest and a point midway between the ASIS and spine coincident with its central long axis.

CENTRING: *Acetabulum*
A vertical central ray, at 90° to the cassette, is directed over the femoral pulse.
Ilium
A vertical central ray, at 90° to the cassette, is directed to a point midway between the ASIS on the raised side and the spine.

Collimation and marker as for previous posterior oblique.

IMAGE EVALUATION

Correct patient identification and anatomical marker included on the radiograph.

Area of interest

Acetabulum

Head and neck of femur and complete outline of acetabulum.

Ilium

Iliac crest, symphysis pubis, sacroiliac joint and ASIS.

Projection

Acetabulum 'en face' and lateral ilium

- Acetabulum demonstrated *'en face'* and ilium demonstrated in profile, with 'opening' of obturator foramen.
- Obturator foramen opened out in comparison to routine AP pelvis.
- Oblique appearance of lumbar vertebrae.

Lateral acetabulum and anteroposterior ilium

- Anterior acetabular rim superimposed on head of femur.
- Ilium demonstrated *'en face'*, with 'closure' of obturator foramen.
- ASIS demonstrated in profile on lateral aspect of ilium.
- Ischial spine demonstrated in profile medial to acetabulum.
- Superimposition of superior and inferior pubic rami.
- Oblique appearance of lumbar vertebrae.

Exposure factors

- kVp sufficient to demonstrate bony trabeculae within the acetabulum through the overlying head of femur and within the ilium, maintaining contrast between the bony pelvis and pelvic viscera.
- mAs should provide adequate image density to demonstrate bony detail within the acetabulum and ilium in contrast to the adjacent soft tissues structures.

No evidence of patient movement.
No artefacts present on the image.

Vertebral column   **5**

ATLANTO-OCCIPITAL JOINTS

RADIOGRAPHIC TECHNIQUE

Anterior obliques (Fig. 5.1)

An 18×24 cm cassette is placed longitudinally in the erect bucky. A lead–rubber cape is applied to the patient's shoulders as radiation protection. The patient is seated with the forehead in contact with the bucky, OMBL (see page 160) and MSP perpendicular to it. The middle of the cassette is coincident with the middle of the inferior orbital margin on the side under examination.

> CENTRING: A horizontal central ray, at 90° to the cassette, is directed to the centre of the bucky. The head is then rotated away from the side under examination until the central ray is coincident with the MSP at the level of the mastoid tip.

Collimate to include base of skull, C2, ramus of mandible and maxillary sinus on the side under examination. Apply a PA anatomical marker within the primary beam. Both sides are examined for comparison.

Lateral

An 18×24 cm cassette is placed longitudinally in the vertical cassette holder. A lead–rubber cape is applied to the patient's shoulders as radiation protection. The patient is erect facing the cassette. The head is turned through 90°, to bring the affected side into contact with the cassette. The MSP of the head is parallel to the cassette. The middle of the cassette is coincident with the mastoid tip.

> CENTRING: A horizontal central ray, at 90° to the cassette, is directed over the mastoid tip.

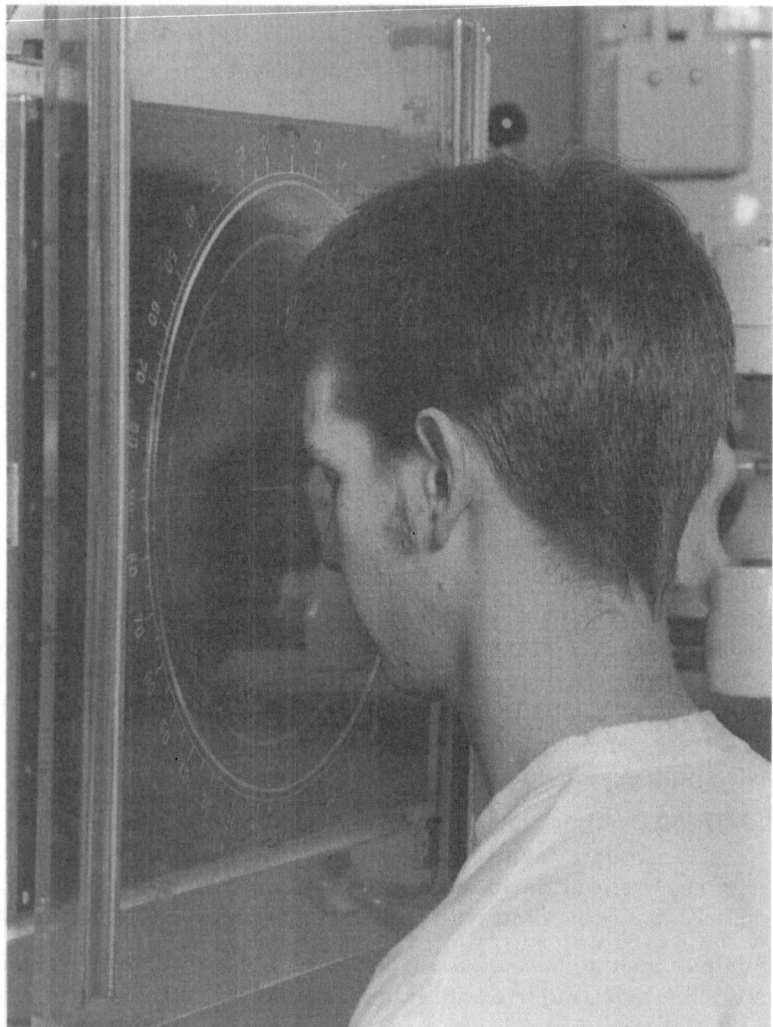

Figure 5.1 Anterior oblique: atlanto-occipital joints.

Collimate to include EAM temporomandibular joints and C1, including spinous process. Apply an AP anatomical marker within the primary beam.

IMAGE EVALUATION

Correct patient identification and anatomical marker included on the radiograph.

Area of interest

Base of occiput and C1.

Projection

Anterior oblique

- Maxillary sinuses projected clear of atlanto-occipital joint under examination.
- Atlanto-occipital joint demonstrated between lateral margin of maxillary sinus and medial margin of body of mandible.

Lateral

- Superimposition of posterior borders of bodies of mandible.
- Superimposition of right and left superior and inferior borders of cervical vertebrae.
- Joint space clearly demonstrated between occiput and C1.

Exposure factors

- kVp sufficient to demonstrate bony trabeculae within C1, maintaining contrast between bony structures and those filled with air.
- mAs to provide adequate image density to demonstrate bony detail in contrast to the air-filled sinuses.

No evidence of patient movement.
No artefacts present on the image.

CERVICAL SPINE

RADIOGRAPHIC TECHNIQUE

Lateral (Fig. 5.2)

A 24×30 cm or 18×24 cm cassette is placed longitudinally in the vertical cassette holder. A lead–rubber apron is applied to the patient's lower abdomen as radiation protection. The patient is erect, with the shoulder of the affected side touching the cassette and the MSP parallel to it. The upper border of the cassette is coincident with the top of the pinna of the ear. The chin is raised to clear the angles of the mandible from the first and second cervical vertebrae. The shoulders are relaxed and the feet slightly separated for stability. The cassette is positioned to include the anterior and posterior soft tissue outlines of the neck.

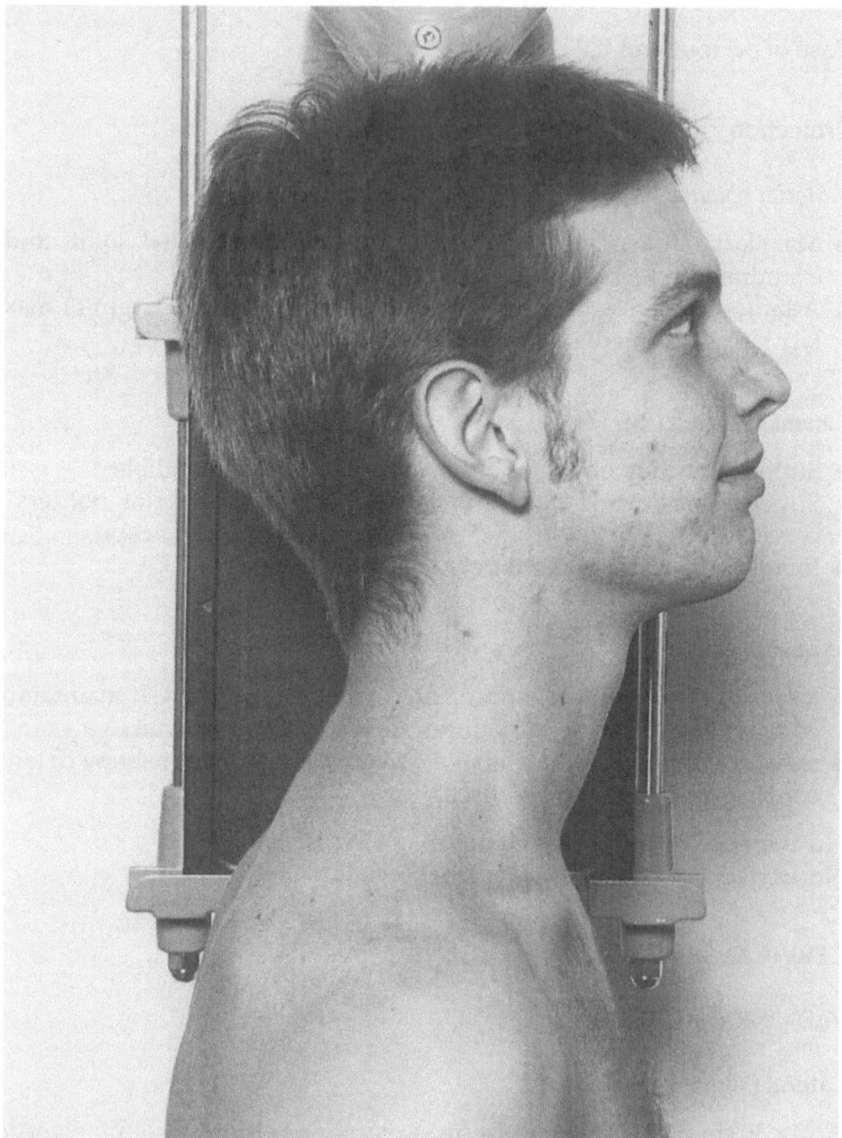

Figure 5.2   Lateral cervical vertebrae.

CENTRING: Using an FFD of 180 cm, a horizontal central ray, at 90° to the cassette, is directed to the middle of the neck at the level of the thyroid eminence.

Collimate to include EAMs, C7/T1 joint space and anterior and posterior

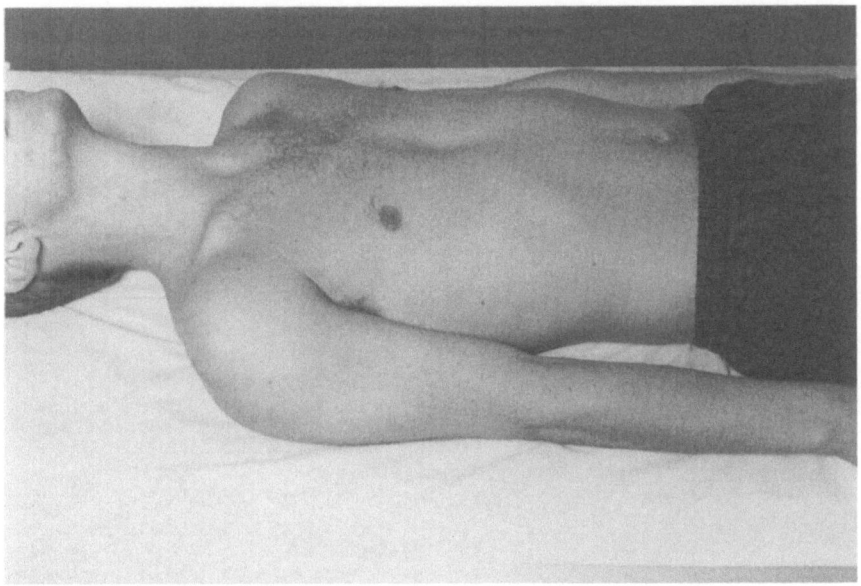

Figure 5.3   AP showing patient position for all AP projections of the vertebral column.

soft tissue outlines of neck. Apply an AP anatomical marker within the primary beam.

Patients with broad muscular shoulders should be given a weight to hold in each hand to assist in projecting the shoulder masses below the level of C7. Exposing the radiograph on arrested expiration will also help.

The soft tissue structures of the anterior neck **must** be included, particularly in cases of trauma, as widening of the retropharyngeal (>5 mm) and retrotracheal (>16 mm) soft tissues is strongly indicative of bony inquiry, even when no bony abnormality is apparent (Grech, 1981).

Special care must be taken with patients following trauma – refer to '**Examination of the spine in cases of trauma**' (p. 158).

Anteroposterior C3–7 (Fig. 5.3)

A 24×30 cm or 18×24 cm cassette is placed longitudinally in the table bucky. The patient lies supine on the table, MSP coincident with and perpendicular to the midline of the table. A lead–rubber sheet is applied to the chest as radiation protection. The upper border of the cassette is level with the external auditory meati and the chin raised to superimpose the symphysis menti over the base of the occiput. The mouth remains closed to maximize clearance of the mandible from C3 on the image.

CENTRING: A vertical central ray, parallel to the line adjoining occiput and symphysis menti, is directed over the MSP, level with the thyroid eminence.

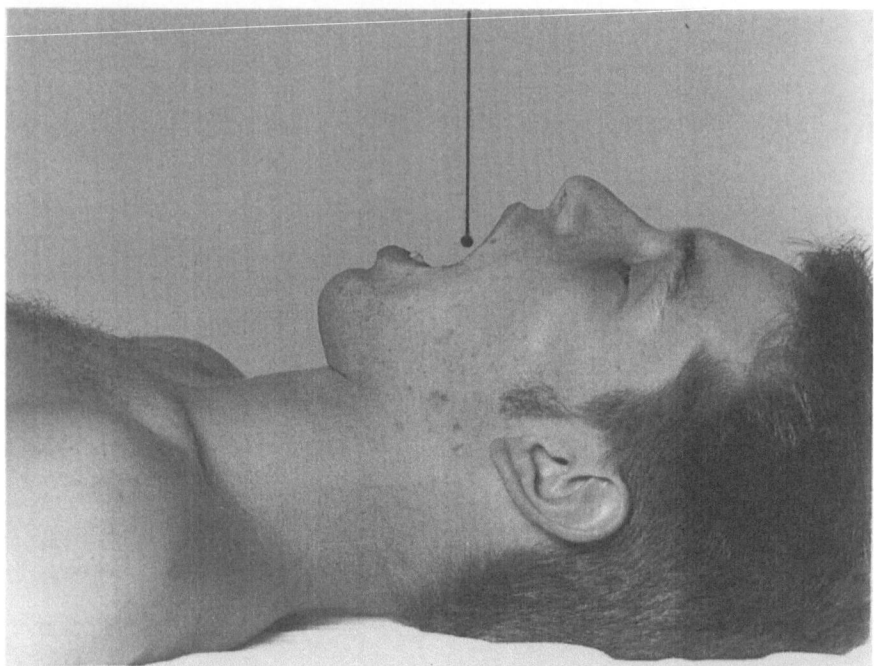

Figure 5.4 AP open-mouth: C1–2.

Collimate to include C2/3 junction, T1 and lateral soft tissues of neck. Apply an AP anatomical marker within the primary beam.

Anteroposterior C1 and 2 (Fig. 5.4)

An 18×24 cm cassette is placed longitudinally in the table bucky. The patient is positioned as for AP C3–7, with the centre of cassette coincident with the upper incisors. The patient is asked to open their mouth slightly and the chin is adjusted to superimpose the lower borders of the upper incisors (gingival margin in edentulous patients) over the base of the occiput.

> CENTRING: A vertical central ray, parallel to the line adjoining the crowns of the upper incisors and occiput, is directed through the open mouth at the level of the lower borders of the upper incisors.

Collimate to include atlanto-occipital joints, C2/C3 joint space and transverse processes. Apply an AP anatomical marker within the primary beam.

Immediately prior to exposure, without moving their head, the patient is asked to open their mouth wide in order to demonstrate C1 and 2 through the open mouth.

AP 3–7 and AP 1 and 2 projections may also be carried out with the patient erect against a vertical bucky.

IMAGE EVALUATION

Correct patient identification and anatomical marker included on the radiograph.

Area of interest

Lateral

EAM, C7/T1 joint space, anterior soft tissue structures of neck and spinous processes.

Anteroposterior C3–7

C2/3 joint space, T1 and transverse processes.

Anteroposterior C1 and 2

Atlanto-occipital and C2/3 joint spaces and transverse processes, through the open mouth.

Projection

Lateral

- No superimposition of angle of mandible over upper vertebrae.
- Superimposition of right and left posterior, superior and inferior borders of vertebral bodies.
- Shoulders projected below level of C7/T1 joint space.

Anteroposterior C3–7

- Base of skull superimposed over lower border of mandible.
- Cervical vertebrae demonstrated down centre of film.
- Spinous processes demonstrated down centre of vertebral bodies.

Anteroposterior C1 and 2

- Base of skull superimposed over lower border of upper teeth (gingival margin in edentulous patients).

- Atlanto-axial joints and odontoid process seen clear of overlying structures.
- Mouth wide open so that lower teeth are superimposed over body of C3.
- Cervical vertebrae demonstrated down centre of film.
- Spinous processes demonstrated down centre of vertebral bodies.

Exposure factors

Lateral

- kVp sufficient to demonstrate the joint space between C7 and T1 and to reduce the subject contrast inherent in this area, providing information of the vertebral bodies, spinous processes and soft tissue structures in the anterior aspect of the neck.
- mAs to provide adequate image density to demonstrate bony detail of the vertebral bodies and spinous processes in contrast to the adjacent soft tissues structures.

Anteroposterior C3–7 and C1 and 2

- kVp sufficient to penetrate the vertebrae, demonstrating bony trabeculae within the bodies and the spinous processes through the bodies, maintaining contrast between the bony and soft tissue structures and air-filled trachea.
- mAs to provide adequate image density to demonstrate bony detail of the cervical vertebrae in contrast to the soft tissues structures of the neck.

No evidence of patient movement.
No artefacts present on the image.

Cervical rib demonstration

If it is suspected that a patient has a cervical rib, a 24×30 cm cassette is used longitudinally and the patient is positioned as for the routine AP cervical spine C3–7. The vertical central ray is directed over the sternal notch and collimation includes C3–T5 and lateral soft tissues of the neck.

OBLIQUE CERVICAL SPINE

RADIOGRAPHIC TECHNIQUE

Anterior oblique (Fig. 5.5)

The right anterior oblique demonstrates the right intervertebral foramina.
The left anterior oblique demonstrates the left intervertebral foramina.

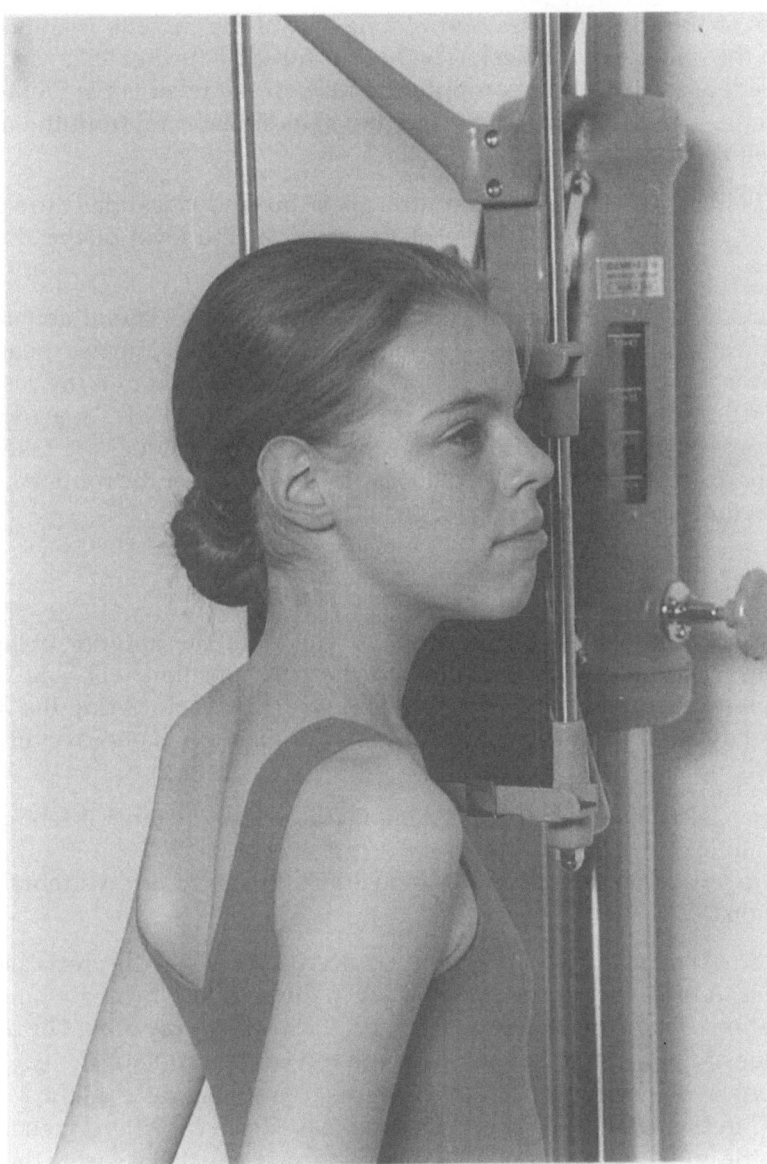

Figure 5.5   Anterior oblique cervical vertebrae.

An 18×24 cm or 24×30 cm cassette is placed vertically in the erect cassette holder. A lead–rubber apron is applied to the patient's lower abdomen as radiation protection. The patient is erect facing the cassette, the upper border of cassette level with the top of the pinna of the ear. The patient is rotated away from the side under examination, until the MSP is at 45° to the cassette. The central long axis of the cassette is coincident with the midline of the neck. The head is turned a further 45° away from the side under examination until the MSP of the head is parallel to the cassette. The chin is raised to clear the mandibular rami from the upper vertebrae.

CENTRING: A horizontal central ray is directed 15° caudally to a point in the middle of the neck, at the level of the thyroid eminence.

Collimate to include atlanto-occipital joints, T1 and lateral soft tissue outlines. Apply an anatomical marker within the primary beam as follows: right anterior oblique – place a Right PA marker on the cassette above the right shoulder; left anterior oblique – place a Left PA marker on the cassette above the left shoulder. Both anterior obliques are taken for comparison. As no grid is used the exposure factors for the routine lateral projection are used, in conjunction with 180 cm FFD.

Posterior oblique

These projections are acceptable alternatives to the anterior obliques; however, it should be remembered that this position will lead to an increased absorbed dose to the thyroid gland. Also, lowering the X-ray tube sufficiently to achieve the 15° cranial angulation may prove difficult at 180 cm FFD.

The right posterior oblique demonstrates the left intervertebral foramina.
The left posterior oblique demonstrates the right intervertebral foramina.

An 18×24 cm or 24×30 cm cassette is placed vertically in the erect cassette holder. A lead–rubber apron is applied to the patient's lower abdomen as radiation protection. The patient is erect, facing the X-ray tube. The upper border of the cassette is level with the top of the pinna of the ear. The patient is rotated away from the side under examination until the MSP is at 45° to the cassette. The central long axis of the cassette is coincident with the midline of the neck. The head is turned a further 45° from the side under examination until the MSP is parallel to the cassette. The chin is raised to clear the mandibular rami from the vertebrae.

CENTRING: A horizontal central ray is directed 15° cranially to a point in the middle of the neck, at the level of the thyroid eminence.

Collimate to include atlanto-occipital joints, T1 and lateral soft tissue outlines. Apply an anatomical marker within the primary beam as follows: right posterior oblique – place a Left AP marker on the cassette above the left shoulder; left posterior oblique – place a Right AP marker on the cassette above the right shoulder. Both posterior obliques are taken for comparison.

OBLIQUES IN CASES OF TRAUMA

Oblique projections of the cervical spine may be requested as a supplementary examination in accident and emergency departments where there is concern over the integrity of the facet joints. AP oblique projections can be undertaken without moving the patient, placing the cassette on the tray beneath the trolley top and angling the X-ray beam 45° across the patient from either side in turn. Rotating the X-ray tube 15° towards the head about the horizontal axis will produce the required cranial angulation. The X-ray beam is directed to the middle of the neck, at the level of the thyroid eminence, on the side nearest the X-ray tube, and the cassette displaced in the opposite direction to accommodate the 45° angulation of the beam. As in the routine posterior oblique projection, the intervertebral foramina and apophyseal joints demonstrated are those on the side remote from the cassette. A grid should only be used if the grid lines can be accurately matched to the direction of the X-ray beam, so preventing grid cut-off. It is easier to work without the grid, using an FFD of 100 cm and selecting the same kVp and up to half the mAs of the routine lateral cervical projection. Both oblique projections are required for comparison.

IMAGE EVALUATION

Correct patient identification and anatomical marker included on the radiograph.

Area of interest

Base of occiput, T1 and lateral soft tissue outlines of neck.

Projection

- Chin raised to clear mandible from upper vertebrae.
- Intervertebral foramina demonstrated slightly elliptically on opposite side of spine to mandible.
- Pedicles of opposite side projected in centre of superior borders of vertebral bodies.
- Spinous processes demonstrated posterior to intervertebral foramina.

- Exaggerated curve of first rib on side under examination, with straightening of rib on opposite side.
- Soft tissue structures of neck demonstrated anterior to vertebral bodies.
- Comparable projections of right and left oblique images.

Exposure factors

- kVp sufficient to demonstrate bony trabeculae within the cervical vertebrae, maintaining contrast between the vertebrae and soft tissue structures of the neck.
- mAs to provide adequate image density to demonstrate bony detail of the cervical vertebrae in contrast to the intervertebral foramina and surrounding soft tissues.

No evidence of patient movement.
No artefacts present on the image.

LATERAL FLEXION AND EXTENSION CERVICAL SPINE

Lateral projections with the cervical spine in flexion and extension will demonstrate the range of movement in the neck and the alignment of the vertebrae. This is particularly useful for assessment of subluxation of C1 and C2, and in these cases the patient's head should be held by the referring clinician.

A 24×30 cm cassette is placed in the erect cassette holder, (a) longitudinally for lateral with extension, and (b) transversely for lateral with flexion. A lead–rubber apron is applied to the patient's lower abdomen as radiation protection. The patient is erect, MSP parallel to the cassette, shoulder in contact with it. The feet are separated for stability. For (a) the neck is extended as far as possible; for (b) the neck is flexed as much as possible. The centre of the cassette is coincident with the middle of the neck, the long axis of the cassette parallel to the long axis of the neck.

> CENTRING: A horizontal central ray, at 90° to the cassette, is directed over a point in the middle of the neck, level with the thyroid eminence.

Collimate to include EAM, C7/T1 joint space and anterior and posterior soft tissue outlines. Apply an AP anatomical marker within the primary beam.

IMAGE EVALUATION

Correct patient identification and anatomical marker included on the radiograph.

Area of interest

EAMs, T1, anterior soft tissue structures of neck and spinous processes.

Projection

- Mandible projected clear of upper vertebrae.
- Superimposition of right and left posterior, superior and inferior borders of vertebral bodies.
- Inclusion of appropriate 'flexion' or 'extension' legends.

Flexion

- Chin pulled in towards chest, with reduction in curve of cervical spine.

Extension

- Chin raised, with exaggeration of curve of cervical spine.

Exposure factors

- kVp sufficient to demonstrate bony trabeculae within the bodies of the cervical vertebrae, maintaining contrast between the vertebrae and soft tissue structures of the neck.
- mAs to provide adequate image density to demonstrate bony detail in contrast to the adjacent soft tissue structures.

No evidence of patient movement.
No artefacts present on the image.

ODONTOID PROCESS

Occasionally it may not be possible to demonstrate the odontoid process, even when the occiput and teeth are correctly superimposed. In these cases, an axial projection is carried out in addition to the routine AP C1 and 2 projection, as the C1–2 joint spaces will not be demonstrated on the axial projection.

RADIOGRAPHIC TECHNIQUE

Axial (Fig. 5.6)

An 18×24 cm cassette is placed longitudinally in the table bucky. The patient lies on the table as for the AP C1 and 2 projection. The chin is raised until the OMBL lies at 45° to the table top. The lower border of the cassette is placed level with the EAMs.

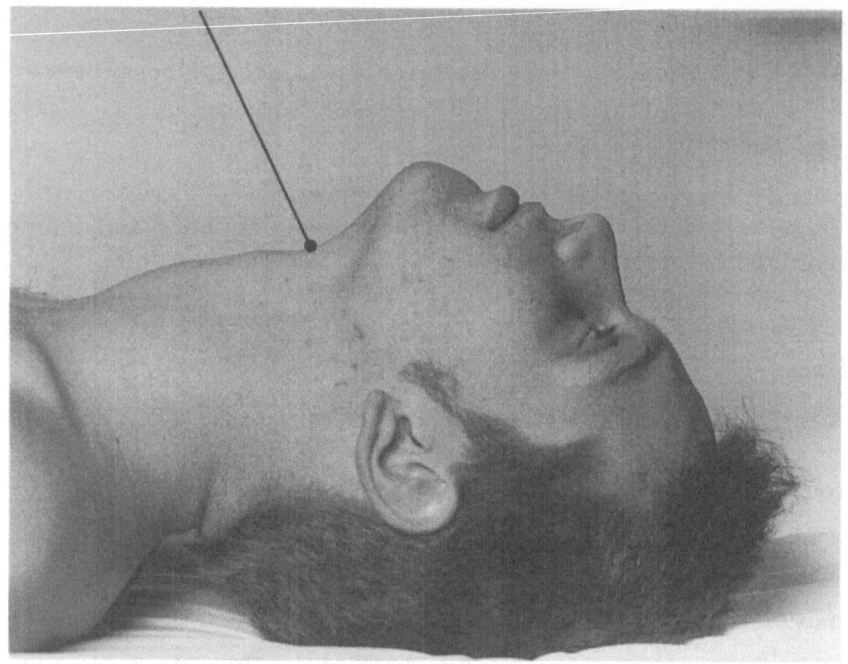

Figure 5.6   Axial projection: odontoid peg.

CENTRING: A vertical central ray is directed 25° cranially to a point midway between the angles of the mandible.

The cassette is displaced cranially so that its centre coincides with the central ray. Collimate to include foramen magnum and odontoid process. Apply an AP anatomical marker within the primary beam.

As extension of the neck is necessary to raise the OMBL to 45°, this projection **must not** be undertaken in cases of trauma.

IMAGE EVALUATION

Correct patient identification and anatomical marker included on the radiograph.

Area of interest

Foramen magnum and C1 and 2.

Projection

- Anterior and posterior arches of C1 demonstrated as a circle, with odontoid process of C2 projected through its centre.
- Mandible projected above, and clear of, C1.

Exposure factors

- kVp sufficient to demonstrate the upper cervical vertebrae through the overlying occiput, maintaining contrast between soft tissue and bony structures.
- mAs to provide adequate image density to demonstrate bony detail of C1 and 2 and the odontoid process in contrast to the adjacent soft tissues structures.

No evidence of patient movement.
No artefacts present on the image.

LATERAL TO DEMONSTRATE CERVICOTHORACIC REGION (Fig. 5.7)

The cervicothoracic region is often inadequately demonstrated on lateral projections of the cervical and thoracic spine, and the following projection is undertaken to demonstrate the area.

An 18×24 cm cassette is placed longitudinally in the erect bucky. A lead–rubber apron is applied to the patient's lower abdomen as radiation protection. The patient is erect with the shoulder in contact with the bucky, MSP parallel to it. The centre of the cassette is level with the heads of the humeri. Without altering the relationship of the MSP to the bucky, the arm nearest the bucky is raised and flexed at the elbow, with the forearm resting across the top of the head, and the shoulder nearest the X-ray tube is lowered as far as possible.

CENTRING: A horizontal central ray, at 90° to the cassette, is directed immediately above the head of the humerus on the side nearest the X-ray tube.

Collimate to include C6, T3, anterior aspect of vertebral bodies and spinous processes. Apply an AP anatomical marker within the primary beam.

Exposure factors and image detail are the main problems in producing diagnostic lateral radiographs of the cervicothoracic region.

Exposure difficulties can be overcome by using an automatic exposure device with the centre chamber selected. If automatic exposure is not available in a vertical bucky, the patient lies on their side on the X-ray table, raising the arm closest to the table and lowering the shoulder of the side nearest the X-ray tube. Selection of approximately 80 kVp will provide adequate penetration of this dense area while keeping scatter production to a minimum. This will help to produce a more detailed image, although it may lead to a relatively high mAs, this factor being under the control of the AED (automatic exposure device). Patient immobilization is therefore essential, as particularly in broad-shouldered

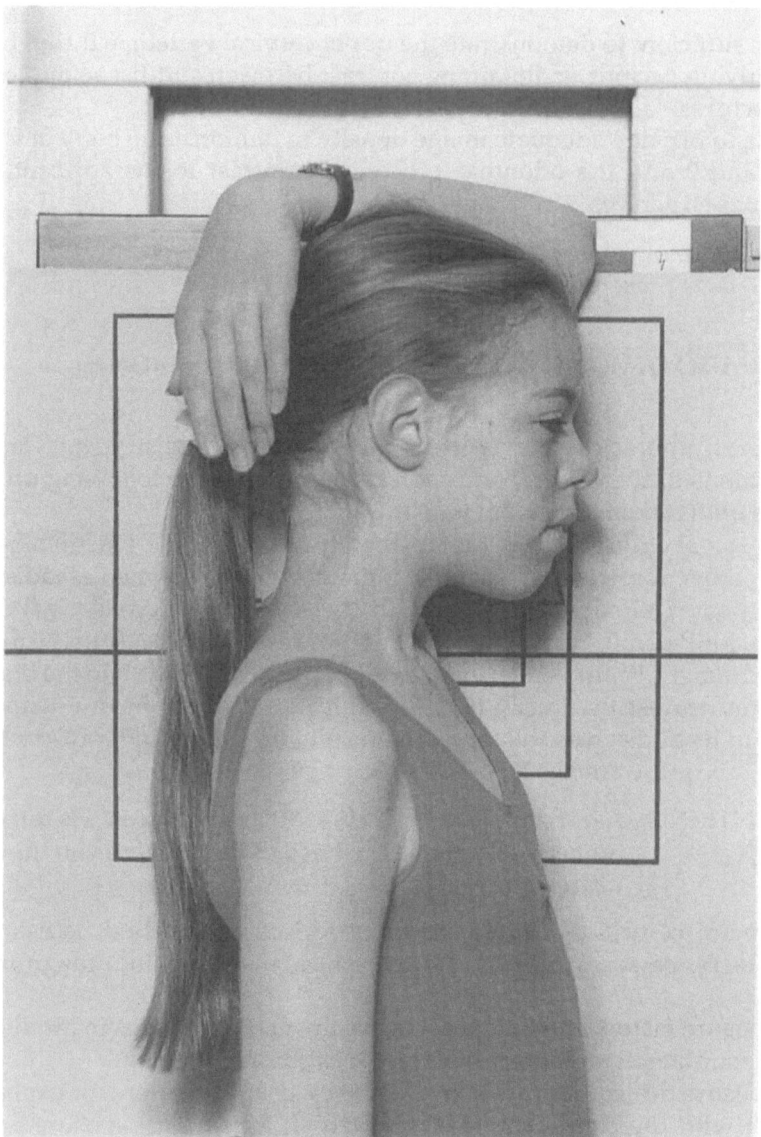

Figure 5.7   Lateral cervicothoracic region.

patients the exposure time may be relatively long for the production of a correctly exposed image.

Strict collimation will significantly improve the quality of the image through a reduction in scatter production. As the temptation is for the radiographer to increase the field size when collimating the X-ray beam after positioning the patient, it is advisable to collimate to within the boundaries of the 18×24 cm cassette before the patient is interposed between it and the X-ray tube.

IMAGE EVALUATION

Correct patient identification and anatomical marker included on the radiograph.

Area of interest

C6, T3, vertebral bodies and spinous processes.

Projection

- Superimposition of right and left posterior, superior and inferior borders of vertebral bodies.
- Superimposition of right and left posterior ribs.
- Vertical separation of right and left shoulder masses, allowing visualization of vertebrae in cervicothoracic region.

Exposure factors

- kVp sufficient to penetrate the shoulder masses and demonstrate bony trabeculae within the vertebral bodies of C6–T3, maintaining contrast between the vertebrae, lungs and air-filled trachea.
- mAs to provide adequate image density to demonstrate bony detail of the vertebral bodies and spinous processes in contrast to the soft tissues of the thorax and neck.

No evidence of patient movement.
No artefacts present on the image.

THORACIC SPINE

RADIOGRAPHIC TECHNIQUE

Anteroposterior (see Fig. 5.3)

An 18×43 cm cassette is placed longitudinally in the table bucky. The patient is supine, arms at their sides and legs extended. A lead–rubber apron is applied to the patient's lower abdomen as radiation protection. The MSP is coincident with, and perpendicular to, the central long axis of the table, ASISs and shoulders equidistant from the table top. The upper

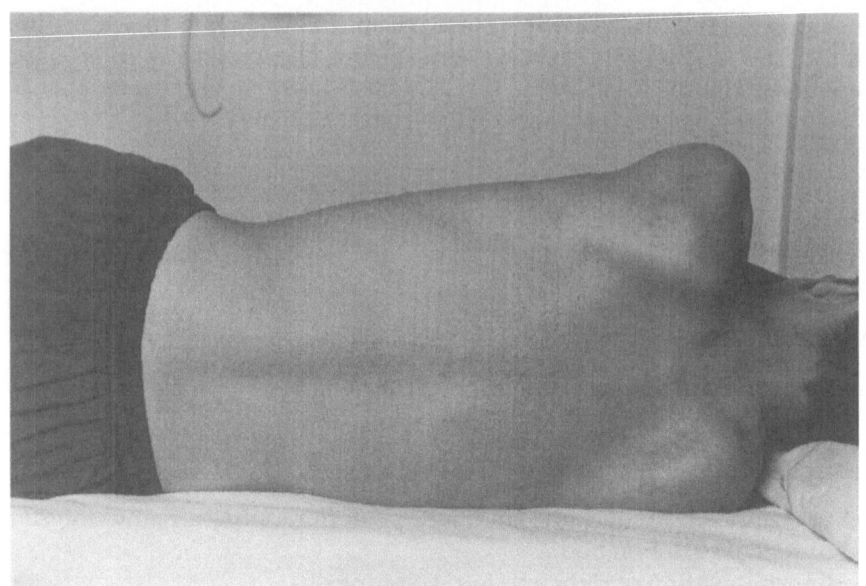

Figure 5.8 Lateral position for thoracic and lumbar spine.

border of cassette is level with the lower border of the thyroid cartilage to ensure that C7 is included on the radiograph.

CENTRING: A vertical central ray, at 90° to the cassette, is directed to a point in the midline and midway between the sternal notch and xiphisternum.

Collimate to include C7, L1 and transverse processes. Apply an AP anatomical marker within the primary beam. Expose on arrested inspiration to demonstrate the maximum number of thoracic vertebrae above the diaphragm.

Lateral (Fig. 5.8)

A 30×40 cm cassette is placed longitudinally in the table bucky. The patient is turned through 90° on to the affected side, with their back to the radiographer. Both arms are raised on to the pillow and the legs are together, with the knees and hips flexed to aid stability. The patient looks forward to avoid rotation of the upper vertebrae. A lead–rubber sheet is placed over the lower abdomen as radiation protection. The upper border of cassette is 2.5 cm above the spinous process of C7 in order to include C7 on the radiograph. The MSP and long axis of the spine, assessed by palpating the spinous processes, are parallel to the table top. A sheet of lead–rubber is placed on the table top behind the patient to absorb some of the scattered radiation produced, thereby improving image quality.

> CENTRING: A vertical central ray, at 90° to the long axis of the spine, is directed to a point level with the sixth thoracic vertebra and 2.5 cm behind the midaxillary line.

Collimate to include C7, L1, anterior vertebral bodies and spinous processes. Apply an AP anatomical marker within the primary beam. Expose on arrested inspiration to demonstrate the maximum number of thoracic vertebrae above the diaphragm or, alternatively, expose on gentle respiration in order to blur out the images of overlying ribs. A low mA and long time should be selected to facilitate this.

If the long axis of the spine is not parallel to the table top, radiolucent pads under the patient's side will correct the position. Alternatively, angling the central ray to pass at 90° to the long axis of the spine will compensate.

In order to demonstrate the range of densities encountered along the length of the thoracic spine on a single image, the following options can be considered.

Anteroposterior projection:

1. use of a higher kVp in conjunction with a lower mAs;
2. wedge aluminium filter with thicker end over the upper thoracic vertebrae will absorb more radiation over this area and produce a more even density over the whole image;
3. flour bag filter placed over the upper thoracic vertebrae will absorb radiation over this area and produce a more even density over the whole image;
4. patient's head at 'anode end' of table will use the anode–heel effect over the upper thoracic vertebrae and even out density on radiograph.

Lateral projection:

1. use of a higher kVp in conjunction with a lower mAs;
2. wedge aluminium filter with thicker end over the lower end of thoracic vertebrae will absorb radiation over this area and even out resulting densities;
3. flour filter placed over lower end of thoracic vertebrae will absorb radiation over this area and even out resulting densities;
4. use of anode–heel effect with patient's trunk at 'anode end' of table.

IMAGE EVALUATION

Correct patient identification and anatomical marker included on the radiograph.

Area of interest

Anteroposterior

C7, L1 and transverse processes.

Lateral

T1/2, L1, anterior borders of vertebral bodies and spinous processes.

Projection

Anteroposterior

- Thoracic vertebrae demonstrated down centre of film.
- Spinous processes demonstrated down centre of vertebral bodies.

Lateral

- Superimposition of posterior, superior and inferior borders of vertebral bodies.
- Superimposition of posterior ribs.
- Upper thoracic vertebrae not obscured by shoulders or upper arms.
- Blurring of images of ribs and lung markings if exposure is made during gentle respiration.

Exposure factors

kVp selected to reduce the subject contrast along the length of the thoracic spine, so enabling all 12 vertebrae to be adequately demonstrated on one image.

- kVp sufficient to demonstrate bony trabeculae in all 12 vertebrae, and the spinous processes through the vertebral bodies in the AP projection, maintaining contrast between the thoracic vertebrae, mediastinum and lung fields.
- mAs to provide adequate image density to demonstrate detail of the vertebrae in contrast to the mediastinum and lungs.

No evidence of patient movement or breathing during the exposure unless breathing technique used for lateral projection.
No artefacts present on the image.

LUMBAR SPINE

RADIOGRAPHIC TECHNIQUE

Anteroposterior (see Fig. 5.3)

A 30×40 cm cassette is placed longitudinally in the table bucky. The patient lies supine, MSP coincident with and perpendicular to the midline of the table. ASISs are equidistant from the table top. The knees are flexed and the plantar aspect of the feet in contact with the table. This reduces the lumbar curve and improves the separation of the vertebral bodies and visualization of the intervertebral joint spaces on the image. The centre of the long axis of the cassette is level with the lower costal margins. A lead–rubber sheet is applied to the lower abdomen with its upper border just below the level of the ASISs – with careful positioning gonad protection can be provided for female, as well as male, patients.

> CENTRING: A vertical central ray, at 90° to the cassette, is directed to a point in the midline, at the level of the lower costal margins.

Collimate to include T12, lower margins of sacroiliac joints, transverse processes and psoas muscle shadows. Apply an AP anatomical marker within the primary beam.

Lateral (see Fig. 5.8)

A 30×40 cm cassette is placed longitudinally in the table bucky. The patient turns on to the affected side, with the hips and knees flexed for stability and arms resting on the pillow. A thin pad between the knees will aid comfort. The MSP and long axis of the spine, assessed by palpating the spinous processes, are parallel to the table top. The centre of the long axis of the cassette is level with the lower costal margin. A lead–rubber sheet is placed on the lateral aspect of the pelvis, just below the level of the ASISs, as radiation protection. A sheet of lead–rubber is placed on the table top behind the patient to absorb some of the scattered radiation produced, improving image quality.

> CENTRING: A vertical central ray, at 90° to the long axis of the spine, is directed to a point 7.5 cm anterior to the spinous process of L3, at the level of the lower costal margin.

Collimate to include T12, first sacral segment, anterior aspect of vertebral bodies and spinous processes. Apply an AP anatomical marker within the primary beam.

If the long axis of the spine is not parallel to the table top, radiolucent pads may be placed under the patient's side to correct the position.

Alternatively, the central ray may be directed to pass at 90° to the long axis of the spine.

For the lateral projection, to assess whether the X-ray beam is correctly centred in the anteroposterior direction, allowing accurate collimation to the anterior vertebral bodies and spinous processes, the longitudinal cross-hair of the light beam should follow the line of the lumbar spine, bisecting the distance between the anterior and posterior aspects of the iliac crest at the level of the ASIS.

Lateral L5/S1 junction (see Fig. 5.8)

An 18×24 cm cassette is placed longitudinally in the table bucky. The patient is positioned as for the lateral lumbar spine L1–5, with the centre of the long axis of the cassette coincident with a point 2.5 cm above the PSISs. An imaginary line adjoining the PSISs will demonstrate the plane of the L5/S1 joint space.

> CENTRING: A vertical central ray, parallel to the line adjoining the PSISs, is directed to a point 7.5 cm anterior to the spinous process of L5, which lies 2.5 cm above the PSISs.

Collimate to include upper border of L5, first sacral segment, vertebral bodies and spinous processes. Apply an AP anatomical marker within the primary beam.

For accurate centring in the lateral L5/S1 projection, centre in the middle of an imaginary triangle made up of the ASIS, PSIS and central point of the top of the iliac crest, approximately 2.5 cm below the midpoint of the iliac crest.

IMAGE EVALUATION

Correct patient identification and anatomical marker included on the radiograph.

Area of interest

Anteroposterior

T12, S1, transverse processes, psoas muscles and sacroiliac joints.

Lateral

T12, S1, anterior borders of the vertebral bodies and the spinous processes.

Lateral L5/S1 junction

L4/5 joint space, S1, anterior borders of the vertebral bodies and spinous processes.

Projection

Anteroposterior

- Lumbar vertebrae demonstrated down centre of film.
- Spinous processes demonstrated down centre of vertebral bodies.
- Visualization of intervertebral joint spaces between L2/3 and L3/4.

Lateral and lateral L5/S1 junction

- Superimposition of right and left posterior, superior and inferior borders of vertebral bodies.
- Superimposition of posterior ribs in the lateral 1–5 projection.
- Superimposition of superior surfaces of ala of sacrum in the lateral L5/S1 projection.

Exposure factors

Anteroposterior

- kVp sufficient to demonstrate bony trabeculae within the vertebrae, and the spinous processes through the vertebral bodies, maintaining contrast between the vertebrae and abdominal viscera.
- mAs to provide adequate image density to demonstrate bony detail in contrast to the soft tissue organs within the abdomen.

Lateral and lateral L5/S1 junction

- kVp sufficient to demonstrate bony trabeculae within all five vertebral bodies through the overlying bony pelvis as well as within the spinous processes, maintaining contrast between the vertebrae and abdominal viscera.
- mAs to provide adequate image density to demonstrate bony detail in contrast to the soft tissue structures of the abdomen.

No evidence of patient movement or breathing during the exposure.
No artefacts present on the image.

POSTERIOR OBLIQUES L1–5

RADIOGRAPHIC TECHNIQUE

The patient is positioned initially as for the oblique projection of the ribs (see Fig. 7.1).

A 30×40 cm or 24×30 cm cassette is placed longitudinally in the table bucky. The patient lies supine, the MSP coincident with and perpendicular to the midline of the table. The centre of the long axis of the cassette is level with the lower costal margins. The trunk is rotated 45° towards the side under examination and radiolucent pads are placed under the trunk and raised shoulder for support.

CENTRING: A vertical central ray, at 90° to the cassette, is directed over a point in the midclavicular line of the raised side, at the level of the lower costal margin.

Collimate to include T12, first sacral segment and transverse processes. Apply an AP anatomical marker within the primary beam and appropriate to the side nearest the cassette. Both sides are taken for comparison.

An alternative method of centring for the oblique projections is described by Francis (1993). For the left posterior oblique projection, lie the patient supine and centre the X-ray beam midway between the MSP and left flank. Rotate the patient 45° towards the left and immobilize in this position. The lumbar vertebrae will now be central to the image. Note that the patient must only rotate: any lateral shift of the body will require them to return to the supine position for recentring.

IMAGE EVALUATION

Correct patient identification and anatomical marker included on the radiograph.

Area of interest

T12, first sacral segment and transverse processes.

Projection

- Parts of lumbar vertebrae described below appear as an image of a 'Scottie dog':
    eye – pedicle;
    nose – transverse process;
    front leg – inferior articular process;
    ear – superior articular process;
    body – lamina.
- If obliquity of patient is correct apophyseal joints (between superior

and inferior articular processes) will be superimposed over centre of superior borders of vertebral bodies.

Exposure factors

- kVp sufficient to demonstrate bony trabeculae within the vertebral bodies, and the pedicles superimposed on the vertebral bodies, maintaining contrast between the lumbar vertebrae and abdominal viscera.
- mAs to provide adequate image density to demonstrate bony detail of the 'Scottie dog' in contrast to the soft tissue abdominal organs.

No evidence of patient movement or breathing during the exposure.
No artefacts present on the image.

LATERAL FLEXION AND EXTENSION LUMBAR SPINE

RADIOGRAPHIC TECHNIQUE

A 30×40 cm cassette is placed longitudinally in the erect bucky. The patient is seated with the affected side in contact with the bucky, MSP parallel to it. The long axis of the spine is coincident with and parallel to the central long axis of the cassette. The middle of the long axis of the cassette is at the level of the lower costal margins.
(a) The patient bends forward, flexing the lumbar spine as much as possible. The arms are extended downwards, the patient holding the legs to aid immobilization.
(b) The patient bends backwards, extending the lumbar spine as much as possible. The hands grip the back of the seat for support.

CENTRING: A horizontal central ray, at 90° to the cassette, is directed 7.5 cm anterior to the spinous process of L3, at the level of the lower costal margins.

Collimate to include T12, first sacral segment, spinous processes and vertebral bodies. Apply an AP anatomical marker within the primary beam.

IMAGE EVALUATION

Correct patient identification and anatomical marker included on the radiograph.

Area of interest

T12, S1, anterior border of the vertebral bodies and spinous processes.

Projection

- Superimposition of the right and left posterior, superior and inferior borders of vertebral bodies.
- Superimposition of posterior ribs.
- Lumbar spine seen to arc forward on flexion and backward on extension projections.
- Inclusion of appropriate 'flexion' or 'extension' legends.

Exposure factors

- kVp sufficient to demonstrate bony trabeculae within all five vertebral bodies through the overlying bony pelvis, as well as within the spinous processes, maintaining contrast between the vertebrae and abdominal viscera.
- mAs to provide adequate image density to demonstrate bony detail in contrast to the soft tissue structures of the abdomen.

No evidence of patient movement.
No artefacts present on the image.

LUMBOSACRAL JUNCTION

RADIOGRAPHIC TECHNIQUE

Anteroposterior (see Fig. 5.3)

An 18×24 cm cassette is placed transversely in the table bucky. The patient lies supine, MSP coincident with and perpendicular to the centre of the table, ASISs equidistant from the table top. The arms are abducted slightly, resting on the table top.

> CENTRING: A vertical central ray is directed 5–15° cranially, to coincide with the L5/S1 joint space, to a point in the midline at the level of the ASISs. Female patients will require a greater beam angulation than males because of their greater sacral angle.

The cassette is displaced cranially until its centre is coincident with the central ray. Collimate to include L5, first sacral segment and sacroiliac joints. Apply an AP anatomical marker within the primary beam.

Posterior oblique (see Fig. 7.1)

An 18×24 cm cassette is placed longitudinally in the table bucky. The patient lies supine, MSP coincident with and perpendicular to the midline of the table. The patient is rotated 45° towards the side under examination and radiolucent pads are placed under the trunk and raised shoulder for support.

> CENTRING: A vertical central ray is directed 5–15° cranially, to a point 7.5 cm medial to the ASIS of the raised side.

The cassette is displaced cranially until its centre is coincident with the central ray. Collimate to include L5, first sacral segment and sacroiliac joints. Apply an AP anatomical marker within the primary beam, appropriate to the side nearest the cassette. Both sides are taken for comparison.

IMAGE EVALUATION

Correct patient identification and anatomical marker included on the radiograph.

Area of interest

L4/5 joint space, first sacral segment and transverse processes.

Projection

Anteroposterior

- Clear visualization of joint space between L5 and S1.
- Spinous processes demonstrated down centre of vertebral bodies and midline of film.

Posterior oblique

- Appearance of 'Scottie dog' as described in oblique lumbar L1–5 projection.
- Demonstration of apophyseal joints (between superior and inferior articular processes) superimposed over centre of superior borders of vertebral bodies.

Exposure factors

- kVp sufficient to demonstrate bony trabeculae within the vertebral bodies and the pedicles superimposed on them, maintaining contrast between the vertebrae and pelvic viscera.

- mAs to provide adequate image density to demonstrate bony detail in contrast to the soft tissues of the abdomen.

No evidence of patient movement.
No artefacts present on the image.

SACRUM

RADIOGRAPHIC TECHNIQUE

Anteroposterior (see Fig. 5.3)

A 24×30 cm cassette is placed longitudinally in the table bucky. The patient lies supine, MSP coincident with and perpendicular to the midline of the table. The ASISs are equidistant from the table top. A lead–rubber sheet is applied to the male gonad area only. The knees are flexed and the plantar aspects of the feet in contact with the table top. This will reduce the lumbar curve and bring the long axis of the sacrum nearer to being parallel to the cassette.

CENTRING: A vertical central ray is directed 5–15° cranially, until at 90° to the long axis of the sacrum, to a point in the midline, midway between the ASISs and upper border of the symphysis pubis. (Female patients will usually require more angulation than males.)

The cassette is displaced cranially until its centre is coincident with the central ray. Collimate to include sacroiliac joints, L5/S1 joint space and sacrococcygeal junction. Apply an AP anatomical marker within the primary beam.

Lateral (see Fig. 5.8)

A 24×30 cm cassette is placed longitudinally in the table bucky. The patient is turned on to the affected side, knees and hips flexed for stability. The arms are placed on the pillow and a small pad is placed between the knees for comfort. The MSP and long axis of the sacrum are parallel to the table top.

CENTRING: A vertical central ray, at 90° to the long axis of the sacrum, is directed to a point midway between the PSISs and coccyx.

Collimate to include L5/S1 joint space, sacrococcygeal junction, sacral promontory and spinous tubercles. Apply an AP anatomical marker within the primary beam.

IMAGE EVALUATION

Correct patient identification and anatomical marker included on the radiograph.

Area of interest

Anteroposterior

L5, sacrococcygeal junction and sacroiliac joints.

Lateral

L5/S1 joint space, sacral promontory and coccyx.

Projection

Anteroposterior

- Spinous processes demonstrated down centre of lower lumbar vertebrae and sacrum.
- Long axis of sacrum coincident with midline of film.

Lateral

- Superimposition of posterior, superior and inferior borders of L5 vertebral body.
- Superimposition of posterior and superior borders of sacrum.
- Superimposition of ala of sacrum.
- Superimposition of heads of femora.

Exposure factors

Anteroposterior

- kVp sufficient to demonstrate the spinous tubercles through body of sacrum and areas of overlap of the ala of the sacrum on the iliac bones, maintaining contrast between the sacrum and pelvic viscera.
- mAs to provide adequate image density to demonstrate bony detail in contrast to the sacroiliac joints and soft tissue organs of the pelvis.

Lateral

- kVp sufficient to demonstrate the sacral promontory through the iliac crests, maintaining contrast between the sacrum, pelvic viscera and soft tissues of the buttocks. kVp needs to be high enough to reduce the subject contrast inherent in the length of the sacrum from the dense sacral promontory to the coccyx.

- mAs to provide adequate image density to demonstrate bony detail throughout the length of the sacrum in contrast to the pelvic organs and surrounding soft tissues.

No evidence of patient movement.
No artefacts present on the image.

COCCYX

RADIOGRAPHIC TECHNIQUE

Anteroposterior (see Fig. 5.3)

An 18×24 cm cassette is placed longitudinally in the table bucky. The patient lies supine on the table with their legs extended, MSP coincident with and perpendicular to the midline of the table. The ASISs are equidistant from the table top.

> CENTRING: A vertical central ray is directed 15° caudally to a point in the midline and 2.5 cm above the upper border of the symphysis pubis.

The cassette is displaced caudally until its centre is coincident with the central ray. Collimate to include sacrococcygeal junction and all coccygeal segments. Apply an AP anatomical marker within the primary beam.

Lateral (see Fig. 5.8)

An 18×24 cm cassette is placed longitudinally in the table bucky. The patient turns on to the affected side, with knees and hips flexed for stability. The arms are placed on the pillow and a small pad is placed between the knees for comfort. The MSP and long axis of the sacrum are parallel to the table top.

> CENTRING: A vertical central ray, at 90° to the long axis of the sacrum, is directed over the palpable coccyx at the base of the spine.

Collimate to include sacrococcygeal junction and all coccygeal segments. Apply an AP anatomical marker within the primary beam.

Visualization of the three segments of the coccyx in the AP projection is usually difficult, particularly when the colon is loaded with faeces. The lateral is the better projection for demonstrating the coccyx, and may be the only projection required in some departmental protocols. As treatment for fractures of the coccyx is rare, some departments do not routinely X-ray the coccyx at all.

IMAGE EVALUATION

Correct patient identification and anatomical marker included on the radiograph.

Area of interest

All coccygeal segments.

Projection

Anteroposterior

- Long axis of coccyx coincident with midline of film.
- Spinous tubercles projected down centre of sacrum.

Lateral

- Superimposition of posterior borders of sacrum and coccyx.
- Superimposition of ischial spines.

Exposure factors

- kVp sufficient to demonstrate bony trabeculae within the coccyx, maintaining contrast between bony structures and the pelvic viscera.
- mAs to provide adequate image density to demonstrate bony detail of the coccyx in contrast to the surrounding soft tissues.

No evidence of patient movement.
No artefacts present on the image.

SACROILIAC JOINTS

RADIOGRAPHIC TECHNIQUE

Posteroanterior

For this projection the patient is in the prone position, as for the prone abdomen (see Fig. 12.2). This projection should be selected in preference to the AP, as the radiation dose to the gonads is reduced through absorption of some of the lower energy radiation by the sacrum.

However, in the PA position utilization of the oblique rays to exactly coincide with the sacroiliac joints is only possible if the FFD is reduced to 18 cm. Even if the shorter FFD could be achieved, reducing the value of mAs required, the great disadvantage is the unacceptable increase in skin dose.

A 24×30 cm cassette is placed transversely in the table bucky. The patient lies prone, MSP coincident with and perpendicular to the midline of the table. The PSISs are equidistant from the table top. The arms rest on the pillow for comfort, with the head turned to the side.

CENTRING: A vertical central ray is directed 5–15° caudally, until at 90° to the long axis of the sacrum, to a point in the midline at the level of the PSISs.

The cassette is displaced caudally until its centre is coincident with the central ray. Collimate to include the sacroiliac joints. Apply a PA anatomical marker within the primary beam.

Anteroposterior (see Fig. 5.3)

A 24×30 cm cassette is placed transversely in the table bucky. The patient lies supine with the knees flexed to reduce the lumbar curve. The arms are slightly abducted, resting at the patient's sides. The MSP is coincident with and perpendicular to the midline of the table. The ASISs are equidistant from the table top.

CENTRING: A vertical central ray is directed 5–15° cranially, until at 90° to the long axis of the sacrum, to a point in the midline, midway between the ASISs.

The cassette is displaced cranially until its centre is coincident with the central ray. Collimate to include the sacroiliac joints. Apply an AP anatomical marker within the primary beam.

Posterior oblique (see Fig. 5.9)

This projection demonstrates the sacroiliac joints more clearly than any other. Both sides are examined for comparison. Left posterior oblique demonstrates the right sacroiliac joint; right posterior oblique demonstrates the left sacroiliac joint.

An 18×24 cm cassette is placed longitudinally in the table bucky. The patient lies supine on the table with the MSP coincident with and perpendicular to the midline of the table. The patient is rotated 15° away from the side under examination and the raised side supported by radiolucent pads. The centre of the cassette is coincident with a point 2.5 cm medial to the raised ASIS.

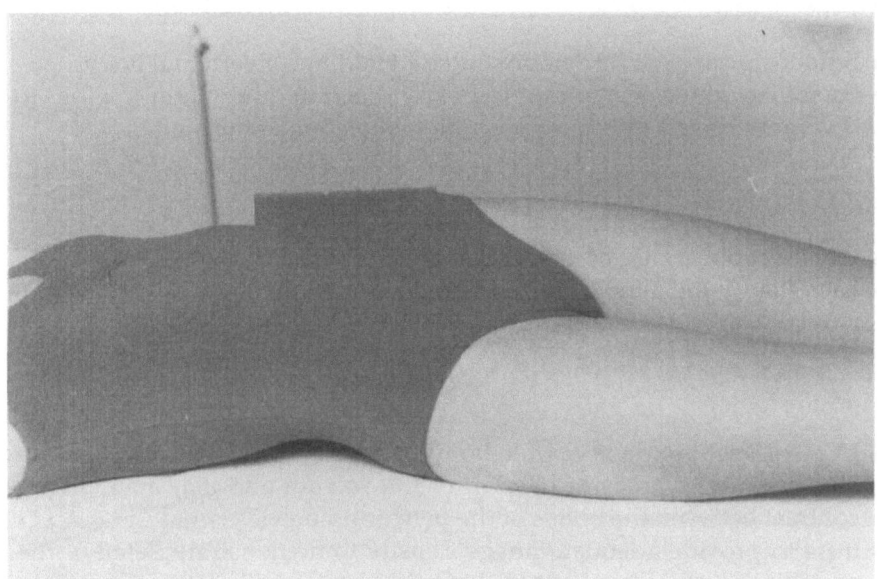

Figure 5.9   Sacroiliac joints – 15° posterior oblique.

CENTRING: A vertical central ray is directed 5–15° cranially, until at 90° to the long axis of the sacrum, to a point 2.5 cm medial to and 2.5 cm below the raised ASIS.

The cassette is displaced cranially until its centre is coincident with the central ray. Collimate to include the sacroiliac joint under examination. Apply an AP anatomical marker within the primary beam.

IMAGE EVALUATION

Correct patient identification and anatomical marker included on the radiograph.

Area of interest

Ala of sacrum and sacroiliac joint(s).

Projection

Posteroanterior

- Spinous process of L5 demonstrated in midline of vertebral body.
- Sacroiliac joints seen partially demonstrated as divergence of X-ray beam approximates direction of the joints.

Anteroposterior

- Spinous process of L5 demonstrated in midline of vertebral body.
- Sacroiliac joints superimposed over sacrum and ilium owing to divergent beam being in opposition to direction of the joints.

Posterior oblique

- Oblique appearance of lower lumbar vertebrae.
- Sacroiliac joint clearly demonstrated owing to vertical central ray passing directly through the joint space.

Exposure factors

- kVp sufficient to demonstrate bony trabeculae within the sacrum and iliac bones and areas of overlap of the sacrum and ilia, maintaining contrast between the bones of the pelvis and pelvic viscera.
- mAs to provide adequate image density to demonstrate detail of the sacroiliac joints in contrast to the pelvic bones and soft tissue organs within the pelvic cavity.

No evidence of patient movement.
No artefacts present on the image.

Radiographic appearances of incorrect positioning (positional faults)

AP projections:
If the patient is rotated, i.e. the MSP is not perpendicular to, or the ASISs equidistant from, the table top, the spinous processes will not be projected down the centre of the vertebral bodies. Rotation towards the left will cause the spinous processes to be projected towards the right-hand side of the vertebral bodies and vice versa.
Lateral projections:
If the long axis of the spine is not parallel to the table top, or the X-ray beam is not directed perpendicular to the long axis of the spine, the superior and inferior borders of the vertebral bodies will not be superimposed and will be projected elliptically.

Before repeating the lateral L5/S1 projection for this fault, inspect the lateral L1–5 and compare the image of the junction to assess whether or not the beam angulation needs to be increased or reduced. If the L5–S1 junction is adequately demonstrated on the lateral L1–5, it may not be necessary to repeat the junction at all.

If the patient is rotated (forwards/backwards) the posterior borders of the vertebral bodies will not be superimposed. To assess whether the patient is rotated forwards or backwards check the images of the ribs, if present. Looking at one pair of ribs, identify which of the pair is the most magnified; this will be the rib remote from the cassette, i.e. the right rib in a left lateral projection. If the magnified rib lies in front of its partner, the patient is rotated forwards, and vice versa.

ERECT PROJECTIONS OF THE SPINE

Erect projections (AP and lateral) may be undertaken in place of any of the routine projections previously described, particularly if the patient's condition is exacerbated, or causes discomfort when lying down, e.g. kyphosis. Considering that the thoracic spine is usually perfectly lateral on a lateral projection of the chest, it makes sense to X-ray the thoracic vertebrae with the patient erect.

Erect projections of the spine, particularly the AP, are frequently requested in children for demonstration of a scoliosis. As affected patients are likely to be X-rayed regularly to assess any corrective treatment, radiation protection in the form of lead–rubber aprons, the recording of previously used exposure factors, short exposure time and high mA selection and fast film–screen combinations, are essential. The PA projection is preferable to the AP as this represents a reduction in dose to the radiosensitive gonads and developing breasts. These projections usually require the demonstration of the entire spine, C1–S1, on a single radiograph – not a problem with young children. With older patients it may be necessary to produce separate radiographs of the upper and lower regions, demonstrating an area of the mid-spine on both images. Selection of a relatively high kVp will assist in reducing the subject contrast along the length of the spine if graduated screens (slower at the upper end and faster at the lower end) are not available.

For the AP projection the shoes are removed and the patient positioned so that the ASISs are equidistant from the cassette. The feet are separated slightly for stability. Collimation should not be excessive in the initial examination, as the extent of the curvature of the spine will be unknown and may be quite severe. Collimation on follow-up examinations should be adjusted accordingly. For the lateral projection, the shoes are removed and the patient positioned so that the apex of the primary curve is towards the cassette and the line adjoining the ASISs is perpendicular to the cassette. The feet are separated slightly for stability and the hands placed on top of the head or holding on to a suitable support.

Supplementary lateral projections may be necessary, angling the X-ray beam into the apex of the curve, in order to demonstrate these vertebrae in as true a lateral projection as possible.

In cases of severe kyphosis routine exposure factors may be inadequate. In the AP projection the area of kyphosis represents an area of increased density, and an increase in kVp is necessary to reduce the marked difference in subject contrast along the length of the thoracic spine. In the lateral projection there will be an exaggeration in the subject contrast between the thoracic vertebrae and lung fields and, similarly, an increase in kVp is required.

Supplementary AP projections may be necessary, angling the X-ray beam into the apex of the curve, in order to demonstrate these vertebrae in as true an AP projection as possible.

An integrated shape imaging system (ISIS) may be found in specialist centres monitoring and treating scoliosis. This does not involve the use of radiation. Spinal radiographs are required initially to demonstrate the cause and extent of the disease, followed by two or three ISIS scans over a 12-month period to monitor the condition. Radiographs may be repeated at the end of a period of treatment to demonstrate any changes in the curvature of the spine.

EXAMINATION OF THE SPINE IN CASES OF TRAUMA

In cases of trauma, when the patient presents supine on a trolley, the lateral projection of any area of the spine is to be undertaken using a horizontal X-ray beam with the cassette supported vertically against the affected side.

For the lateral cervical spine the cassette is supported against the lateral aspect of the shoulder. With the brakes applied to the trolley, and no movement of the neck, the arms are pulled downwards by a suitably protected medical officer during the exposure in order to include the C7/T1 joint space on the radiograph. In severely injured patients the lateral projection should be undertaken first and examined by the medical officer, who will decide whether the patient can be moved for further basic projections.

For examinations of the thoracic and lumbar spines the AP projections are obtained by placing a gridded cassette on the tray beneath the trolley top. The patient must not be turned to lie on their side and so the lateral projection is undertaken utilizing a horizontal beam directed perpendicularly to a gridded cassette, which is supported vertically against the patient's affected side. In order to include the spinous processes on the image, the cassette should be pushed down into the trolley mattress or supported against the mattress edge, in a suitable stand. An increase in FFD, and therefore exposure (mAs), will be necessary to compensate for any increase in OFD that this projection may cause.

In order to eliminate the problems of grid cut-off, the AP projections of the cervical spine may be undertaken without the use of a grid. As this is an area of relatively low volume and density, and as modern generators and film–screen systems allow the selection of suitably low exposure factors, the amount of scatter produced is not sufficient to cause a detrimental effect on image quality. In addition, the reduction in radiation dose to the thyroid gland and orbits suggests that AP projections of the cervical spine should routinely be carried out without the use of a grid/bucky, except when the patient is extremely large or fine detail is essential (Robinson, 1995). This does not hold true for the thoracic and lumbar regions, where density of the structures and scatter production dictate that a grid should be used.

POSTEROANTERIOR PROJECTIONS

Although it is not currently common practice, the anterior curvature of the cervical and lumbar spines would suggest that the PA could be the projection of choice over the AP. In this position the divergence of the X-ray beam would more closely follow the direction of the intervertebral joint spaces, thus demonstrating them more clearly on the PA radiograph. A perceived problem with this method is the magnification and unsharpness associated with the increased OFD, although a compensatory increase in FFD (and consequently mAs) will reduce this effect. However, Colleran (1994) states that magnification in the PA projection is insufficient to cause a serious loss in image quality and, considering the superior detail provided over the sacrum, sacroiliac joints, intervertebral joint spaces, pedicles and transverse processes, recommends its adoption as routine in place of the AP projection of the lumbar spine.

Skull 6

INTRODUCTION

All radiographic examinations of the skull are based on a set of basic positions which use easily located surface markings and lines/baselines which are determined by drawing an imaginary line between two surface markings.

SURFACE MARKINGS

Glabella: The slight bulge in the middle of the forehead, between and slightly above the eyebrows.

EOP: External occipital protuberance. Found posteriorly and inferiorly, in the middle of the occiput.

EAM: External auditory meatus. The 'ear hole', which transmits sound from the outside to the eardrum.

Nasion: Depression at the top of the nasal bone at its junction with the frontal bone.

Other surface markings used include the inferior orbital margin, the outer canthus of the eye, the mastoid process, the angle of the mandible and the temporomandibular joint.

LINES AND BASELINES USED IN SKULL RADIOGRAPHY

Orbitomeatal baseline (OMBL) A line connecting the outer canthus of the eye with the EAM. This is most commonly used when examining patients on a table, trolley or Schonander-type skull unit.

Anthropological baseline Extends from the inferior orbital margin to the upper margin of the EAM. Used most commonly in conjunction with isocentric skull units. It makes an angle of 10° with the OMBL.

Auricular line Passes through the EAM at 90° to the anthropological baseline.

Median sagittal plane (MSP) Divides the skull and body vertically into left and right sides. Used extensively in radiographic techniques for many areas of the body.

Interpupillary line Joins the centre of the orbits or pupils and is at 90° to the MSP.

Infraorbital line Connects the inferior orbital margins.

BASIC POSITIONS UPON WHICH ALL RADIOGRAPHIC EXAMINATIONS OF THE SKULL ARE BASED

Occipitofrontal (OF) (Fig. 6.1)

The patient is positioned with the forehead in contact with the bucky, and for most projections the OMBL and MSP are perpendicular to the cassette. Variations in this projection involve using cranial or caudal tube

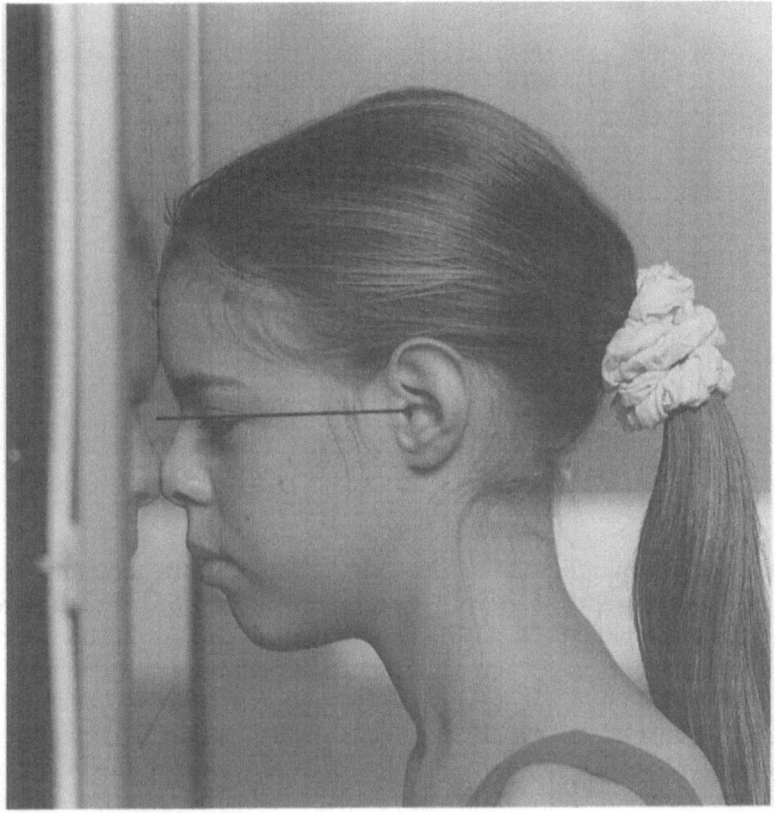

Figure 6.1   Occipitofrontal.

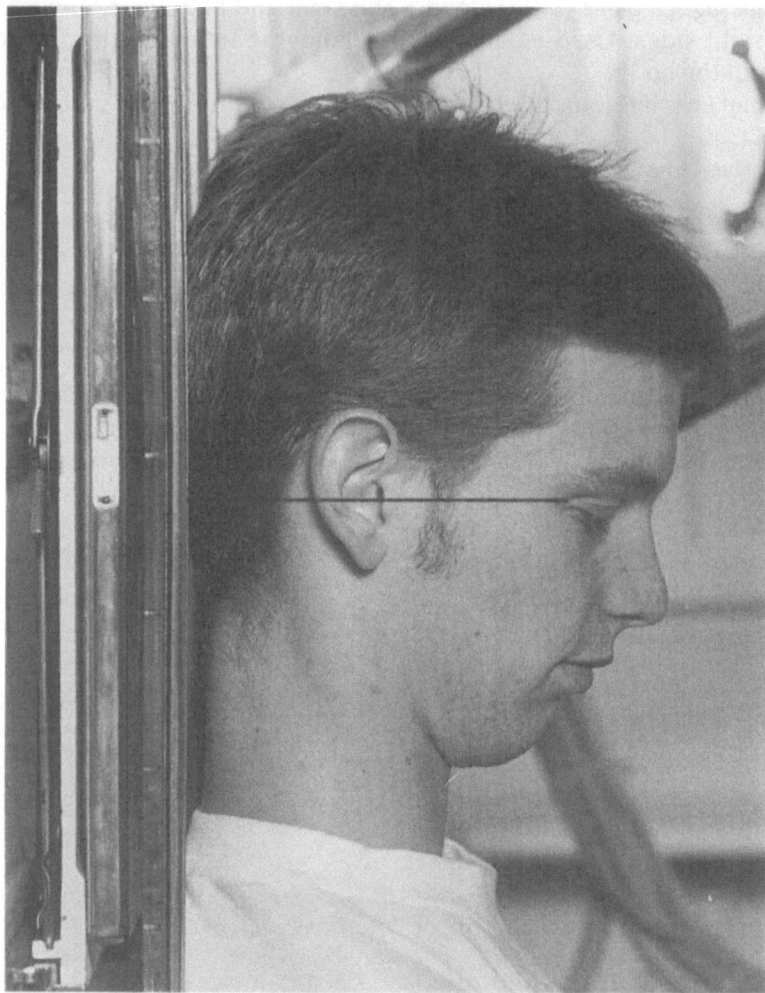

Figure 6.2 Fronto-occipital.

angulations, raising/lowering the chin to alter the relationship of the OMBL to the cassette, or altering the relationship of the MSP to the bucky.

It is common practice to ask the patient to place their nose and forehead in contact with the bucky when commencing positioning. Remember that the OMBL will not necessarily be perpendicular to the cassette, as differences in nose size and shape will affect position. The patient will often think that their nose should remain in contact with the bucky at all costs, and it is sometimes more difficult to alter the OMBL as a result. Asking them to place their forehead only in contact with the bucky will avoid this problem.

Whether using a dedicated skull unit or a vertical bucky, accurate positioning can be achieved by placing the forehead in contact with the unit so that the MSP is coincident with the vertical central line of the bucky. Adjust the chin to bring the OMBL into the correct position in relation to the cassette and then, after instructing the patient to keep their neck still, rotate them from the shoulders until the central vertical light runs down the centre of the spine. As long as the MSP remains central to the bucky, this is an easy and accurate way to position the patient, and this technique can be used in reverse when positioning for the FO projection.

Fronto-occipital (FO) (Fig. 6.2)

The patient is positioned with the occiput in contact with the bucky. Usually the MSP and OMBL are perpendicular to the bucky, but variations can be made in the same ways as for the OF projection.

Occipitomental (OM) (Fig. 6.3)

The patient sits facing the bucky with the chin in contact with it. The OMBL is raised to make an angle with a line perpendicular to the bucky. This angle varies according to examination requirements, and is typically 30° or 45°. Relationship of the MSP to the bucky can be varied according to examination requirements, but is most often perpendicular.

It is common practice to ask the patient to place their nose and chin in contact with the bucky when commencing positioning. The OMBL most often lies at approximately 30° in this position, and is therefore inappropriate for 45° projections of the sinuses and facial bones. For these the chin only should be placed in contact with the bucky.

Accurate patient positioning can be achieved using the method described above for OF projection. Position can also be assessed by the radiographer looking down at the patient's face as they are positioning from behind.

Lateral (Fig. 6.4)

The lateral aspect of the head is in contact with the bucky, with the MSP parallel to the cassette. Variations in this projection involve tube angulation or lateral tilt of the head.

Submentovertical (SMV) (Fig. 6.5)

The patient faces the X-ray tube and extends their neck until the vertex of the skull is in contact with the bucky. The OMBL is parallel to the cassette. Variations include cranial or caudal tube angulation.

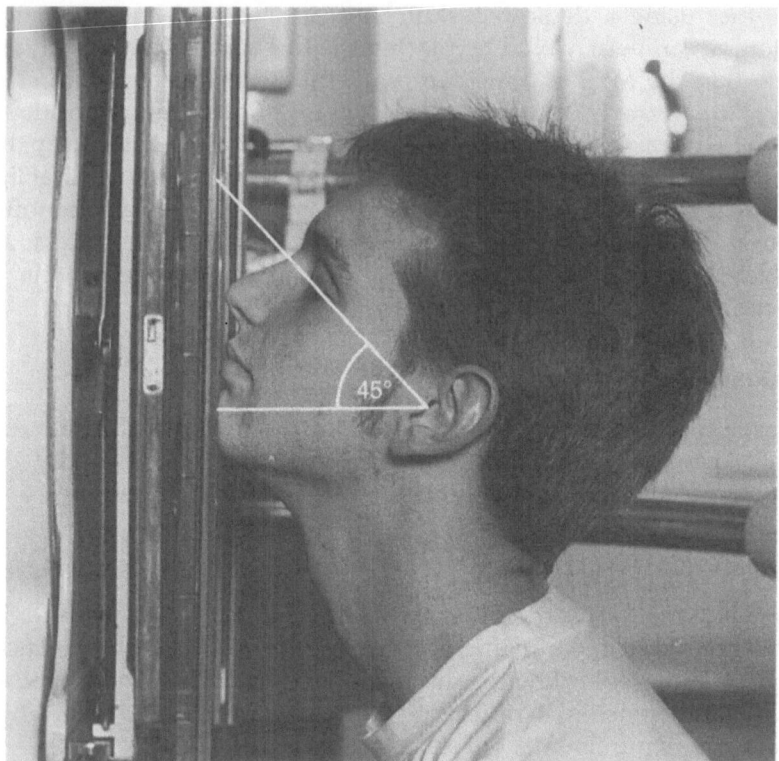

Figure 6.3 Occipitomental. 45°.

The basic projections described for the skull cover the range used by imaging departments. Examination protocols are agreed by discussing radiologists' preferences and the equipment available. Modifications to the series will be implemented according to the patient's ability to cooperate (Gallagher, 1993).

Successful positioning of the skull is highly dependent upon the confidence and control of the radiographer. Students who are new to the techniques often feel uncomfortable when handling the face and head, owing to the intimate nature of close eye and tactile contact. Asking the patient to close their eyes throughout positioning may help put both radiographer and patient at ease. Additionally, patients often watch the radiographer walk away to make the exposure, thus risking movement which may affect positioning. Closing the eyes will also avoid this.

As the neck provides extensive movement of the head in three planes, the inexperienced often have difficulty in achieving the correct positions of OMBL and MSP at the same time. The solution lies in the handling of the patient's head during positioning; to do this effectively the fingers

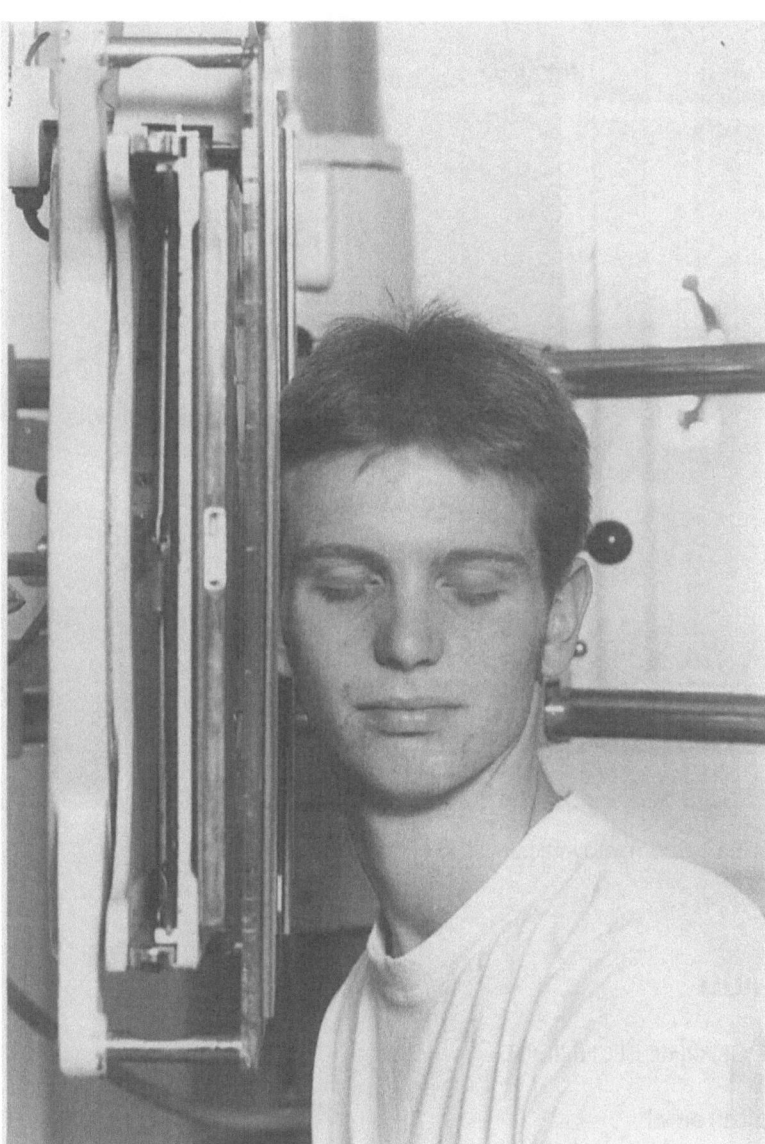

Figure 6.4 Lateral.

should be spread out to provide a large area of firm yet gentle control, enabling the radiographer to position the MSP and OMBL simultaneously.

The following descriptions are for conventional skull radiography; isocentric skull techniques are described in a later section. The criteria for image evaluation are the same for each method.

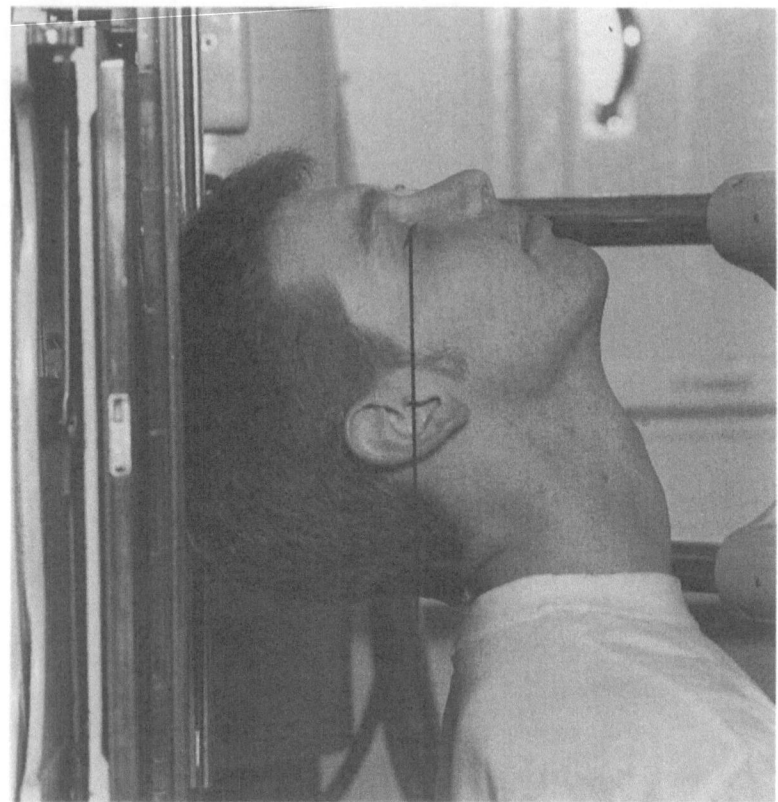

Figure 6.5 Submentovertical.

CRANIUM

RADIOGRAPHIC TECHNIQUE

Occipitofrontal

A 24×30 cm cassette is placed longitudinally in the erect bucky. The patient is seated facing the bucky, with their forehead in contact with it. The glabella is coincident with the centre of the cassette. The OMBL is perpendicular to the cassette, the MSP coincident with and perpendicular to its central long axis.

> CENTRING: The X-ray beam is directed to project the upper border of the petrous portion of the temporal bone to the required level:

90° to cassette will ensure that the upper border of the petrous temporal bone is level with the superior orbital margins;

10° caudal angulation will project the upper border of the petrous temporal bone midway through the orbits;

20° caudal angulation will project the upper border of the petrous temporal bone level with inferior orbital margins.

A horizontal central ray is directed to a point in the midline, above the EOP, to emerge through the glabella.

The height of the centring point above the EOP will vary according to the degree of angulation, but the emergent beam will always pass through the glabella.

Collimate to include vertex of skull, maxillae and parietal bones. Place a PA anatomical marker within the primary beam.

In cases of injury, when a patient is supine on a casualty trolley, it is necessary to carry out a fronto-occipital projection instead of the OF described above. To achieve the required projection, angulation must be applied cranially instead of caudally, with the X-ray beam centred over the glabella.

Fronto-occipital 30°, 'Towne's' or half-axial

A 24×30 cm cassette is placed longitudinally in the erect bucky. The patient is seated facing the X-ray tube with the occiput in contact with the bucky. The upper border of the cassette is level with the vertex of the skull. The OMBL* is perpendicular to the cassette, the MSP coincident with and perpendicular to its central long axis.

CENTRING: A horizontal central ray, at 90° to the cassette, is directed 30° caudally to a point in the midline above the glabella, to pass 2 cm above the level of the EAMs.

Collimate to include vertex of skull, maxillae and parietal bones. Apply an AP anatomical marker within the primary beam.

*Positioning the OMBL at 90° to the cassette in the FO position can be difficult for many patients. Asking them to press the back of the neck, rather than the back of the head, into the bucky will bring the OMBL more easily into the required position. For patients unable to do this, forward angulation of the top of the bucky (approximately 20°) will help, as shown in Figure 6.6. It is important to maintain 30° caudal angulation between the central ray and the OMBL.

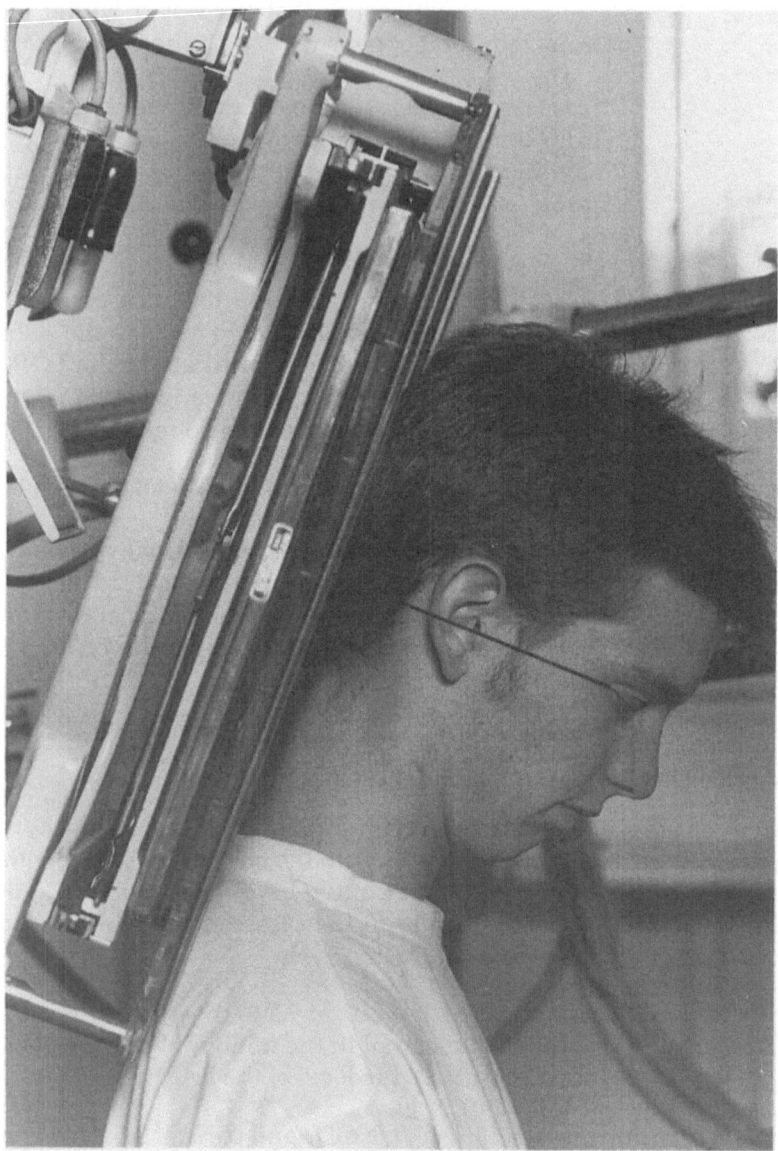

Figure 6.6   Fronto-occipital with bucky tilt to aid positioning.

This method can be employed for any fronto-occipital projection, and bucky angulation can be replaced by a gridded cassette supported at an angle for supine trauma cases. Alternatively, the cassette can be left horizontal and a radiolucent pad placed behind the head to ensure that the OMBL is perpendicular to the cassette and/or the angle of the central ray increased. The conventional 'Towne's' projection already causes distortion of the cranium, with magnification unsharpness of the major portion of the vault and temporal bones. Increasing the OFD or beam angulation will exaggerate these effects, and although during examination of the occiput these areas are of secondary importance, plain radiography of the mastoids, temporomandibular joints and petrous temporal all include 'Towne's' as part of the examination routine, and need to be produced with minimal unsharpness. Bearing this in mind, the implementation of extra angulation or 'padding' should be avoided whenever possible and only used as a last resort.

Lateral

A 24×30 cm cassette is placed transversely in the erect bucky. The patient is seated facing the bucky and their head turned through 90° to bring the affected side into contact with it. The MSP is parallel to the cassette, the interpupillary line perpendicular to it. The top of the cassette is 5 cm above the vertex of the skull, its central long axis coincident with the EAMs.

> CENTRING: A horizontal central ray, at 90° to the cassette, is directed to a point midway between the glabella and the EOP.

Collimate to include vertex and base of skull, glabella and EOP. Place an AP anatomical marker within the primary beam.

Elderly patients often find it impossible to achieve or maintain the required position when erect against a conventional skull unit. To assist in accurate positioning the bucky can be tilted until parallel to the MSP, maintaining the correct tube angulation in relation to the MSP and cassette.

Horizontal beam lateral

This is an adaptation of the lateral skull technique, useful when the patient's condition allows no alternative. This project **must** be used in all cases of trauma.

A 24×30 cm gridded cassette is selected. The patient lies supine with their shoulders relaxed and hands at their sides. The head is raised on to a radiolucent rectangular pad to ensure that the occiput will be included on the radiograph. The cassette rests on its short edge on the trolley top and is placed in contact with the affected side of the patient's head. The cassette is perpendicular to the table top, its long edge 5 cm above the vertex of the skull, supported by means of pads and sandbags. The MSP is parallel to the cassette and the interpupillary line perpendicular to it.

> CENTRING: A horizontal central ray, at 90° to the cassette, is directed midway between the EOP and the glabella, to the centre of the grid.

Collimation and marker as for conventional lateral projection.

The use of the horizontal beam for the lateral projection of the traumatized skull can prove beneficial to diagnosis, in addition to safe practice and patient care, particularly with regard to patients who also have spinal injuries. Where the radiographic appearances of bony outlines suggest otherwise, the presence of air–fluid levels can indicate bony damage (World Health Organization, 1985).

Submentovertical

A 24×30 cm cassette is placed longitudinally in the erect bucky. The patient sits facing the X-ray tube on a stool placed halfway between the tube and the bucky. With support from the radiographer the patient leans back, raising the chin until the vertex of the skull can be placed in contact with the bucky. The middle of the long axis of the cassette is level with the EAMs. The OMBL is parallel to the cassette, the MSP coincident with and perpendicular to its central long axis. The patient holds on to the chair for support.

> CENTRING: A horizontal central ray, at 90° to the OMBL, is directed 5° towards the face, midway between the angles of the mandible.

Collimate to include occiput, parietal bones and outline of nose. Apply an AP anatomical marker within the primary beam.

If the patient cannot lift the chin and extend the neck sufficiently to bring the OMBL parallel to the cassette, the bucky of the skull unit can be tilted until this is achieved. Ensure that the correct tube angulation is maintained in relation to the OMBL.

IMAGE EVALUATION

Correct patient identification and anatomical marker included on the radiograph.

Area of interest

Occipitofrontal

Outer table of skull around its circumference, maxillae and base of skull.

Fronto-occipital 30°, 'Towne's' or half-axial

Outer table of skull around its circumference and upper third of mandibular rami.

Lateral

Outer table of skull around its circumference and sphenoid sinus.

Submentovertical

Outer table of skull in occipital and parietal regions and outline of nose.

Projection

Occipitofrontal

- Equidistance of lateral borders of orbits, or innominate lines, to outer table of skull.
- MSP coincident with midline of film.
  Central ray 90° to cassette
- Superior border of petrous ridge coincident with superior orbital margin.
  10° caudal angulation
- Superior border of petrous ridge projected halfway down orbit.
  20° caudal angulation
- Superior border of petrous ridge coincident with inferior orbital margin.

Fronto-occipital 30°, 'Towne's' or half-axial

- Dorsum sellae and posterior clinoid processes projected through centre of foramen magnum.
- MSP coincident with midline of film.

Lateral

- Superimposition of right and left sides of floors of anterior and posterior cranial fossae.
- Superimposition of right and left sides of inner table of skull.
- Superimposition of right and left anterior and posterior clinoid processes and floor of pituitary fossa.
- Superimposition of anterior margins of sphenoid bone.

Submentovertical

- MSP coincident with midline of film.
- Symmetry of right and left halves of skull, with foramen magnum projected centrally.
- Odontoid process of C2 projected as a circle through anterior portion of foramen magnum.
- Angles of mandible projected clear of petrous temporal ridge.

Exposure factors

Occipitofrontal

- kVp sufficient to demonstrate the sagittal and lambdoid sutures over the skull vault and structures of the middle and inner ear within the petrous ridge through the centre of the orbits, maintaining contrast between the skull vault and dense petrous ridge.
- mAs to provide adequate image density to demonstrate bony detail of the skull vault in contrast to the air-filled sinuses.

Fronto-occipital 30°, 'Towne's' or half-axial

- kVp sufficient to demonstrate the internal occipital crest over the skull vault and structures of the middle and inner ear within the petrous ridge, maintaining contrast between these two areas.
- mAs to provide adequate image density to demonstrate bony detail over all areas of the skull vault in contrast to the dense petrous ridge.

Lateral

- kVp sufficient to demonstrate the coronal and lambdoid sutures over the skull vault and the external auditory meati through the dense petrous ridge, maintaining contrast between these two areas.
- mAs to provide adequate image density to demonstrate bony detail over all areas of the skull vault in contrast to the vascular markings and air-filled sinuses.

Submentovertical

- kVp sufficient to demonstrate the structures of the internal auditory meati within the petrous temporal bone, maintaining contrast between the dense petrous ridge, the cranium and the air-filled sinuses.
- mAs to provide adequate image density to demonstrate detail of the foramina in the base of the skull and the IAMs within the petrous bone

in contrast to the bones of the cranium and face and air-filled sinuses and mastoids.

No evidence of patient movement.
No artefacts present on the film.

Positional faults

Occipitofrontal – 0°, 10° or 20° angulation:
If the relationship between the X-ray beam and the cassette is correct but the chin is raised, the upper border of the petrous portion of the temporal bone (petrous ridge) will appear too low in relation to the outline of the orbit. The chin should be lowered to bring the OMBL perpendicular to the cassette.

If the relationship between the X-ray beam and the cassette is correct but the chin is too low, the upper border of the petrous ridge will appear too high in relation to the outline of the orbit. The chin should be raised to bring the OMBL perpendicular to the cassette.

FO 30°/'Towne's'/half-axial:
If the tube angulation is correct but the chin is raised, the foramen magnum will appear small, or be absent, with the dorsum sellae appearing above it. The chin should be lowered to bring the OMBL perpendicular to the bucky.

If the tube angulation is correct but the chin lowered too much, the arch of C1 will be seen in the lower portion of the foramen magnum and the dorsum sellae will not be visible. The chin should be raised to bring the OMBL perpendicular to the bucky.

Occipitofrontal and fronto-occipital projections:
Rotation of the head (about the MSP) is characterized by a difference in the distances seen between the lateral orbital margins, or innominate lines, and the lateral aspects of the skull vault. The side demonstrating the shorter distance is the side to which the head is turned.

Lateral:
Rotation of the head about the MSP is characterized by the horizontal separation of the right and left sides of the inner table of the skull, the anterior margins of the sphenoid bone and the anterior and posterior clinoid processes.

Tilting of the head about the coronal plane is characterized by the vertical separation of the right and left sides of the floors of the pituitary and anterior and posterior cranial fossae.

Submentovertical:
If the chin is not raised sufficiently to bring the OMBL parallel to the cassette, the mandible will be seen below the maxillary sinuses and the image of the odontoid peg will be elongated rather than appearing as a circle in the anterior aspect of the foramen magnum.

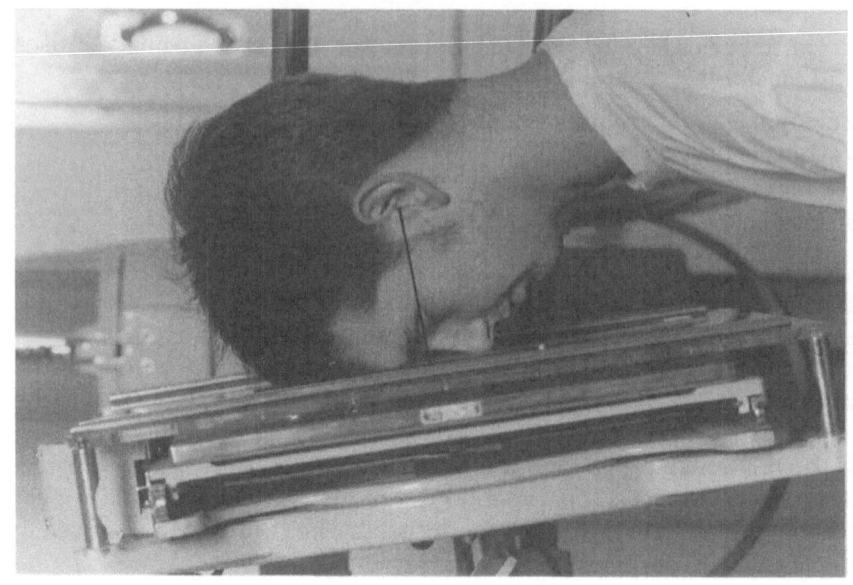

(b)

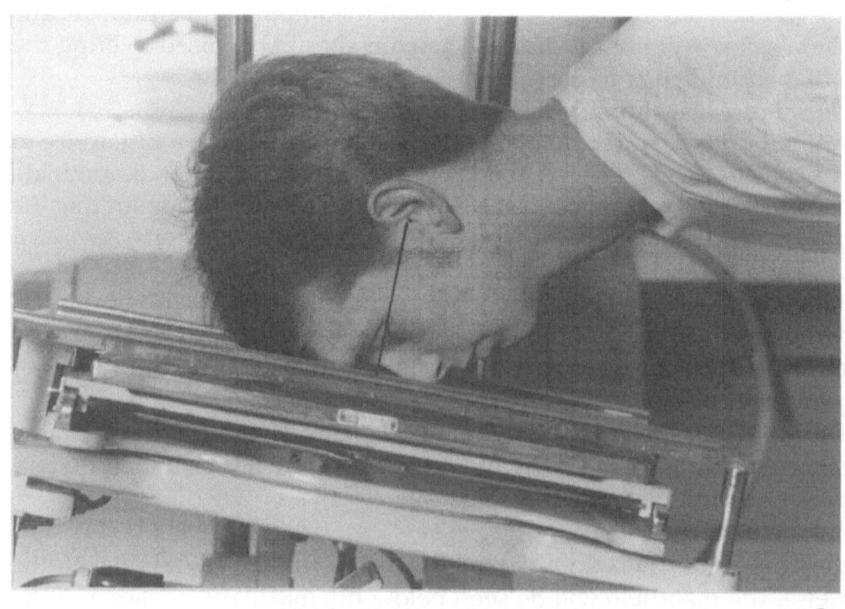

(a)

Figure 6.7 Occipitofrontal. (a) To show frontal sinuses. (b) To show sphenoid sinuses and posterior ethmoids.

PARANASAL SINUSES

It is extremely important to examine the paranasal sinuses with the patient erect, always using a horizontal central ray. This will ensure that fluid levels within the sinuses are adequately demonstrated or excluded.

RADIOGRAPHIC TECHNIQUE

Occipitomental

This will demonstrate the maxillary sinuses, with the frontal sinuses in evidence (although distorted and magnified). If the patient's mouth is open during exposure the sphenoid sinus will be seen through the mouth.

An 18×24 cm cassette is placed longitudinally in the erect bucky. The patient is seated facing the bucky. The chin is raised until the OMBL is 45° from the horizontal, and placed in contact with the bucky. The centre of the long axis of the cassette is level with the inferior orbital margins. The MSP is coincident with and perpendicular to the central long axis of the cassette, EAMs equidistant from the bucky.

CENTRING: A horizontal central ray, at 90° to the cassette, is directed over the midline of the occiput to emerge at the level of the inferior orbital margins.

Collimate to include the frontal and maxillary sinuses. Apply a PA anatomical marker within the primary beam.

If, after viewing the OM projection, it is suspected that the sinuses are fluid filled, the projection can be repeated with a lateral tilt of the patient's head. If fluid is present, fluid levels will remain horizontal in relation to the floor, whereas other pathologies, e.g. polyps, will remain in the same position in relation to the sinus.

Occipitofrontal to demonstrate frontal sinuses (Fig. 6.7a)

The upper border of the erect bucky of the skull unit is angled 10° towards the patient. An 18×24 cm cassette is placed longitudinally in the bucky. The patient is seated facing the bucky, their forehead in contact with it and the OMBL perpendicular to it, i.e. raised 10° from the horizontal. The centre of the cassette is coincident with the nasion. The MSP is perpendicular to the cassette, EAMs equidistant from it.

CENTRING: A horizontal central ray, at 10° to the OMBL, is directed over a point in the midline of the occiput to emerge through the nasion.

Collimate to include the frontal and anterior ethmoid sinuses. Apply a PA anatomical marker within the primary beam.

In the absence of a dedicated skull unit, when the bucky cannot be angled, the patient's chin (OMBL) should be raised through 10° and the head supported with a small radiolucent pad between the bucky and the forehead.

Occipitofrontal to demonstrate maxillary and anterior ethmoid sinuses (see Fig. 6.1)

An 18×24 cm cassette is placed longitudinally in the erect bucky. The patient is seated facing the bucky, their forehead in contact with it and the OMBL perpendicular to it. The centre of the long axis of the cassette is level with the inferior orbital margins. The MSP is coincident with and perpendicular to the central long axis of the cassette, EAMs equidistant from the bucky.

> CENTRING: A horizontal central ray, at 90° to the cassette, is directed over the midline of the occiput to emerge at the level of the inferior orbital margins.

Collimate to include all paranasal sinuses. Apply a PA anatomical marker within the primary beam.

The sphenoid and posterior/middle ethmoid sinuses will be superimposed. Frontal sinuses appear foreshortened and small frontal sinuses may not be demonstrated at all.

Occipitofrontal to demonstrate sphenoid and posterior/middle ethmoid sinuses (Fig. 6.7b)

The upper border of the erect bucky of the skull unit is angled 10° away from the patient. An 18×24 cm cassette is placed longitudinally in the bucky. The patient is seated facing the bucky, their forehead in contact with it and the OMBL perpendicular to it, i.e. lowered 10° from the horizontal. The centre of the cassette is coincident with the nasion. The MSP is perpendicular to the cassette, EAMs equidistant from it.

> CENTRING: A horizontal central ray, at 10° to the OMBL, is directed over the midline of the occiput to emerge through the nasion.

Collimate to include the sphenoid and posterior/middle ethmoid sinuses. Apply a PA anatomical marker within the primary beam.

In the absence of a dedicated skull unit, when the bucky cannot be angled, the patient's chin (OMBL) should be lowered through 10° and the head supported with a small radiolucent pad between the bucky and the chin.

Lateral (see Fig. 6.4)

An 18×24 cm cassette is placed longitudinally in the erect bucky. The patient sits facing the bucky, the head turned through 90° to bring the affected side into contact with it. The MSP is parallel to the cassette and the interpupillary line perpendicular to it. The centre of the cassette is coincident with a point midway along the OMBL.

> CENTRING: A horizontal central ray, at 90° to the cassette, is directed to a point halfway along the OMBL.

Collimate to include frontal, sphenoid, ethmoid and maxillary sinuses. Apply an AP anatomical marker within the primary beam.

Lateral postnasal space

The postnasal space is examined in order to demonstrate the soft tissues of the pharynx and, in particular, to assess possible adenoid enlargement.

The patient is positioned as for lateral sinuses, with the upper border of the cassette level with the glabella.

> CENTRING: A horizontal central ray, at 90° to the cassette, is directed to a point 2.5 cm behind and 5 cm below the outer canthus of the eye.

Collimate to include the maxillary sinuses and pharynx. Apply an AP anatomical marker within the primary beam.

As movement of the tongue during exposure may cause unsharpness, the patient is asked to keep the tongue in contact with the roof of the mouth.

IMAGE EVALUATION

Correct patient identification and anatomical marker included on the radiograph.

Area of interest

Occipitomental and occipitofrontal

Those sinuses which each of the individual projections is intended to demonstrate.

Lateral

All paranasal sinuses.

Lateral postnasal space

All paranasal sinuses and pharynx.

Projection

Occipitomental

- Symmetry of right- and left-sided facial structures, with equidistance of innominate lines to lateral margins of orbits.
- MSP coincident with midline of film.
- Upper border of petrous ridge coincident with lower border of maxillary antra.

Occipitofrontal

- Symmetry of right- and left-sided facial structures.
- MSP coincident with midline of film.
  To demonstrate frontal sinuses
- Upper border of petrous ridge projected halfway down orbits.
  To demonstrate maxillary and anterior ethmoid sinuses
- Upper border of petrous ridge coincident with superior orbital margin.
  To demonstrate sphenoid and posterior/middle ethmoid sinuses
- Upper border of petrous ridge projected above superior orbital margin.
- Sphenoid and posterior/middle ethmoid sinuses demonstrated between upper borders of petrous ridge.
- Dorsum sella projected slightly above sphenoid sinuses.

Lateral sinuses and postnasal space

- Superimposition of right- and left-sided facial structures.
- Superimposition of right and left sides of floors of pituitary and anterior cranial fossae.
- Superimposition of right and left anterior and posterior clinoid processes and anterior margins of sphenoid bone.

Exposure factors

Paranasal sinuses

- kVp sufficient to penetrate vault of skull and facial bones to demonstrate the full extent of the paranasal sinuses, maintaining contrast between the air-filled sinuses, bony structures and surrounding soft tissues.
- mAs to provide adequate image density to demonstrate detail of the

air-filled sinuses in contrast to the adjacent bones and soft tissue structures.

Lateral postnasal space

- kVp sufficient to demonstrate bony trabeculae within the mandible, maintaining contrast between the air-filled sinuses and pharynx and the facial bones.
- mAs to provide adequate image density to demonstrate retropharyngeal soft tissue detail in contrast to the air-filled oro- and nasopharynx and bony facial structures.

No evidence of patient movement.
No artefacts present on the image.

Positional faults

Occipitomental:
Rotation of the head (about the MSP) is characterized by a difference in the distances seen between the innominate lines and lateral orbital margins. The side demonstrating the shorter distance is the side to which the head is turned.

If the relationship between the X-ray beam and the cassette is correct but the chin is raised, the upper border of the petrous ridge will appear below the inferior margin of the maxillary antra, with excessive foreshortening of the orbits and superimposition of the teeth/alveolar margins over the maxillary sinuses. The chin should be lowered to bring the OMBL to 45° to the cassette.

If the relationship between the X-ray beam and the cassette is correct but the chin is too low, the upper border of the petrous ridge will appear within the maxillary antra. The chin should be raised to bring the OMBL to 45° to the cassette.

Occipitofrontal:
As for the skull (see p. 173).

FACIAL BONES

RADIOGRAPHIC TECHNIQUE

Occipitomental

A 24×30 cm cassette is placed longitudinally in the erect bucky. The patient is seated facing the bucky. The chin is raised until the OMBL makes an angle of 45° to the horizontal, and placed in contact with the bucky. The centre of the long axis of the cassette is level with the nostrils.

The MSP is perpendicular to and coincident with the central long axis of the cassette.

> CENTRING: *Occipitomental*
> A horizontal central ray, at 90° to the cassette, is directed to the midline of the occiput to emerge level with the alae of the nostrils.
> *Occipitomental 30°*
> A horizontal central ray, at 90° to the cassette, is angled 30° caudally to a point in the midline of the occiput to emerge level with the alae of the nostrils.

The cassette is displaced until its centre coincides with the central ray. Collimate to include orbits, zygomas, maxilla and mandible. Apply a PA anatomical marker within the primary beam.

Lateral

A 24×30 cm cassette is placed longitudinally in the bucky. The patient is seated facing the bucky, the head turned through 90° to bring the affected side into contact with it. The middle of the cassette is coincident with a point 2.5 cm below the outer canthus of the eye. The MSP is parallel to the cassette.

> CENTRING: A horizontal central ray, at 90° to the cassette, is directed to a point 2.5 cm below the outer canthus of the eye.

Collimate to include orbits, maxillae, zygomas, mandible and temporomandibular joints. Apply an AP anatomical marker within the primary beam.

In cases of trauma the lateral projection **must** be carried out using a horizontal beam – the patient may be erect or supine. In this way fluid levels within the sinuses, which are indicative of bony injury, will be demonstrated.

In cases of trauma it is likely that the patient will need to be examined supine on a trolley. In this case, the following modified projections are undertaken in place of the OM and OM 30°.

Mento-occipital (Fig. 6.8)

A 24×30 cm gridded cassette is placed longitudinally beneath the patient's head. If the patient's condition allows, the chin is raised until the OMBL is 45° to the cassette. The centre of the long axis of the cassette is level with the nostrils. The MSP is coincident with and perpendicular to the central long axis of the cassette.

> CENTRING: A vertical central ray, at 45° to the OMBL, is directed to a point in the midline and level with the alae of nostrils.

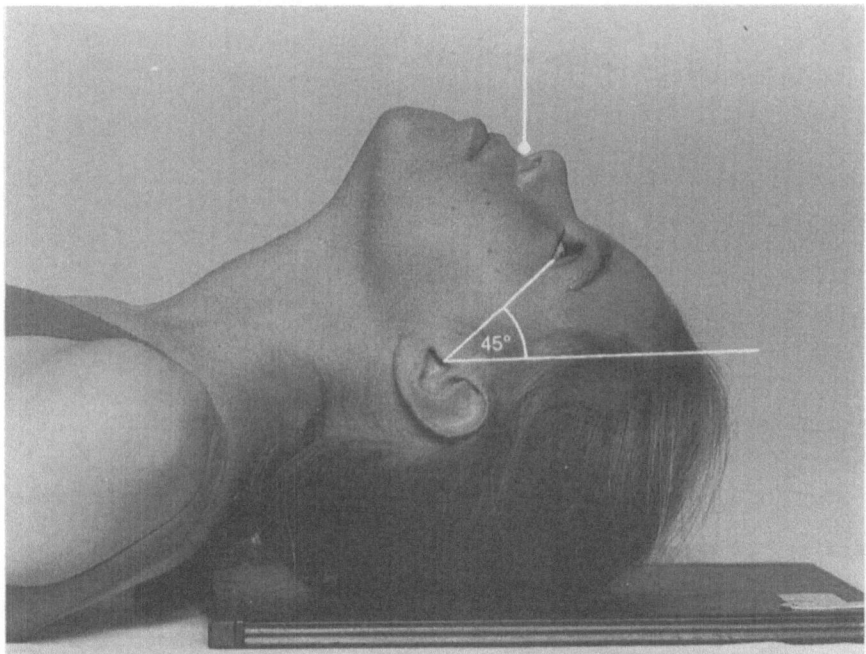

Figure 6.8   Mento-occipital.

Collimation as for routine OM facial bones. Apply an AP anatomical marker within the primary beam.

Mento-occipital 30° (Fig. 6.9) (After Ponsford and Clements, 1991)

The patient remains supine. If the patient's condition allows, the head is raised on a small rectangular radiolucent pad. The shoulders are relaxed down and the chin lowered until the OMBL is as near vertical as the patient can manage. The MSP is perpendicular to the trolley top. A 24×30 cm gridded cassette, resting on its short edge on the trolley top, is placed in contact with the vertex of the skull. The cassette is parallel to the OMBL, its central long axis perpendicular to and coincident with the MSP. The cassette is supported with pads/sandbags.

> CENTRING: A horizontal central ray is initially directed at 90° to the OMBL and then angled 20° towards the floor and centred over the symphysis menti.

Collimation as for routine OM facial bones. Apply an AP anatomical marker within the primary beam.

The advantage of this projection over the reverse OM 30° is the reduction in image distortion and magnification.

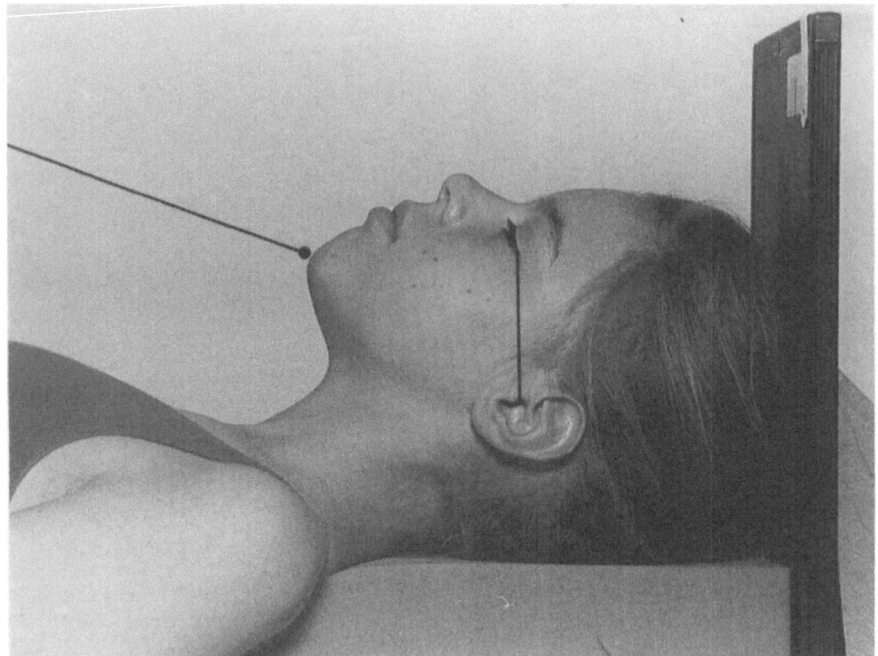

Figure 6.9 Modified mento-occipital.

IMAGE EVALUATION

Correct patient identification and anatomical marker included on the radiograph.

Area of interest

Occipitomental and mento-occipital

Superior borders of orbits and frontal sinus, mandible and zygomas.

Lateral

Frontal sinus and floor of anterior cranial fossa, mandible, nose and soft tissue outlines of the face.

Projection

Occipitomental and mento-occipital

- MSP coincident with midline of film.

- Equidistance of lateral borders of orbits to lateral margins of skull.
- Superior border of petrous ridge coincident with inferior margin of maxillary sinuses.

Occipitomental 30° and mento-occipital 30°

- MSP coincident with midline of film.
- Equidistance of lateral borders of orbits to lateral margins of skull.
- Coronoid processes of mandible projected clear of, and below, zygomatic processes of maxillae.
- Odontoid process of C2 demonstrated through foramen magnum below symphysis menti.
- Demonstration of infraorbital foramina through superior aspect of maxillary sinuses.

Lateral

- Superimposition of right and left facial structures, mandible and floor of anterior cranial fossa.

Exposure factors

Occipitomental and mento-occipital

- kVp sufficient to demonstrate the floor of maxillary sinuses and areas of overlap of the zygoma and mandible on the bones of the skull, maintaining contrast between the facial bones and air-filled sinuses.
- mAs to provide adequate image density to demonstrate bony detail of the facial bones in contrast to the air-filled sinuses and surrounding soft tissues.

Lateral

- kVp sufficient to demonstrate areas of overlap of the left and right facial structures, maintaining contrast between the facial bones, air-filled sinuses and soft tissue outlines of the face and neck.
- mAs to provide adequate image density to demonstrate bony detail in contrast to the air-filled sinuses and soft tissue outlines.

No evidence of patient movement.
No artefacts present on the image.

ZYGOMATIC ARCHES

RADIOGRAPHIC TECHNIQUE

The zygomatic arches can be seen adequately on occipitomental projections, but are inadequately demonstrated in the lateral. A 'Towne's' or SMV projection will demonstrate the degree of depression of the fractured fragments.

Fronto-occipital 30°/'Towne's'

An 18×24 cm cassette is placed transversely in the erect bucky. The patient is seated facing the X-ray tube with the back of the head in contact with the bucky. The OMBL is perpendicular to the cassette, the MSP coincident with and perpendicular to its central short axis. The upper border of the cassette is level with the EOP.

> CENTRING: A horizontal central ray, parallel to the OMBL, is directed 30° caudally to a point above the glabella to pass through the zygomatic arches.

Collimate to include zygomatic arches and surrounding soft tissues. Apply an AP anatomical marker within the primary beam.

Submentovertical

An 18×24 cm cassette is placed transversely in the erect bucky. The patient is seated facing the X-ray tube on a stool which is placed midway between the tube and the bucky. With support from the radiographer the patient leans back, raising the chin, until the vertex of the skull can be placed in contact with the bucky. The OMBL is parallel to the cassette, the MSP coincident with and perpendicular to its central short axis. The centre of the short axis of the cassette is level with the EAMs.

> CENTRING: A horizontal central ray, at 90° to the OMBL, is directed midway between and 2.5 cm anterior to the angles of the mandible.

Collimate to include zygomatic arches and surrounding soft tissues. Apply an AP anatomical marker within the primary beam.

Exposure factors should be much lower than those selected for the routine OF 30° and SMV cranium projections, as the density in the region of the zygomatic arches is very low by comparison.

IMAGE EVALUATION

Correct patient identification and anatomical marker included on the radiograph.

Area of interest

Left and right zygomatic arches.

Projection

Fronto-occipital 30°

- Symmetry of left and right mandibular rami about midline.
- Zygomatic arches demonstrated in profile lateral to mandibular rami.

Submentovertical

- Symmetry of lateral skull margins about nasal septum.
- Zygomatic arches demonstrated in profile lateral to outer margins of skull.

Exposure factors

- kVp sufficient to demonstrate bony detail within the zygomatic arches, but not within the mandible or skull, maintaining contrast between the zygomas and air-filled sinuses and soft tissues of the face.
- mAs to provide adequate image density to demonstrate the zygomatic arches in contrast to the soft tissues of the face.

No evidence of patient movement.
No artefacts present on the image.

NASAL BONES

RADIOGRAPHIC TECHNIQUE

Occipitomental

An 18×24 cm cassette is placed longitudinally in the erect bucky. The patient is seated with their back to the X-ray tube. The chin is raised until the OMBL is 45° to the horizontal, and placed in contact with the bucky. The MSP is coincident with and perpendicular to the central long axis of the cassette. The centre of the cassette is coincident with the nasal bones.

> CENTRING: A horizontal central ray, at 90° to the cassette, is directed to the midline of the occiput to emerge through the nasal bones.

Collimate to include nasal bones and anterior nasal spine. Apply a PA anatomical marker within the primary beam.

Lateral

An 18×24 cm cassette is placed longitudinally in the erect cassette holder. The patient is seated facing the cassette, the head turned through 90° to bring the affected side into contact with it. The middle of the cassette is coincident with the nasal bones. The MSP is parallel to the cassette.

CENTRING: A horizontal central ray, at 90° to the cassette, is directed over the centre of the nose.

Collimate to include nasal bones, anterior nasal spine and surrounding soft tissues. Apply an AP anatomical marker within the primary beam.

IMAGE EVALUATION

Correct patient identification and anatomical marker included on the radiograph.

Area of interest

Occipitomental

Nasal cavity, medial portion of maxillary sinuses, inferior portion of the frontal sinuses and upper incisors.

Lateral

Nasal bones, anterior nasal spine and soft tissue outlines.

Projection

Occipitomental

- MSP coincident with midline of film.
- Symmetry of right and left facial structures.
- Superior border of petrous ridge coincident with lower border of maxillary antra.

Lateral

- Superimposition of lateral borders of orbits.
- Nasal bones and inferior nasal spine projected clear of maxillae.

Exposure factors

Occipitomental

- kVp sufficient to demonstrate the nasal bones within the nasal cavity, maintaining contrast between the nasal bones and the air-filled nasal cavity and maxillary sinuses.
- mAs to provide adequate image density to demonstrate the bony nasal septum in contrast to the surrounding air-filled structures.

Lateral

- kVp sufficient to demonstrate the trabeculae within the nasal bone, maintaining contrast between the bony septum and surrounding soft tissues.
- mAs to provide adequate image density to demonstrate bony detail in contrast to the soft tissue structures.

No evidence of patient movement.
No artefacts present on the image.

ORBITS

RADIOGRAPHIC TECHNIQUE

Occipitomental

This OM projection varies slightly from Figure 6.3 since the OMBL lies at 30° rather than at 45° to the bucky. An 18×24 cm cassette is placed transversely in the erect bucky. The patient is seated facing the bucky. The chin is raised until the OMBL is at 30° to the horizontal, and placed in contact with the bucky. The MSP is perpendicular to the cassette. The centre of the cassette is coincident with the midpoint between the orbits.

> CENTRING: A horizontal central ray, at 90° to the cassette, is directed to the midline of the occiput to emerge in the centre of the interpupillary line.

Collimate to include orbits and maxillary sinuses. Apply a PA anatomical marker within the primary beam.

Lateral

An 18×24 cm cassette is placed longitudinally in the erect bucky. The patient is seated facing the bucky, the head rotated through 90° to bring the affected side into contact with it. The centre of the cassette is coincident with the outer canthus of the eye. The MSP is parallel to the cassette.

CENTRING: A horizontal central ray, at 90° to the cassette, is directed over the outer canthus of the eye.

Collimate to include orbits and maxillary sinuses. Apply an AP anatomical marker within the primary beam.

The commonest indications for radiography of the orbits are injury and demonstration of intraocular foreign body (IOFB). A 'blowout' fracture of the orbital floor, classically caused by a blow to the orbital rim, causes herniation of orbital soft tissue into the sinus below, and is seen as a semicircle or 'teardrop' of soft tissue in the roof of the maxillary antrum. There will also be interruption of the bony floor of the orbit, although this is not always obvious. Inclusion of the maxillary sinuses on the image is essential, as the presence of fluid within the sinus can confirm a fracture of the orbital floor. If the patient cannot be examined erect then a supine mento-occipital projection is produced (as described previously for facial bones), in addition to a horizontal beam lateral projection. This will demonstrate the presence of any fluid levels, thus indicating bony injury.

When demonstration of an intraorbital foreign body is required (IOFB) two OM projections are taken – with the eyes raised and eyes lowered. Alternatively, the eyes can be moved to the left and right. Laterals are also taken with the eyes raised and lowered. The appropriate legends must be included on each image. Good practice involves the use of cassettes which are reserved exclusively for this examination. They are kept, unloaded, in the darkroom. Prior to each use the screens are cleaned, so as to minimize the presence of artefacts which may mimic IOFBs on the resultant images, and loaded before use.

IMAGE EVALUATION

Correct patient identification and anatomical marker included on the radiograph.

Area of interest

Outline of bony orbits and maxillary sinuses.

Projection

Occipitomental

- Symmetry of left and right facial structures.
- Superior border of petrous bone projected halfway down maxillary antra.
- Clear visualization of entire outline of bony orbit.

Lateral

● Superimposition of outlines of right and left bony orbits.

Exposure factors

Occipitomental

● kVp sufficient to demonstrate the lower portion of the maxillary antra through the overlying petrous bone.

Occipitomental and lateral

● kVp sufficient to demonstrate the bony trabeculae within the frontal and facial bones, maintaining contrast between the bony orbit, frontal bone and air-filled sinuses.
● mAs to provide adequate image density to demonstrate the outline of the bony orbit in contrast to the frontal bone and air-filled frontal, maxillary and ethmoid sinuses.

No evidence of patient movement.
No artefacts present on the image.

MANDIBLE

RADIOGRAPHIC TECHNIQUE

Posteroanterior

Positioning of the head is as for a basic OF skull, but since the beam does not travel through the occiput or frontal bone the projection is termed PA rather than OF.

For optimum detail a bucky/grid is used as the cervical vertebrae overlie the mandible in the PA projection.

An 18×24 cm cassette is placed longitudinally in the erect bucky. The patient is seated facing the bucky, with their forehead in contact with it. The OMBL is perpendicular to the cassette, the MSP coincident with and perpendicular to its central long axis. The middle of the long axis of the cassette is level with the angles of the mandible.

> CENTRING: A horizontal central ray, at 90° to the cassette, is directed to a point in the midline of the neck at the level of the angles of the mandible.

Collimate to include temporomandibular joints, rami and bodies of mandible and symphysis menti. Apply a PA anatomical marker within the primary beam.

Lateral

For optimum detail a bucky/grid is used as the right and left halves of the mandible are superimposed in the lateral projection.

An 18×24 cm cassette is placed longitudinally in the erect bucky. The patient is seated facing the bucky, the head turned through 90° to bring the affected side into contact with it. The chin is raised slightly to clear the mandible from the upper cervical vertebrae and shoulder. The centre of the cassette is coincident with the angles of the mandible. The MSP is parallel to the cassette.

> CENTRING: A horizontal central ray, at 90° to the cassette, is directed over the angle of the mandible nearest the X-ray tube.

Collimate to include temporomandibular joints, angles of mandible and symphysis menti. Apply an AP anatomical marker within the primary beam.

Lateral oblique (Fig. 6.10)

Both lateral obliques are carried out as contrecoup fractures (those occurring on the opposite side to the impact as a result of transmitted force) of the mandible are common.

Sufficient detail can be obtained without the use of a bucky/grid, since the object of the lateral oblique projection is to show each side of the mandible in turn, clear of overlying structures. As the shoulders can be placed underneath the erect cassette holder, positioning of the patient is much easier than when trying to achieve the same position with the patient's shoulders up against a large bucky.

An 18×24 cm cassette is placed transversely in the erect cassette holder. The patient is seated with the side under examination in contact with the cassette, MSP parallel to it. The centre of the cassette is coincident with the angles of the mandible. Without rotating the head, the vertex of the skull is tilted 15° towards the cassette, resting on the cassette for stability. The chin is raised to clear the mandibular condyles from the cervical vertebrae.

> CENTRING: A horizontal central ray is angled 10° cranially, to a point midway between the angles of mandible.

The cassette is displaced cranially until its centre is coincident with the central ray. Collimate to include temporomandibular joint, angle of mandible and symphysis menti on the side under examination. Apply an AP anatomical marker within the primary beam.

A common problem with this projection when examining large patients is the superimposition of the shoulder mass over the mandible. This can be avoided by moving the shoulder nearest the X-ray tube backwards,

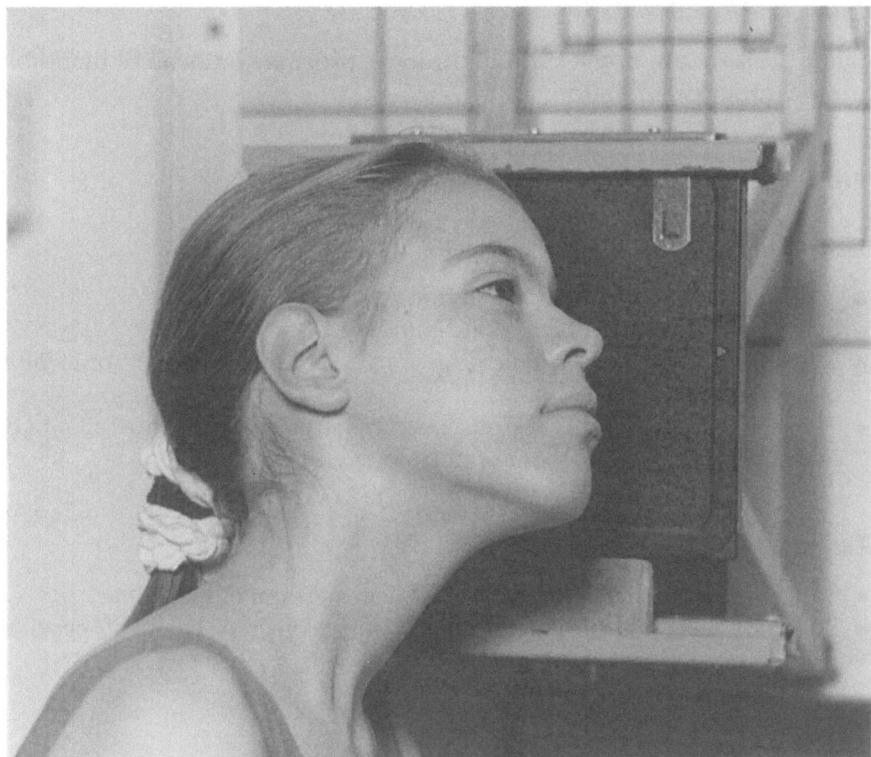

Figure 6.10   Lateral oblique for mandible. Cassette displaced cranially owing to cranial angulation of beam.

with a slight rotation of the trunk, while maintaining the correct position of the head.

Orthopantomography (OPT) is a useful method of demonstrating the mandible in its entirety. An OPT may replace or supplement conventional mandible projections.

IMAGE EVALUATION

Correct patient identification and anatomical marker included on the radiograph.

Area of interest

Posteroanterior

Bodies, rami and heads of mandible.

Lateral and lateral oblique

Symphysis menti, body, ramus, coronoid process and head of mandible of side under examination.

Projection

Posteroanterior

- MSP coincident with midline of film.
- Symmetry of right and left mandibular rami.
- Superior border of petrous ridge projected just above supraorbital margins.
- Temporomandibular joints obscured by superimposition of heads of mandible on inferior border of petrous ridge.

Lateral

- Superimposition of right and left bodies and rami of mandible.
- Posterior borders of mandibular rami projected clear of cervical vertebrae.

Lateral oblique

- Side remote from cassette projected above side closer to it, enabling clear visualization of body, ramus, coronoid process and head of mandible of side under examination.
- Partial superimposition of right and left bodies of mandible at symphysis menti.
- Posterior border of mandibular ramus projected clear of cervical vertebrae.

Exposure factors

- kVp sufficient to demonstrate bony detail of the areas of mandible under examination through overlying bone, maintaining contrast between the mandible, air-filled trachea and soft tissue structures of the mouth and neck.
- mAs to provide adequate image density to demonstrate bony detail of those areas of the mandible under examination in contrast to soft tissue and air-filled structures.

No evidence of patient movement.
No artefacts present on the image.

Positional faults

Lateral oblique:
If the tube angulation or head tilt are not sufficient there will be inadequate separation of the right and left sides of the mandible, and the temporomandibular joint on the side under examination will not be demonstrated. If the chin is not raised sufficiently, the temporomandibular joint and posterior ramus on the side under examination will be superimposed over the cervical spine.

SPECIALIZED SKULL PROJECTIONS

PITUITARY FOSSA

RADIOGRAPHIC TECHNIQUE

Lateral

An 18×24 cm cassette is placed longitudinally in the erect bucky. The patient is seated facing the bucky, the head rotated through 90° to bring the affected side into contact with it. The middle of the cassette is coincident with the squamous portion of the temporal bone. The MSP is parallel to the cassette.

> CENTRING: A horizontal central ray, at 90° to the cassette, is directed 2.5 cm perpendicularly above a point 2.5 cm anterior to the EAM along the OMBL.

Collimate to include the anterior and posterior clinoid processes, pituitary fossa and sphenoid sinus. Apply an AP anatomical marker within the primary beam.

Occipitofrontal

An 18×24 cm cassette is placed longitudinally in the erect bucky. The patient is seated facing the bucky, the forehead in contact with it. The OMBL is perpendicular to the cassette, the MSP coincident with and perpendicular to its central long axis.
(a) *To demonstrate the floor of the pituitary fossa*
The middle of the cassette is coincident with the nasion.

> CENTRING: A horizontal central ray is directed 20° caudally in the midline of the occiput to emerge through the nasion.

(b) *To demonstrate posterior clinoid processes*
The middle of the cassette is 7.5 cm above the nasion.

> CENTRING: A horizontal central ray is directed 30° cranially in the midline of the neck to pass through the level of the EAMs.

Collimate to include (a) floor of pituitary fossa through sphenoid and ethmoid sinuses and lesser wings of sphenoid, or (b) dorsum sellae and posterior clinoid processes within foramen magnum. Apply a PA anatomical marker within the primary beam.

IMAGE EVALUATION

Correct patient identification and anatomical marker included on the radiograph

Area of interest

Lateral

Anterior and posterior clinoid processes, pituitary fossa, sphenoid sinus and dorsum sellae.

Occipitofrontal to demonstrate floor of pituitary fossa

Lesser wing of sphenoid and sphenoid and ethmoid sinuses.

Occipitofrontal to demonstrate posterior clinoid processes

Foramen magnum, posterior clinoid processes and dorsum sellae.

Projection

Lateral

- Superimposition of right and left sides of floors of sella turcica and anterior cranial fossa.
- Superimposition of right and left anterior and posterior clinoid processes.

Occipitofrontal to demonstrate floor of pituitary fossa

- MSP coincident with midline of film.
- Superior border of petrous ridge superimposed on inferior orbital margin.
- Medial borders of orbits equidistant from nasal septum.
- Floor of pituitary fossa demonstrated through ethmoid sinuses.

Occipitofrontal to demonstrate posterior clinoid processes

- MSP coincident with midline of film.
- Dorsum sellae and posterior clinoid processes demonstrated through centre of foramen magnum.

Exposure factors

- kVp sufficient to demonstrate the specific parts of the pituitary fossa through the overlying bony structures, maintaining contrast between the pituitary fossa, air-filled sinuses, cranium and sphenoid bone.
- mAs to provide adequate image density to demonstrate detail of the pituitary fossa in contrast to the air-filled sinuses, cranium and sphenoid bone.

No evidence of patient movement.
No artefacts present on the image.

TEMPOROMANDIBULAR JOINTS

RADIOGRAPHIC TECHNIQUE

Fronto-occipital 30°

An 18×24 cm cassette is placed transversely in the erect bucky. The patient is seated facing the X-ray tube with the back of the head in contact with the bucky. The OMBL is perpendicular to the cassette, MSP coincident with and perpendicular to its central short axis. The upper border of the cassette is level with the EOP. The mouth is opened to open up the temporomandibular joints.

> CENTRING: A horizontal central ray, parallel to the OMBL, is directed 30° caudally to a point above the glabella to emerge at the level of the EAMs.

Collimate to include mastoid air cells and condyles of mandible. Apply an AP anatomical marker within the primary beam.

The temporomandibular joints are seen just below the mastoid air cells, on the lateral extremes of the vault. The mouth should be open during exposure, to bring the condyles of the mandible forward. This may cause the patient to lift the chin slightly and raise the OMBL, so care must be taken to check the OMBL immediately before exposure.

This projection can be carried out as an OF with 30° cranial angulation, centring below the EOP so that the X-ray beam passes through the level of the EAMS.

Lateral oblique

An 18×24 cm cassette is placed longitudinally in the erect bucky. The patient is seated facing the bucky, the head rotated through 90° until the side under examination is in contact with it. The centre of the cassette is coincident with the temporomandibular joint. The MSP is parallel to the cassette.

> CENTRING: A horizontal central ray is directed 25° caudally to a point above the temporomandibular joint nearest the tube, to emerge through the temporomandibular joint in contact with the bucky.

Collimate to include temporomandibular joint and mandibular condyle under examination. Apply an AP anatomical marker within the primary beam. Both sides are examined for comparison.

Routinely, two exposures are made of each side: with mouth open and mouth closed. Legends are included to identify the different projections. Further projections may also be required with the back teeth clenched.

Orthopantomography offers an alternative method of imaging the temporomandibular joints.

IMAGE EVALUATION

Correct patient identification and anatomical marker included on the radiograph.

Area of interest

Fronto-occipital 30°

Both temporomandibular joints and mandibular condyles.

Lateral oblique

Temporomandibular joint of side under examination.

Projection

Fronto-occipital 30°

- MSP coincident with midline of film.
- Symmetry of mandibular rami about the MSP.

- Posterior clinoid processes and dorsum sellae projected through centre of foramen magnum.
- Heads of mandible and temporomandibular joints projected clear of temporal bone owing to mouth being open during exposure.

Lateral oblique

- Temporomandibular joint under examination clearly demonstrated in front of EAM, with no superimposition of TMJ of opposite side, which is projected off the image.
- Mandibular fossa of temporal bone demonstrated in centre of film.
- 'mouth open'/'mouth closed'/'teeth clenched' legends included as appropriate.

Exposure factors

- kVp sufficient to demonstrate head of mandible and mandibular fossa through the overlying skull, maintaining contrast between the head of mandible and air-filled mastoids and sinuses.
- mAs to provide adequate image density to demonstrate detail of the head of mandible in contrast to the temporomandibular joint space and mastoid air cells.

No evidence of patient movement.
No artefacts present on the image.

MASTOID AIR CELLS

The quantity of mastoid air cells will vary from patient to patient, with some appearing to have hardly any air cells at all.

RADIOGRAPHIC TECHNIQUE

Fronto-occipital 30°

An 18×24 cm cassette is placed transversely in the erect bucky. The patient is seated facing the X-ray tube with the back of the head in contact with the bucky. The OMBL is perpendicular to the cassette, the MSP coincident with and perpendicular to its central short axis. The upper border of the cassette is level with the EOP.

CENTRING: A horizontal central ray, parallel to the OMBL, is directed 30° caudally to a point above the glabella to emerge through the level of the EAMs.

Collimate to include temporal bone and mastoid processes. Apply an AP anatomical marker within the primary beam.

Mastoid air cells are demonstrated at the extreme lateral ends of the petrous temporal bone, above the temporomandibular joints.

This projection can be carried out as an OF with 30° cranial angulation, centring below the EOP with the X-ray beam passing through the level of the EAMs.

Lateral oblique

An 18×24 cm cassette is placed longitudinally in the erect bucky. The patient is seated facing the bucky, the head rotated through 90° to bring the side under examination into contact with it. The pinna of the ear is folded forward and held in place by the head being in contact with the bucky. The centre of the cassette is coincident with the mastoid processes. The MSP is parallel to the cassette.

CENTRING: A horizontal ray is directed 25° caudally to a point above the mastoid process nearest the X-ray tube, to emerge through the mastoid process nearest the cassette.

Collimate to include temporal bone and mastoid process of side under examination. Apply an AP anatomical marker within the primary beam. Both sides are examined for comparison.

The air cells under examination will be demonstrated behind and above the EAM.

Profile (posterior oblique) (Fig. 6.11)

An 18×24 cm cassette is placed longitudinally in the erect bucky. The patient is seated facing the X-ray tube with the back of their head in contact with the bucky. With the OMBL and MSP perpendicular to the cassette the head is rotated through 30°, away from the side under examination. The centre of the cassette is coincident with the mastoid process remote from the cassette.

CENTRING: A horizontal central ray is directed 25° caudally to the mastoid process remote from the cassette.

Collimate to include the mastoid air cells and mastoid process. Apply an

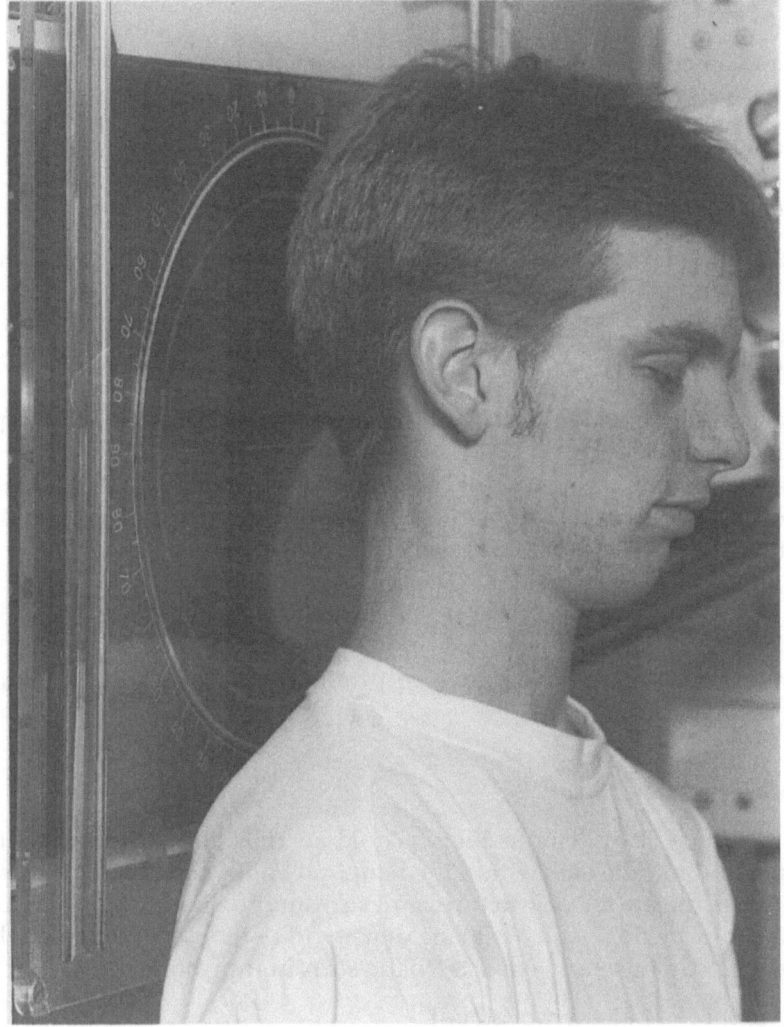

Figure 6.11   Mastoids: profile.

AP anatomical marker within the primary beam. Both sides are examined for comparison.

IMAGE EVALUATION

Correct patient identification and anatomical marker included on the radiograph.

Area of interest

Mastoid air cells within petrous bone and mastoid process.

Projection

Fronto-occipital 30°

- Dorsum sellae and posterior clinoid processes projected through centre of foramen magnum.

Lateral oblique

- Mastoid air cells demonstrated in centre of film, posterior to temporomandibular joint and EAM.
- Head of mandible and mastoid air cells of opposite side projected below those under examination, with no superimposition of one on the other.
- Pinna of ear folded forward so as not to obscure image of air cells.

Profile (posterior oblique)

- Mastoid process demonstrated in profile free of overlying skull and facial structures.

Exposure factors

- kVp sufficient to demonstrate mastoid air cells and structures of the inner and middle ears within the temporal bone, maintaining contrast between the air-filled structures and surrounding bone.
- mAs to provide adequate image density to demonstrate fine detail of the mastoid air cells in contrast to the surrounding bone.

No evidence of patient movement.
No artefacts present on the image.

INTERNAL AUDITORY MEATI

Examination of this region is to assess the size of the meatus in order to demonstrate or exclude any erosion, usually caused by an acoustic neuroma. Plain radiography of the petrous portion of temporal bone is carried out less frequently than previously, since the introduction of MRI, which is preferred not only for radiation protection reasons but also for its capacity to demonstrate the neuroma at a much earlier stage than plain radiography or tomography, both of which will only confirm neuroma after expansion of the meatus has occurred. Unfortunately, although MRI is becoming more widely available, it is not yet available to all and plain radiography may still be the first, or only, option.

Tomographic examination of the area is sometimes used instead of plain radiography but it should be remembered that tomographic 'cuts' are required at 2 mm intervals through a depth of approximately 2 cm, making a total of 10–12 exposures. Immobilization of the patient is paramount if they are to remain perfectly still throughout the examination.

The OF projection demonstrates both meati, semicircular canals and vestibules within the petrous portion of the temporal bone and through the orbits, whereas the 'Towne's' projection shows a less defined image of both meati exiting the petrous portions of temporal bones halfway along their upper borders. The anterior oblique projections demonstrate each individual set of semicircular canal, vestibule and meatus within the petrous portion of temporal bone.

RADIOGRAPHIC TECHNIQUE

Occipitofrontal 5°

An 18×24 cm cassette is placed transversely in the erect bucky. The patient is seated facing the bucky with their forehead in contact with it. The OMBL and MSP are perpendicular to the cassette. The centre of the cassette is coincident with the nasion.

> CENTRING: A horizontal central ray is directed 5° caudally to the midline of the occiput to emerge through the nasion.

Collimate to include superior, inferior and lateral borders of orbits. Apply a PA anatomical marker within the primary beam.

Previously, this projection was commonly undertaken as a fronto-occipital. The increased distance of the orbits from the film results in their magnification on the image, theoretically allowing clearer visualization of the IAMs within them. However, owing to the significant increase in radiation dose to the eyes, this method is no longer acceptable in practice.

Fronto-occipital 30°/'Towne's'/half-axial

An 18×24 cm cassette is placed transversely in the erect bucky. The patient is seated facing the X-ray tube with the back of the head in contact with the bucky. The chin is lowered until the OMBL is perpendicular to the cassette, MSP coincident with and perpendicular to its central short axis. The upper border of the cassette is level with the EOP.

> CENTRING: A horizontal central ray, parallel to the OMBL, is directed 30° caudally to a point above the glabella to pass through the level of the EAMs.

Collimate to include the temporal bones. Apply an AP anatomical marker within the primary beam.

The 'Towne's' projection can be carried out as an OF with 30° cranial angulation, centring below the EOP with the X-ray beam passing through the level of the EAMs.

Anterior oblique (Fig. 6.12)

An 18×24 cm cassette is placed longitudinally in the erect bucky. The patient is seated facing the bucky with their forehead in contact with it and the MSP and OMBL perpendicular to it. The centre of the cassette is coincident with the middle of the inferior orbital margin on the side under examination. The head is rotated through 45°, away from the side under examination, and rested against the bucky.

> CENTRING: A horizontal central ray is directed 12° cranially to a point midway between the EOP and EAM nearest the tube, to emerge midway along the OMBL of the side nearest the bucky.

Collimate to include the temporal bone of the side under examination. Apply a PA anatomical marker within the primary beam. Both sides are examined for comparison.

This is essentially an OF position, with the head subsequently rotated through 45° to bring the petrous portion of the temporal bone of the side under examination parallel to the cassette. The angle the petrous portion of the temporal bone makes with the MSP can vary between 40° and 54° (Ballinger and Merrill, 1991; Lewis, 1984), depending on the individual. Lewis' research suggests that 56% of subjects will still require positioning with 45° rotation, whereas those with more elongated heads (in the AP direction) require a 50° turn and those with circular or foreshortened heads (AP direction) require a turn of 40°.

IMAGE EVALUATION

Correct patient identification and anatomical marker included on the radiograph.

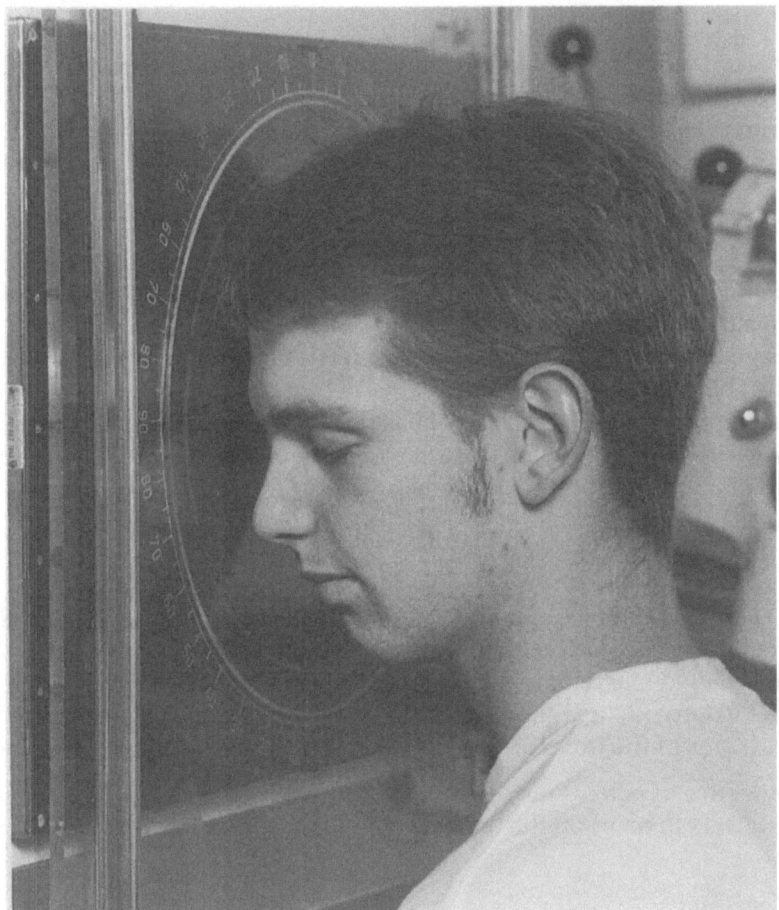

Figure 6.12   Anterior oblique to show right internal auditory meatus.

Area of interest

Petrous portions of temporal bones.

Projection

Occipitofrontal 5°

- Superior border of petrous ridge projected one-quarter of the way down orbits.
- Vestibules of IAMs equidistant from lateral margins of orbits.

Fronto-occipital 30°

- Dorsum sellae and posterior clinoid processes of sella turcica projected through centre of foramen magnum.
- Structures of inner and middle ears demonstrated below arcuate eminence.

Anterior oblique

- Mastoid air cells of side under examination projected lateral to semicircular canals.
- Image of occiput of opposite side (seen with internal occipital protuberance) bisects mastoid air cells.
- Images of right and left sides of base of skull are aligned horizontally.
- Structures of inner and middle ears demonstrated below arcuate eminence, superior to head of mandible.

Exposure factors

- kVp sufficient to demonstrate the structures of the inner and middle ears within the petrous temporal bone, maintaining contrast between the air-filled mastoids and the dense petrous bone.
- mAs to provide adequate image density to demonstrate detail of the structures of the inner and middle ears in contrast to the dense bone.

No evidence of patient movement.
No artefacts present on the image.

Positional faults

Incorrect rotation of the head will result in a foreshortened meatus; if the internal occipital crest crosses the meatus or semicircular canals, rotation has not been sufficient.

OPTIC FORAMINA

RADIOGRAPHIC TECHNIQUE

Anterior oblique (Fig. 6.13)

This is basically an OM projection with obliquity to bring the foramen perpendicular to the cassette.

An 18×24 cm cassette is placed longitudinally in the erect bucky. The patient is seated facing the bucky. The chin is raised until the OMBL is at 30° to the cassette, and placed in contact with the bucky. The MSP is

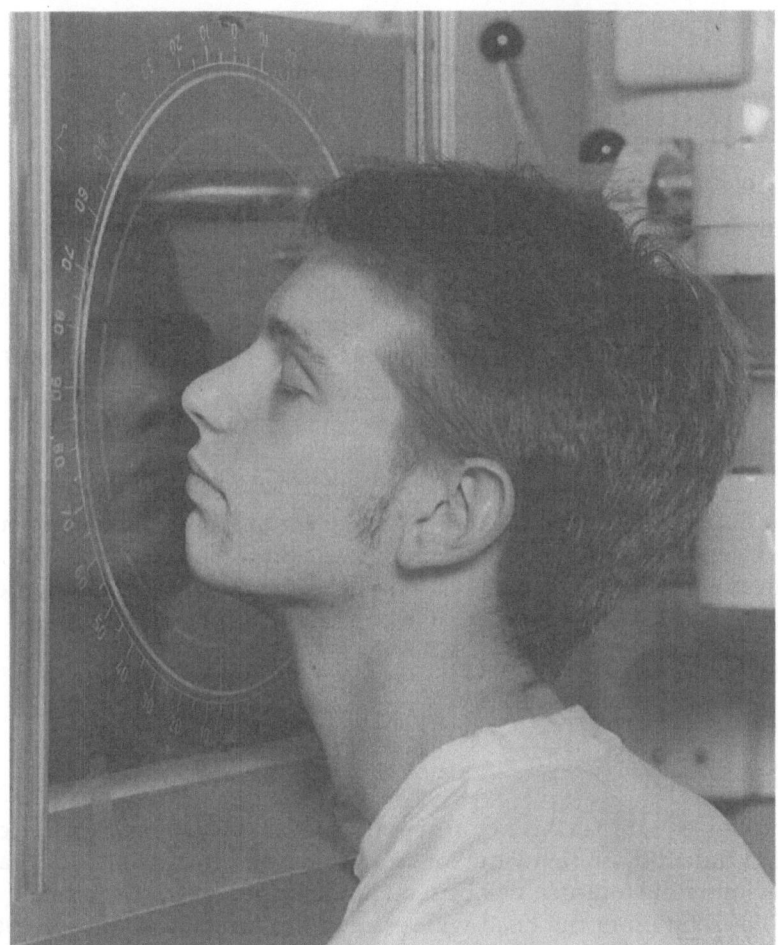

Figure 6.13 Anterior oblique to show right optic foramen.

perpendicular to the cassette, the centre of the cassette coincident with the midpoint between the orbits. The head is rotated through 30°, away from the side under examination.

CENTRING: A horizontal central ray, at 90° to the cassette, is directed over a point 7.5 cm above and 7.5 cm behind the EAM on the side nearest the X-ray tube, to emerge through the lower outer quadrant of the orbit nearest the bucky.

Collimate to include bony outline of orbit under examination. Apply a PA anatomical marker within the primary beam. Both sides are examined for comparison.

IMAGE EVALUATION

Correct patient identification and anatomical marker included on the radiograph.

Area of interest

Complete bony outline of orbit.

Projection

• Optic foramen is demonstrated as a circle, medial to lateral border of orbit and approximately halfway down orbit.

Exposure factors

• kVp sufficient to demonstrate the optic foramen, maintaining contrast between the foramen, bony orbit and air-filled sinuses.
• mAs to provide adequate image density to demonstrate the optic foramen within the bony orbit in contrast to the air-filled sinuses.

No evidence of patient movement.
No artefacts present on the image.

Positional faults

If the chin (OMBL) is raised too high the foramen will be seen in the lower half of the orbit, or below the inferior orbital rim. If the chin is not raised sufficiently the foramen will be seen in the upper half of the orbit.

Over-rotation of the head will result in the foramen being seen at the outer rim, or outside the lateral orbital margin. Under-rotation of the head will result in the foramen being seen in the medial half of the orbit.

Incorrect positioning will result in inadequate demonstration of the foramen, which will be seen as an ellipse rather than the required circle.

JUGULAR FORAMINA

RADIOGRAPHIC TECHNIQUE

Submentovertical

An 18×24 cm cassette is placed transversely in the erect bucky. The patient is seated facing the X-ray tube on a stool which is placed midway between the tube and the bucky. With support from the radiographer the patient leans back, raising the chin until the vertex of the skull can be placed in contact with the bucky. The upper border of the cassette is placed level with the outer canthus of the eye. The OMBL is parallel to the cassette, the MSP coincident with and perpendicular to its central short axis.

CENTRING: A horizontal central ray is directed 20° caudally to a point midway between the EAMs.

Collimate to include angles of mandible, symphysis menti and foramen magnum. Apply an AP anatomical marker within the primary beam.

IMAGE EVALUATION

Correct patient identification and anatomical marker included on the radiograph.

Area of interest

Lower border of symphysis menti, foramen magnum and angles of mandible.

Projection

- MSP coincident with midline of film.
- Odontoid process of C2 demonstrated through foramen magnum.
- Mandible projected clear of jugular foramina and superimposed on petrous temporal bone.
- Jugular foramina demonstrated symmetrically on either side of midline, midway between odontoid process and angles of mandible.

Exposure factors

- kVp sufficient to demonstrate the odontoid process through the overlying occiput, maintaining contrast between the jugular foramina and surrounding bone.
- mAs to provide adequate image density to demonstrate the jugular foramina within the base of the skull.

No evidence of patient movement.
No artefacts present on the image.

ISOCENTRIC TECHNIQUES

The versatility of isocentric units makes them an ideal addition to any accident and emergency department, enabling the production of accurate, reproducible occipitofrontal projections on the seriously injured patient. When an injured patient arrives in the X-ray department on a trolley, fronto-occipital projections are frequently carried out using a conventional overcouch X-ray tube. This results in a higher radiation dose to the radiosensitive lenses of the eyes for what are often substandard radiographs. This is particularly the case with the 'Towne's' projection, where excessive beam angulation, needed to compensate for patient position, leads to gross elongation of the image of the cranium. Image distortion in the 'Towne's' is not a problem on the isocentric unit, as the X-ray beam will always be perpendicular to the cassette, no matter what the degree of angulation applied. With an isocentric skull unit the patient remains supine on being transferred to the X-ray table and the skull unit C-arm moves around their head. With angulation possible about the horizontal and vertical axes, beam direction can be achieved to simulate movement or rotation of the patient's head, while the patient remains supine. The only consideration in using the isocentric unit is that the patient's condition allows them to be moved from the trolley on to the X-ray table, which is obviously not possible in the case of spinal injuries. Once on the X-ray table, a patient with serious multiple injuries can be examined speedily and accurately using the isocentric unit around the head and the general overcouch tube (and bucky) for AP and horizontal beam lateral projections of the trunk and limbs.

THE ISOCENTRIC UNIT

Figure 6.14 shows the 'Orbix' isocentric unit, manufactured by Siemens. Other manufacturers also supply isocentric units.

TERMINOLOGY

The following terms are used throughout the isocentric technique descriptions.

Tube position

Lateral – the support column is positioned at the side of the X-ray table, at 90° to its long axis.
Medial – the support column is positioned at the end of the X-ray table, in line with its central long axis.
AP – the C-arm is vertical (0°) with the X-ray tube above the table and the cassette holder below.
PA – the C-arm is vertical (0°) with the cassette holder above the table and the X-ray tube below.
Horizontal – the C-arm is horizontal (90°) with the X-ray tube at one side of the table and the cassette holder on the other.

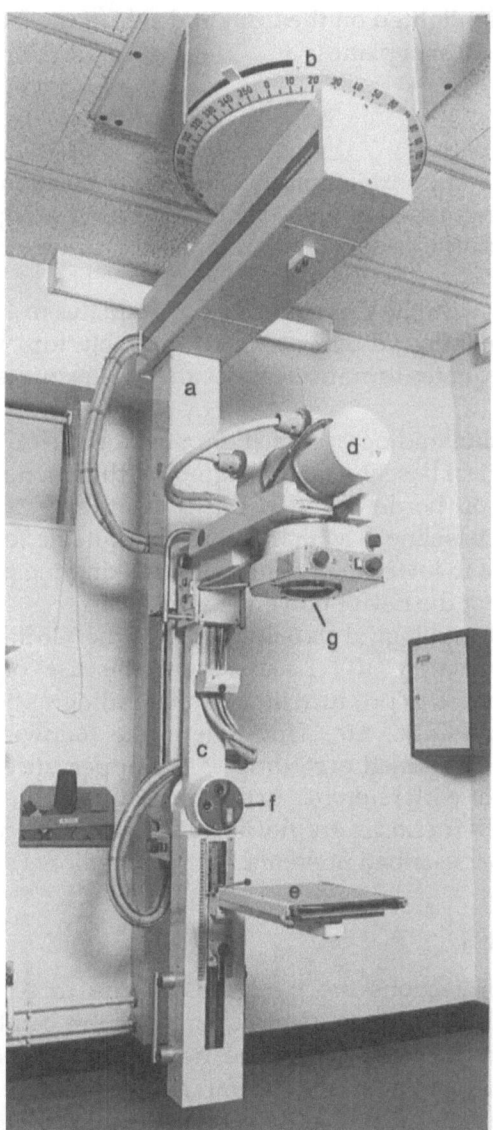

Figure 6.14   The 'Orbix' isocentric unit. a, support column; b, support column scale; c, C-arm; d, X-ray tube; e, cassette holder; f, horizontal and vertical positional lights; g, light beam diaphragm and central positional light.

Positional lights

Central – that highlighted on the patient's face in the sagittal plane.
Horizontal – that highlighted on the side of the face in the coronal plane.

Vertical – that highlighted on the front and side of the face, at 90° to both the sagittal and coronal planes.

Angulations

C-arm – with the support column in the lateral position this equates to cranial/caudal angulation of the X-ray beam. With the support column in the medial position this equates to the patient turning their head to the left or right.

Support column – with the C-arm vertical this equates to a lateral tilt of the head, MSP remaining vertical at 90° to the table top. With the C-arm horizontal this equates to cranial/caudal angulation of the X-ray beam.

In isocentric skull radiography patient position can be described using the anthropological baseline (a line adjoining the inferior orbital margin and the superior border of the EAM) or the OMBL. Use of the anthropological baseline is actually more comfortable for the patient, as they do not have to lower their chin so far, making the position easier to hold and reducing the risk of movement.

With the anthropological baseline vertical the OMBL will be raised through approximately 10°, necessitating the use of different tube angulations in order to produce images that radiographers recognize as OF 0°/10°/20° or FO 30° etc. Throughout the following descriptions, projections will be named according to the appearances of the images produced and not with reference to the angulation of the X-ray beam.

Image evaluation criteria are not included in this section as they are identical to those described previously for conventional skull techniques.

START POSITIONS

All isocentric projections are variations of the three basic positions described below. With the patient supine the unit can be angled in all directions around the head to produce the required projection.

With the X-ray tube in the lateral AP position, ensure that the angulation scales are set at 0° and the cassette holder is at the end of the C-arm. The cassette holder should always be moved to the end of the C-arm between projections to prevent damage to the equipment or patient while the tube position/angulation is being altered.

PATIENT POSITION

A sheet of lead–rubber is placed on the table top to correspond with the area that will be covered by the patient's shoulders and upper thorax. The patient lies supine on the X-ray table with the head resting in a

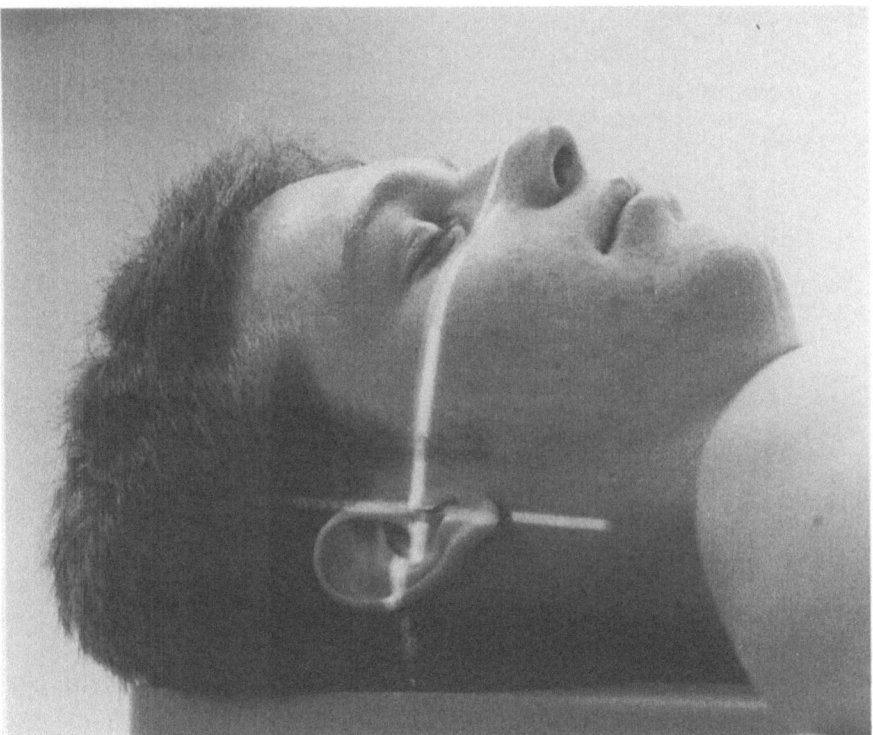

Figure 6.15   Skull start position.

radiolucent skull pad on the head extension board. The table is raised to the correct working height for the isocentric unit.

Skull (Fig. 6.15)

The MSP of the head and body is perpendicular to the midline of the table, coincident with the central positional light. The chin is positioned to bring the anthropological baseline vertical, coincident with the vertical positional light. The height of the isocentric unit is altered to bring the horizontal positional light through the centre of the EAM.

Facial (Fig. 6.16)

The skull pad is removed and the head rested on the extension board. The MSP of the head and body is perpendicular to the midline of the table, coincident with the central positional light. The chin is raised to bring the OMBL to an angle of 45° to the horizontal. (This can be measured by bringing the horizontal positional light to pass directly through the EAM,

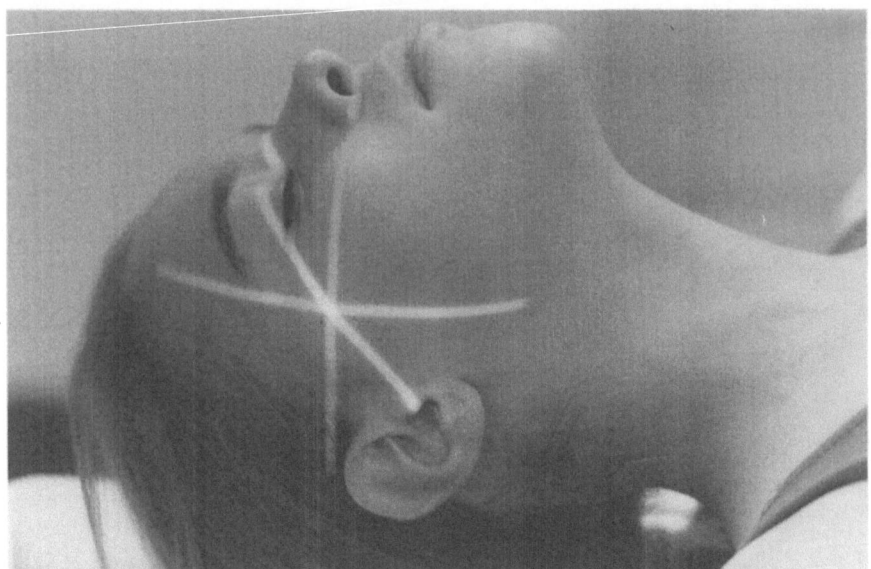

Figure 6.16 Facial start position.

directing the X-ray beam 45° caudally and then raising the chin until the OMBL coincides with the light beam on the side of the face. The X-ray tube is then taken back to the vertical AP position.) The height of the isocentric unit is altered so that the horizontal positional light is level with the outer canthus of the eye.

Submentovertical (Fig. 6.17)

Use a 'stepped' headrest (if available) for easier positioning. The skull pad is removed and the head rested on the extension board. The MSP of the head and body is perpendicular to the midline of the table, coincident with the central positional light. The chin is raised and the neck flexed to bring the OMBL as close to the horizontal as possible. The table is moved to bring the vertical positional light through the EAM. The height of the isocentric unit is altered to bring the horizontal positional light through the centre of the EAM.

CRANIUM

START POSITION – SKULL

The table is moved caudally to bring the vertical central ray over the glabella. Using the iris diaphragm, collimate to include vertex of skull, maxillae and parietal bones.

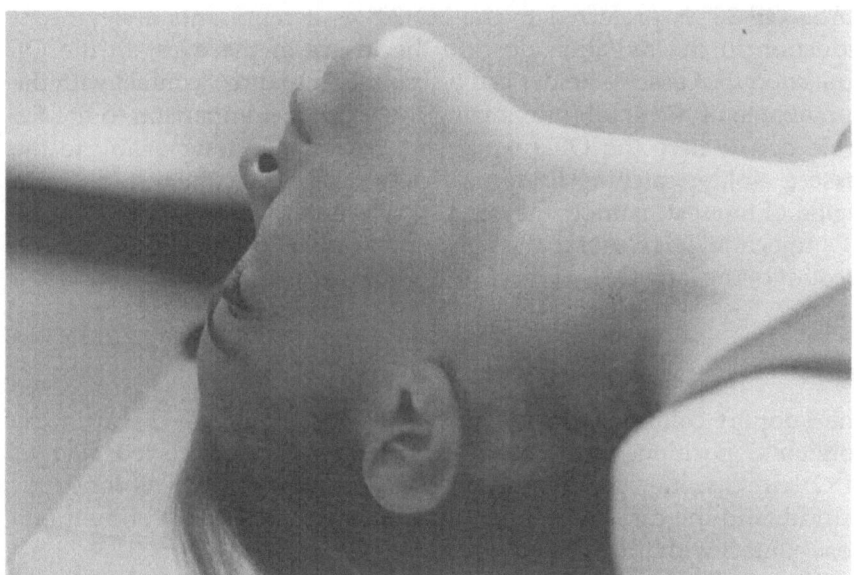

Figure 6.17 Submentovertical start position.

Occipitofrontal

The support column is in the lateral position and the C-arm in the PA position. A 24×30 cm cassette is placed in the cassette holder with its long axis parallel to the MSP. Affix a PA anatomical marker within the primary beam.

BEAM ANGULATION: C-arm –
Equivalent of OF 0° – the X-ray beam is directed 10° cranially.
Equivalent of OF 10° – the X-ray beam remains vertical (0°).
Equivalent of OF 20° – the X-ray beam is directed 10° caudally.

The cassette is brought into close contact with the frontal region of the skull.

Occipitofrontal 30°/'Towne's'/half-axial

The support column is in the lateral position and the C-arm in the PA position. A 24×30 cm cassette is placed in the cassette holder with its long axis parallel to the MSP. Affix a PA anatomical marker within the primary beam.

BEAM ANGULATION: C-arm – the X-ray beam is directed 40° cranially.

The cassette is brought into close contact with the frontal region of the skull.

The OF 30° is preferred to the FO 30° as it represents a significant reduction in the radiation dose to the lenses of the eyes. In the OF projection the cassette holder can be brought into direct contact with the frontal area of the skull, minimizing the OFD, in comparison to the FO projection, where the OFD would be unavoidably long owing to the cassette holder catching underneath the table. Even though the main region of interest, namely the occiput, is remote from the film in the OF 30° projection, it is closer to the film than it would be in the FO 30°, taking account of the long OFD.

Lateral

The support column is in the medial position and the C-arm in the horizontal position, with the cassette holder at the affected side. A 24×30 cm cassette is placed in the cassette holder with its long axis vertical, and the cassette holder moved along the C-arm to bring it into close contact with the affected side of the head.

Affix an AP anatomical marker within the primary beam. Using the iris diaphragm, collimate to include vertex of skull, base of occiput, glabella and EOP.

Submentovertical

Start position

The support column is in the lateral position and the C-arm in the AP position. A 24×30 cm cassette is placed in the cassette holder with its long axis parallel to the MSP. Affix an AP anatomical marker within the primary beam.

BEAM ANGULATION: C-arm – The X-ray beam is directed at 90° to the OMBL and then a further 5° cranially.

The cassette is brought into close contact with the underside of the head support. Using the iris diaphragm, collimate to include outline of entire skull.

FACIAL BONES

START POSITION

The table is moved to bring the vertical central ray over the midline at the level of the alae of the nose.

Using the iris diaphragm, collimate to include superior orbital margins, mandible, zygomas and lateral soft tissue outlines.

Occipitomental

The support column is in the lateral position and the C-arm in the PA position. A 24×30 cm cassette is placed in the cassette holder with its short axis parallel to the MSP. Affix a PA anatomical marker within the primary beam.

> BEAM ANGULATION: C-arm – OM – the X-ray beam remains vertical (0°).
> OM 30° – the X-ray beam is directed 30° caudally.

The cassette holder is moved along the C-arm to bring the film into close contact with the face. (Orienting the cassette with its short axis parallel to the MSP minimizes the unavoidable OFD in the OM 30° projection.)

Lateral

The support column is in the medial position and the C-arm in the horizontal position, with the cassette holder at the affected side. A 24×30 cm cassette is placed in the cassette holder with its long axis vertical. The cassette holder is moved along the C-arm to bring it into close contact with the affected side of the face.

Affix an AP anatomical marker within the primary beam. Using the iris diaphragm, collimate to include superior orbital margins, mandible, nose and soft tissue outlines.

ZYGOMATIC ARCHES

Submentovertical

Start position

The support column is in the lateral position and the C-arm in the PA position. An 18×24 cm cassette is placed in the cassette holder with its short axis parallel to the MSP. Affix a PA anatomical marker within the primary beam.

> BEAM ANGULATION: C-arm – The X-ray beam is directed at 90° to the OMBL.

The height of the isocentric unit is altered so that the central X-ray beam passes midway along the zygomatic arches. The cassette is brought into close contact with the chin. Using the rectangular diaphragm, collimate to include zygomatic arches.

Occipitofrontal 30°/'Towne's'/half-axial

Start position – skull

The support column is in the lateral position and the C-arm in the PA position. An 18×24 cm cassette is placed in the cassette holder with its short axis parallel to the MSP. Affix a PA anatomical marker within the primary beam.

BEAM ANGULATION: C-arm – The X-ray beam is directed 40° cranially.

The height of the isocentric unit is altered so that the central X-ray beam passes midway along the zygomatic arches. The cassette is brought into close contact with the frontal region of the skull. Using the rectangular diaphragm, collimate to include zygomatic arches.

PARANASAL SINUSES

With the C-arm in the horizontal position, the patient is examined erect, sitting facing the 18×24 cm cassette holder. The OM, lateral and lateral postnasal space projections are produced in exactly the same way as the conventional sinus techniques described earlier. For the OF projections, in order to demonstrate any fluid levels within the sinuses the isocentric unit must remain horizontal and the patient's chin be raised or lowered in order to produce the correct relationship between the OMBL and the X-ray beam. The patient is immobilized in the required position by placing a radiolucent sponge pad between the cassette holder and the forehead/chin.

MANDIBLE

START POSITION – SKULL

The table is moved to bring the vertical central ray over the midline at the level of the angles of the mandible. The height of the isocentric unit is altered to bring the horizontal positional light through the angle of the mandible. Using the iris diaphragm, collimate to include symphysis menti and temporomandibular joints.

Posteroanterior

The support column is in the lateral position and the C-arm in the PA position. An 18×24 cm cassette is placed in the cassette holder with its long axis parallel to the MSP. Affix a PA anatomical marker within the primary beam.

BEAM ANGULATION: C-arm – The X-ray beam is directed 10° cranially.

The cassette is brought into close contact with the face.

Lateral

The support column is in the medial position and the C-arm in the horizontal position, with the cassette holder at the affected side. An 18×24 cm cassette is placed in the cassette holder with its long axis vertical. Affix an AP anatomical marker within the primary beam. The cassette is brought into close contact with the side of the face.

Lateral oblique

With the support column in the medial position and the C-arm in the AP position, the patient is displaced *to each side of the midline in turn*, so that the central positional light passes through the angle of the mandible of the side under examination. The C-arm is turned to the horizontal position with the cassette holder at the side under examination. An 18×24 cm cassette is placed in the cassette holder with its long axis vertical. Affix an AP anatomical marker within the primary beam.

BEAM ANGULATION: C-arm – the X-ray beam is directed 10° upwards. (This prevents the X-ray tube head hitting the table top when the second angle is applied.)
Support column – rotated to direct the X-ray beam 25° cranially.

The cassette is brought into close contact with the side of the face.

PITUITARY FOSSA

START POSITION – SKULL

The table is moved to bring the vertical central ray over the midline 2.5 cm superior to the level of the EAMs. The height of the isocentric unit is altered to bring the horizontal positional light 2.5 cm anterior to the EAM.

Using the iris diaphragm, collimate to a diameter of approximately 10 cm to include the sella turcica.

Lateral

The support column is in the medial position and the C-arm in the horizontal position. An 18×24 cm cassette is placed in the cassette holder with its long axis vertical. Affix an AP anatomical marker within the primary beam. The cassette is brought into close contact with the side of the head.

Occipitofrontal 30°/'Towne's'/half-axial

The support column is in the lateral position and the C-arm in the PA position. An 18×24 cm cassette is placed in the cassette holder with its long axis parallel to the MSP. Affix a PA anatomical marker within the primary beam.

BEAM ANGULATION: C-arm – The X-ray beam is directed 40° cranially.

The cassette is brought into close contact with the frontal region of the skull.

Occipitofrontal 20°

The support column is in the lateral position and the C-arm in the PA position. An 18×24 cm cassette is placed in the cassette holder with its long axis parallel to the MSP. Affix a PA anatomical marker within the primary beam.

BEAM ANGULATION: C-arm – The X-ray beam is directed 10°caudally.

The cassette is brought into close contact with the face.

TEMPOROMANDIBULAR JOINTS

These projections are usually undertaken with the mouth both wide open and closed, and may also be repeated with the teeth clenched.

START POSITION – SKULL

The table is moved to bring the vertical central ray over the midline at the level of the temporomandibular joints. The height of the isocentric unit is altered to bring the horizontal positional light through the joints.

Occipitofrontal 30°/'Towne's'/half-axial

Using the rectangular diaphragm, collimate to include the lateral margins of skull and the proximal halves of the mandibular rami.

The support column is in the lateral position and the C-arm in the PA position. An 18×24 cm cassette is placed in the cassette holder with its short axis parallel to the MSP. Affix a PA anatomical marker within the primary beam.

BEAM ANGULATION: C-arm – The X-ray beam is directed 40° cranially.

The cassette is brought into close contact with the frontal region of the skull.

Lateral oblique

With the support column in the medial position and the C-arm in the AP position the patient is displaced *to each side of the midline in turn*, so that the central positional light passes through the temporomandibular joint of the side under examination. The C-arm is turned to the horizontal position, with the cassette holder at the side under examination. An 18×24 cm cassette is placed in the holder with its long axis vertical. Affix an AP anatomical marker within the primary beam.

BEAM ANGULATION: Support column – rotated to direct the X-ray beam 25° caudally.

Using the iris diaphragm, collimate to a diameter of approximately 10 cm to include the joint under examination. The cassette is brought into close contact with the side of the face.

MASTOID AIR CELLS

START POSITION – SKULL

The table is moved to bring the vertical central ray over the midline at the level of the EAMs. The height of the isocentric unit is altered to bring the horizontal positional light through the EAMs.

Occipitofrontal 30°/'Towne's'/half-axial

Using the rectangular diaphragm, collimate to include lateral margins of skull and proximal halves of mandibular rami.

The support column is in the lateral position and the C-arm in the PA position. An 18×24 cm cassette is placed in the cassette holder with its short axis parallel to the MSP. Affix a PA anatomical marker within the primary beam.

BEAM ANGULATION: C-arm – The X-ray beam is directed 40° cranially.

The cassette holder is brought into close contact with the frontal region of the skull.

Lateral oblique

With the support column in the medial position and the C-arm in the AP position the patient is displaced *to each side of the midline in turn*, so that the central positional light passes through the mastoid air cells of the side under examination. The C-arm is turned to the horizontal position, with the cassette holder at the side under examination. An 18×24 cm cassette is placed in the cassette holder with its long axis vertical. Affix an AP anatomical marker within the primary beam.

BEAM ANGULATION: Support column – The X-ray beam is directed 25° caudally.

The cassette holder is brought into close contact with the side of the face. Using the iris diaphragm, collimate to a diameter of approximately 15 cm to include the mastoid air cells under examination.

INTERNAL AUDITORY MEATI

START POSITION – SKULL

The table is moved to bring the vertical central ray over the midline at the level of the EAMs. Using the rectangular diaphragm, collimate to include bony outlines of orbits.

Occipitofrontal 5°

The support column is in the lateral position and the C-arm in the PA position. An 18×24 cm cassette is placed in the cassette holder with its short axis parallel to the MSP. Affix a PA anatomical marker within the primary beam.

BEAM ANGULATION: C-arm – The X-ray beam is directed 5° cranially.

The cassette is brought into close contact with the face.

Occipitofrontal 30°/'Towne's'/half-axial

The support column is in the lateral position and the C-arm in the PA position. An 18×24 cm cassette is placed in the cassette holder with its short axis parallel to the MSP. Affix a PA anatomical marker within the primary beam.

> BEAM ANGULATION: C-arm – The X-ray beam is directed 40° cranially.

The cassette is brought into close contact with the frontal region of the skull.

Anterior oblique

With the support column in the medial position and the C-arm in the AP position the patient is displaced *to either side of the midline in turn*, to bring the central positional light over the centre of the orbit of the side under examination. An 18×24 cm cassette is placed in the holder with its long axis parallel to the MSP.

Using the iris diaphragm, collimate to a diameter of approximately 10 cm to include the petrous ridge of the side under examination.

The C-arm is moved into the PA position.

> BEAM ANGULATION: C-arm – the X-ray beam is directed 45° towards the side under examination.
> Support column – rotated to direct the X-ray beam 25° cranially.

The cassette is brought into close contact with the orbit on the side under examination. Affix a PA anatomical marker within the primary beam.

OPTIC FORAMINA

START POSITION – SKULL

The table is moved to bring the vertical central ray over the midline and half-way down the orbits. The height of the isocentric unit is altered to bring the horizontal positional light to the level of the outer canthus of the eye.

With the support column in the medial position and the C-arm in the AP position, the patient is displaced *to each side of the midline in turn*, to bring the central positional light through the centre of the orbit under examination.

Using the iris diaphragm, collimate to include the outline of the bony orbit. The C-arm is turned into the PA position.

An 18×24 cm cassette is placed in the cassette holder with its long axis parallel to the MSP. Affix a PA anatomical marker within the primary beam.

BEAM ANGULATION: C-arm – the X-ray beam is directed 40° towards the side under examination.
Support column – rotated to direct the X-ray beam 25° caudally.

The cassette is brought into close contact with the orbit under examination. (The film should approach the three-point landing position, with the chin, nose and cheek of the side under examination in close proximity to the cassette.)

JUGULAR FORAMINA

START POSITION – SMV

The support column is in the lateral position and the C-arm in the AP position. An 18×24 cm cassette is placed in the cassette holder with its short axis parallel to the MSP. Affix an AP anatomical marker within the primary beam.

BEAM ANGULATION: C-arm – The X-ray beam is directed at 90° to the OMBL and then 20° caudally to pass in the midline through the level of the EAMs.

Using the rectangular diaphragm, collimate to angles of mandible and symphysis menti.

The cassette is brought into close contact with the underside of the head support.

Bony thorax

7

RIBS

RADIOGRAPHIC TECHNIQUE

The main reason for radiographic examination of the ribs is to exclude the presence of a pneumothorax caused by a fractured rib penetrating the underlying lung. The fact that the ribs are fractured is of secondary importance. For this reason a chest X-ray must always be carried out and in many departmental protocols this is the only projection required following injury to the ribs.

The first to sixth ribs are demonstrated in their entirety on the routine PA chest projection, but the lateral aspect of the bony thorax and ribs 7–12 are inadequately demonstrated. Oblique projections will demonstrate all ribs, although some magnification and distortion will occur.

Posterior oblique (Fig. 7.1)

A 30×40 cm cassette is placed longitudinally in the table bucky. The patient is supine, the MSP perpendicular to the table top. The midclavicular line of the affected side is coincident with the midline of the table. The patient is rotated 45° towards the affected side and supported with radiolucent pads. The arm of the affected side is raised, resting on the pillow, and the knee of the unaffected side flexed to aid stability. A lead–rubber apron is applied to the patient's lower abdomen as radiation protection.

Upper ribs

The upper edge of the cassette is positioned level with C7.

> CENTRING: A vertical central ray is directed over the sternal notch and then angled caudally until it is coincident with the centre of the cassette.

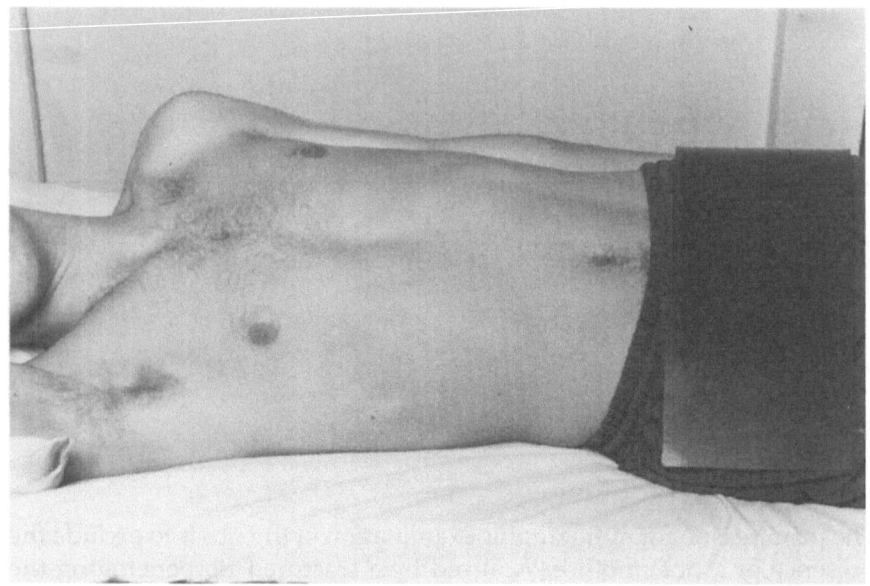

Figure 7.1   45° posterior oblique ribs (right).

Collimate to include ribs 1–7. Apply an AP anatomical marker within the primary beam. Exposure is made on arrested inspiration. This action, in conjunction with the caudal angulation, will demonstrate the maximum number of ribs above the level of the diaphragm.

Lower ribs

The lower border of the cassette is placed level with the lower costal margin.

> CENTRING: A vertical central ray is directed over the midline of the patient, at the level of the lower costal margin, and then angled cranially until it is coincident with the centre of the cassette.

Collimate to include ribs 7–12. Apply an AP anatomical marker within the primary beam. Exposure is made on arrested expiration. This action, in conjunction with the cranial angulation, will demonstrate the maximum number of ribs below the level of the diaphragm.

When examining upper or lower ribs, the kVp selected should be sufficient to reduce the subject contrast between the radiodense heart or upper abdomen and radiolucent lung fields. A relatively high kVp – at least 70 – will reduce image contrast, demonstrating the full length of the ribs through both areas on a single image.

IMAGE EVALUATION

Correct patient identification and anatomical marker included on the radiograph.

Area of interest

Upper ribs

Full length of ribs 1–7 demonstrated above diaphragm.

Lower ribs

Full length of ribs 7–12 demonstrated below diaphragm.

Projection

- Ribs are 'flattened out', showing full length of each individual rib.
- Oblique appearance of vertebral column.
- Arms abducted clear of rib cage.
- Heart projected over lung field.

Upper ribs

- Adequate inspiration to demonstrate eighth rib above level of diaphragm.

Lower ribs

- Adequate expiration to demonstrate eighth rib below level of diaphragm.

Exposure factors

Upper ribs

kVp selected to reduce the difference in subject contrast between the heart and lung fields, so allowing visualization of the ribs in both of these areas.

Lower ribs

kVp selected to maintain optimum contrast in order to visualize the ribs superimposed on the upper abdominal viscera.

Upper and lower ribs

- kVp sufficient to demonstrate bony trabeculae within the ribs through the overlying shadows of the heart, mediastinum, diaphragm and upper abdominal organs, maintaining contrast between the bony thorax, air-filled lungs, mediastinum and surrounding soft tissues.
- mAs to provide adequate image density to demonstrate bony detail in contrast to the lungs and mediastinum.

No evidence of patient movement or breathing during the exposure.
No artefacts present on the image.

STERNUM

RADIOGRAPHIC TECHNIQUE

Lateral

A 24×30 cm cassette is placed longitudinally in the erect bucky (a gridded cassette may be used in a vertical stand). A lead–rubber apron is applied to the patient's lower abdomen as radiation protection. The patient is erect with their shoulder against the bucky, MSP parallel to it. If standing, the feet are separated for stability. The centre of the cassette is coincident with a point midway between the sternal notch and xiphisternum. The hands are clasped behind the back and the shoulders drawn back.

CENTRING: A horizontal central ray, at 90° to the cassette, is directed midway between the sternal notch and the xiphisternum.

Collimate to include entire sternum, allowing for the forward movement of the ribcage during inspiration. Apply an AP anatomical marker within the primary beam. Exposure is made on arrested inspiration.

Left anterior oblique (Fig. 7.2)

A 24×30 cm cassette is placed lengthwise in the table bucky. The patient lies prone, MSP perpendicular to and coincident with the midline of the table. The middle of the long axis of the cassette is at the level of T6. The right arm is raised on to the pillow and the head turned to the right. The right side is raised through 30° and supported with radiolucent pads. A lead–rubber sheet is applied to the patient's lower abdomen as radiation protection.

CENTRING: A vertical central ray, at 90° to the cassette, is directed to a point 7.5 cm lateral to the spinous process of T6, on the raised side.

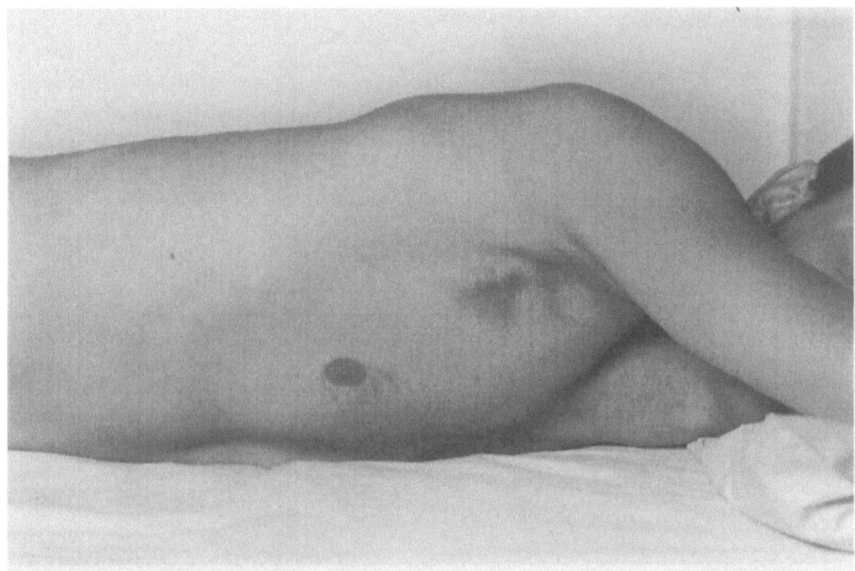

Figure 7.2 Left anterior oblique: sternum.

Collimate to include sternum and sternoclavicular joints. Apply a right PA anatomical marker within the primary beam to correspond with the right-hand side of the patient. Exposure is made during gentle respiration, using a low mA and long time selection, to blur out the images of overlying lung markings and ribs.

Anterior oblique – alternative method (Fig. 7.3)

This technique is very easy to carry out, but only on mobile patients whose hip joints are approximately level with the table top.

A 24×30 cm cassette is placed transversely in the table bucky with a right PA anatomical marker applied to the right side of the short axis of the cassette. The vertical X-ray beam is angled 30° along the table towards its left-hand end and the FFD set at 100 cm. Centre to the middle of the cassette and collimate to within its borders. The patient stands facing the table and bends forward to place the anterior aspect of the chest in contact with the table top. A lead–rubber apron is applied to the patient's lower abdomen as radiation protection. The patient is positioned with the MSP perpendicular to the table top and coincident with the central long axis of the cassette. A point midway between the sternal notch and xiphisternum, at the level of T6, is coincident with the midpoint of the cassette.

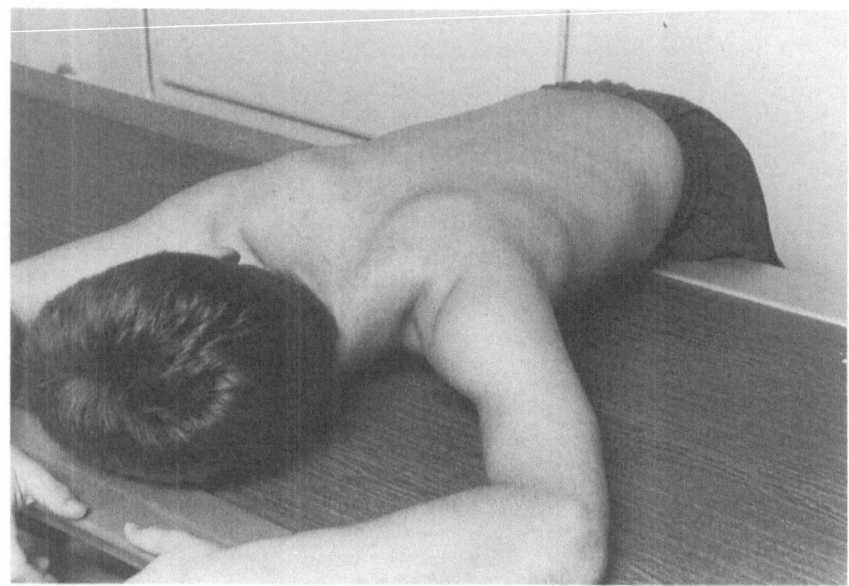

Figure 7.3 Sternum – patient prone.

CENTRING: When the patient is in the correct position the central X-ray beam will be directed to a point 7.5 cm to the right of the spinous process of T6.

Collimate to include sternum and sternoclavicular joints. Exposure is made on gentle respiration, with exposure conditions as described above.

This alternative projection may be carried out with the patient erect facing a gridded cassette in a vertical holder. The grid lines **must** run horizontally in order to avoid grid cut-off, and therefore it may be necessary to use a 30×40 cm cassette.

IMAGE EVALUATION

Correct patient identification and anatomical marker included on the radiograph.

Area of interest

Manubrium sterni, body of sternum and xiphisternum.

Projection

Lateral

• Superimposition of right and left borders of sternum.

- Superimposition of medial ends of clavicles.
- Demonstration of joint spaces between manubrium, body and xiphisternum.

Anterior oblique

- Sternum projected over lung field, to the right of vertebral column.
- Joint spaces visible between manubrium, body and xiphisternum.
- Oblique appearance of vertebral column.
- Blurring of ribs and lung markings owing to exposure being made during gentle respiration.

Exposure factors

Lateral

kVp selected to demonstrate detail of the sternum over the density range from manubrium to xiphisternum.

- kVp sufficient to demonstrate bony trabeculae within the sternum, maintaining contrast between the sternum and the air-filled lungs.
- mAs to provide adequate image density to demonstrate bony detail of the sternum in contrast to the air-filled lungs.

Anterior oblique

- kVp sufficient to demonstrate bony trabeculae within the sternum through the overlying image of the heart, maintaining contrast between the bony thorax and air-filled lungs.
- mAs to provide adequate image density to demonstrate bony detail of the sternum in contrast to the lungs and mediastinum.

No evidence of patient movement. Breathing movement may be seen on anterior oblique.
No artefacts present on the image.

STERNOCLAVICULAR JOINTS

RADIOGRAPHIC TECHNIQUE

Anterior oblique (Fig. 7.4)

An 18×24 cm cassette is placed in the erect cassette holder. A lead–rubber apron is applied to the patient's lower abdomen as radiation protection. The patient is erect facing the cassette, with the sternal notch coincident with the middle of the cassette and the MSP perpendicular to it. The

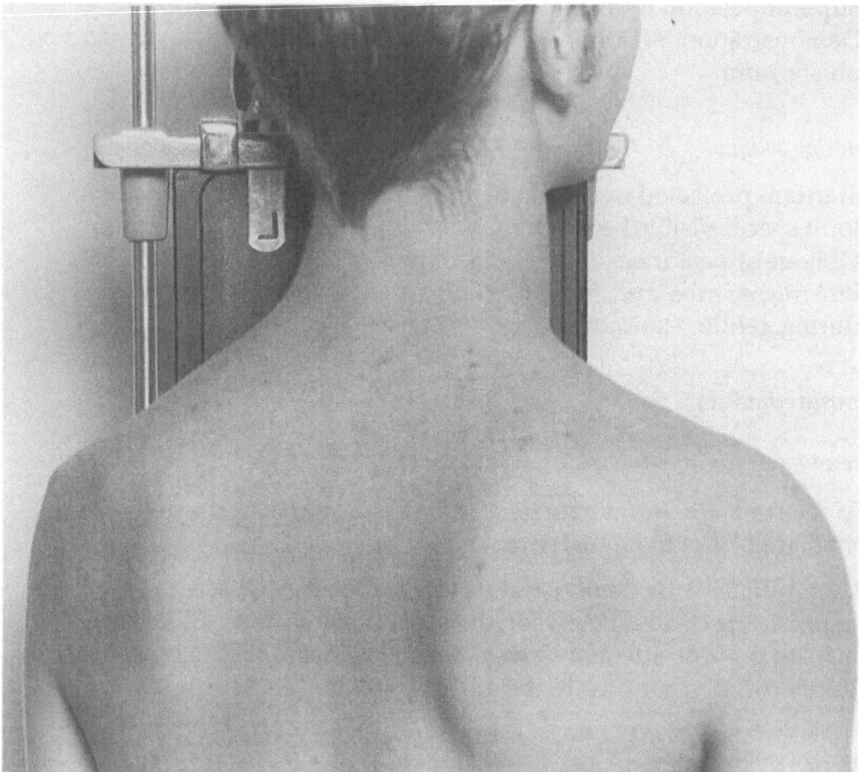

Figure 7.4 Anterior oblique: left sternoclavicular joint.

patient is turned away from the side under examination until the MSP is 45° to the cassette.

> CENTRING: A horizontal central ray, at 90° to the cassette, is directed over a point 10 cm lateral to the spinous process of T4, on the side furthest from the cassette.

Collimate to include manubrium sterni and both sternoclavicular joints. Apply a PA anatomical marker, appropriate to the side in contact with the cassette, within the primary beam. Both sides are examined for comparison.

This projection can alternatively be carried out in the prone position.

Lateral

An 18×24 cm cassette is placed in the erect cassette holder. A lead–rubber apron is applied to the patient's lower abdomen as radiation protection. The patient is erect, with the MSP parallel to the cassette. The middle of the cassette is coincident with the sternoclavicular joints. The hands are clasped behind the back and the shoulders drawn back in order to bring the sternoclavicular joints into profile.

  CENTRING: A horizontal central ray, at 90° to the cassette, is directed
      over the medial ends of the clavicles.

Collimate to include the medial ends of clavicles, sternoclavicular joints and manubrium sterni. Apply an AP anatomical marker within the primary beam.

IMAGE EVALUATION

Correct patient identification and anatomical marker included on the radiograph.

Area of interest

Manubrium sterni and medial ends of clavicles.

Projection

Anterior oblique

- Clear visualization of joint under examination, i.e. closest to spine.
- Joint further away from spine obscured by superimposition of medial end of clavicle on manubrium sterni.

Lateral

- Superimposition of sternoclavicular joints.
- Superimposition of medial ends of clavicles.
- Shoulders pulled back so as not to obscure sternoclavicular joints.

Exposure factors

- kVp sufficient to demonstrate the medial ends of clavicles, sternum and intervening joint spaces, maintaining contrast between the bony structures, air-filled lungs and mediastinum.
- mAs to provide adequate image density to demonstrate soft tissue information of the sternoclavicular joints in contrast to the clavicles, sternum, lungs and mediastinum.

No evidence of patient movement.
No artefacts present on the image.

Respiratory system 8

CHEST

When examining the chest, the PA projection is preferable to the AP for a number of reasons.

1. As the heart is closer to the film magnification is reduced, enabling a more accurate assessment of the heart size. Magnification of the image of the heart is further reduced by using an FFD of 180 cm.
2. The images of the scapulae are more effectively cleared from the lung fields on the resultant image.
3. The PA projection facilitates compression of the breast masses, particularly in female patients. This has a twofold effect on reducing radiation dose:
   - compression of the breasts against the cassette reduces the thickness of tissue to be irradiated, especially in the region of the lung bases/costophrenic angles, allowing a reduction in exposure factors for the production of a correctly exposed image;
   - as the exposure factors and volume of tissue are reduced less scattered radiation is produced, not only reducing patient dose, but also improving image quality.
4. Radiation dose to anterior radiosensitive structures, e.g. the thyroid gland, breasts and lenses of the eyes, is reduced as the lower energy radiation is absorbed by the posterior structures of the thorax.
5. The risk of producing a lordotic image is greatly reduced.

It is common practice to use a lead–rubber waist apron for radiation protection of the gonad region during radiography of the chest. Departmental protocols differ as to whether the apron should be applied to the anterior or posterior aspect of the patient's abdomen when undertaking a PA projection. Posterior application is probably the convention, but an increasing school of thought is that the greater risk is from secondary radiation being scattered back on to the patient from the walls and equipment behind the cassette. The same argument applies to application of the apron for the lateral projection, with the convention being to apply the apron to the side facing the X-ray tube.

RADIOGRAPHIC TECHNIQUE

Posteroanterior (Fig. 8.1)

A lead–rubber apron is applied to the patient's lower abdomen as radiation protection. A 35×35 cm or 35×43 cm cassette is placed in a vertical cassette holder, either longitudinally or transversely according to patient build. The patient stands facing the cassette with the anterior aspect of the chest in contact with it. The feet are separated slightly for stability. The MSP is coincident with and perpendicular to the central long axis of the cassette, the medial ends of the clavicles equidistant from it. The chin is raised and rested on the upper edge of the cassette, which is positioned above the lung apices to include the first ribs on the radiograph. The elbows are flexed and the backs of the hands rested on the sides of the pelvis. The elbows are carefully pressed forwards to assist in projecting the scapulae clear of the lung fields.

> CENTRING: 1. A horizontal central ray is directed 5° caudally to a point in the midline of the posterior aspect of the patient at the level of T6.
> 2. A horizontal central ray, at 90° to the cassette, is directed to a point in the midline of the posterior aspect of the patient at the level of T6.

Collimate to include C7, lung apices, diaphragms, costophrenic angles and lateral rib margins. Apply a PA anatomical marker within the primary beam. Expose on arrested full inspiration.

The practice of centring a horizontal central beam at the level of T4, still routine to some radiographers, should be discontinued (Day, 1994) and has therefore not been described in this text. Of the two centring points described above, (1) should be routinely employed, with (2) being used in cases of suspected or follow-up pleural effusion. The slight caudal angle employed in (1) allows for the demonstration of the maximum volume of lung tissue above the diaphragm without elongation of the lung fields, and also enables the radiographer to collimate accurately to the lung apices and bases (i.e. the limits of the cassette), including the costophrenic angles, without irradiating the patient's head. This leads to a reduction in primary and secondary radiation dose and an improvement in image quality through the production of less scatter.

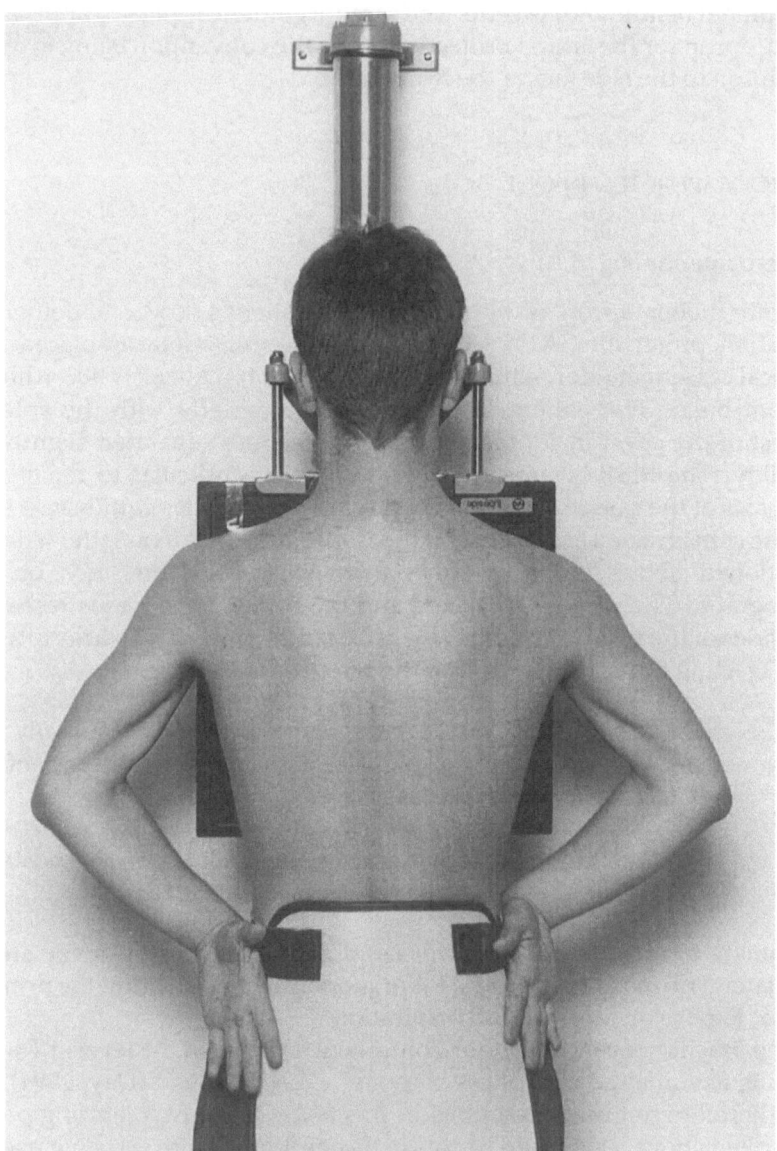

Figure 8.1 PA erect chest.

Anteroposterior

The AP projection will be necessary when the back of the wheelchair does not fold down and the patient's condition will not allow him or her to stand or be transferred on to a suitable seat for a PA projection. Patients who should remain on a trolley or in bed will also need to be examined AP.

If the patient is to remain in a wheelchair, pads/pillows should be used to sit them as upright as possible. If the patient is in bed or on a trolley he or she is supported using a large 45° sponge placed between the cassette and the angled back support.

With the patient erect the maximum amount of lung tissue will be demonstrated because of the effects of gravity on the abdominal organs, and the more vertical position will make it easier for the patient to inflate the lungs fully. Erect examination is more suitable in order that fluid levels are demonstrated, if present. However, the very sick or unconscious patient will need to be examined supine. In the supine position the cassette should be placed directly underneath the patient, rather than on a cassette tray, in order to reduce image magnification, particularly of the heart.

For AP projections of the chest the FFD is an important factor in keeping image magnification and geometric unsharpness to a minimum. With the patient sitting in a wheelchair there is usually no problem in achieving an FFD of 180 cm. With the patient supine the maximum FFD attainable, up to 180 cm, should be used by raising the X-ray tube to the top of the tube column and lowering the height of the bed/trolley if possible.

Lordotic appearances of an AP chest are common when using a horizontal/vertical X-ray beam. These appearances can be reduced by directing the beam 10–15° caudally.

Anteroposterior – erect (Fig. 8.2)

A 35×35 cm or 35×43 cm cassette is selected and may be used either longitudinally or transversely, according to patient build. The patient is seated with the posterior aspect of the chest in contact with the cassette, which is supported as described above. A lead–rubber sheet is placed across the lower abdomen as radiation protection. The upper border of the cassette is positioned above the lung apices to include the first ribs on the radiograph. The MSP is coincident with and perpendicular to the central long axis of the cassette, the medial ends of the clavicles equidistant from it. The chin is raised and the arms internally rotated and abducted slightly to clear the scapulae from the lung fields. They are then rested on the trolley sides, chair arms or pillows placed on the bed on either side of the patient.

CENTRING: (1) A horizontal central ray is directed 10–15° caudally to a point midway between the sternal notch and xiphisternum.

(2) A horizontal central ray, at 90° to the cassette, is directed midway between the sternal notch and xiphisternum.

Collimate to include C7, lung apices, diaphragms, costophrenic angles and lateral rib margins. Apply an AP anatomical marker within the primary beam. Expose on arrested full inspiration.

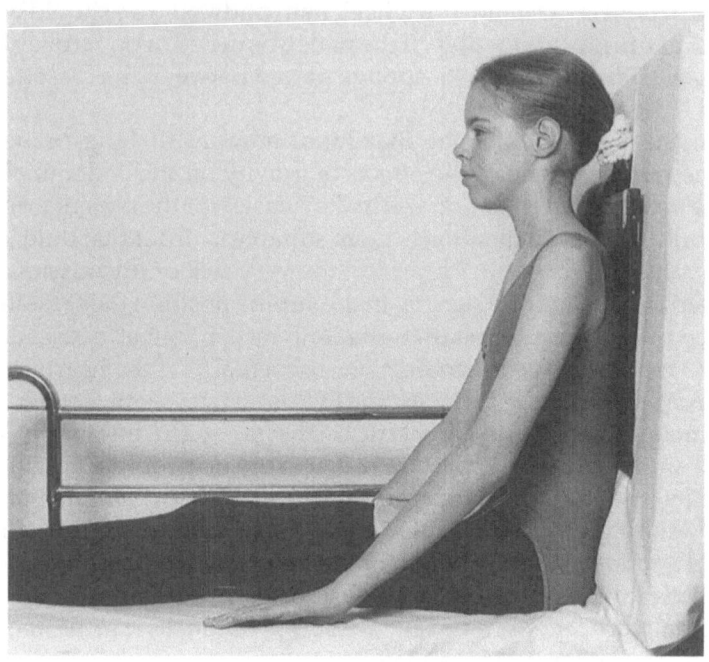

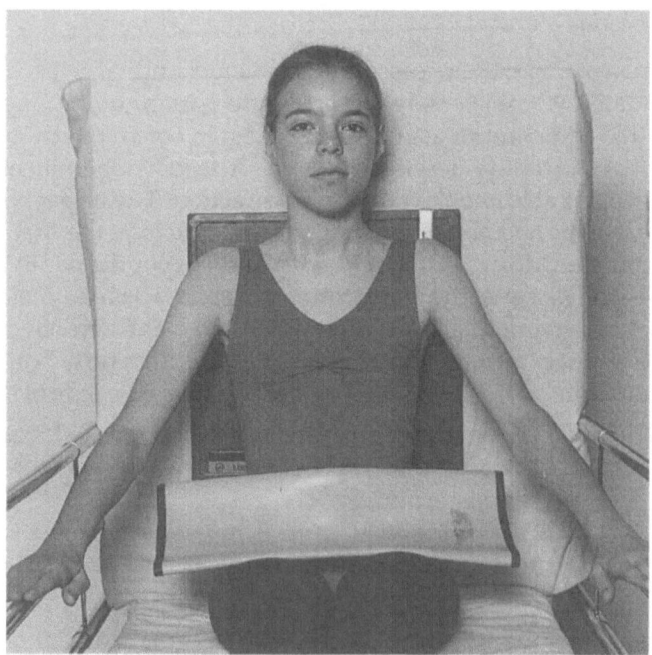

Figure 8.2 AP erect chest.

As discussed in the PA projection, of the two centring points described above, (1) should be routinely employed, with (2) being used in cases of suspected or follow-up pleural effusion. Method (1) will assist in projecting the clavicles below the apices of the lungs, reducing the lordotic appearance of the image and making it more comparable with the PA projection.

Anteroposterior – supine

A lead–rubber sheet is placed across the lower abdomen as radiation protection. The patient's upper body is lifted until a 35×35 cm or 35×43 cm cassette can be placed under their back, either longitudinally or transversely according to patient build. Any monitors or tubes attached to the patient should be handled with care and cleared from the area of interest wherever possible. The posterior aspect of the patient's chest is brought into contact with the cassette. The upper border of the cassette is positioned above the lung apices to include the first ribs on the radiograph. The MSP is coincident with and perpendicular to the central long axis of the cassette, the medial ends of the clavicles equidistant from it. The chin is raised and the arms internally rotated and abducted slightly.

CENTRING: A vertical central ray is directed 10–15° caudally to a point midway between the sternal notch and xiphisternum.

Collimate to include C7, lung apices, diaphragms, costophrenic angles and lateral rib margins. Apply an AP anatomical marker within the primary beam. Expose on arrested full inspiration.

Lateral decubitus

In the very ill patient, in order to demonstrate pleural effusion, a lateral decubitus projection with the patient lying on the affected side is undertaken. The horizontal central ray is directed to the level of T6, at 90° to the cassette. Any fluid present will collect against the lateral thoracic wall. The patient should not lie on the unaffected side as the fluid may be obscured by mediastinal structures.

Lateral (Fig. 8.3)

A lead–rubber apron is applied to the patient's lower abdomen as radiation protection. A 35×43 cm cassette is placed longitudinally in the erect chest stand. The patient stands with the affected side against the cassette, with the MSP parallel to it. The feet are separated slightly for stability. The centre of the cassette is coincident with a point in the

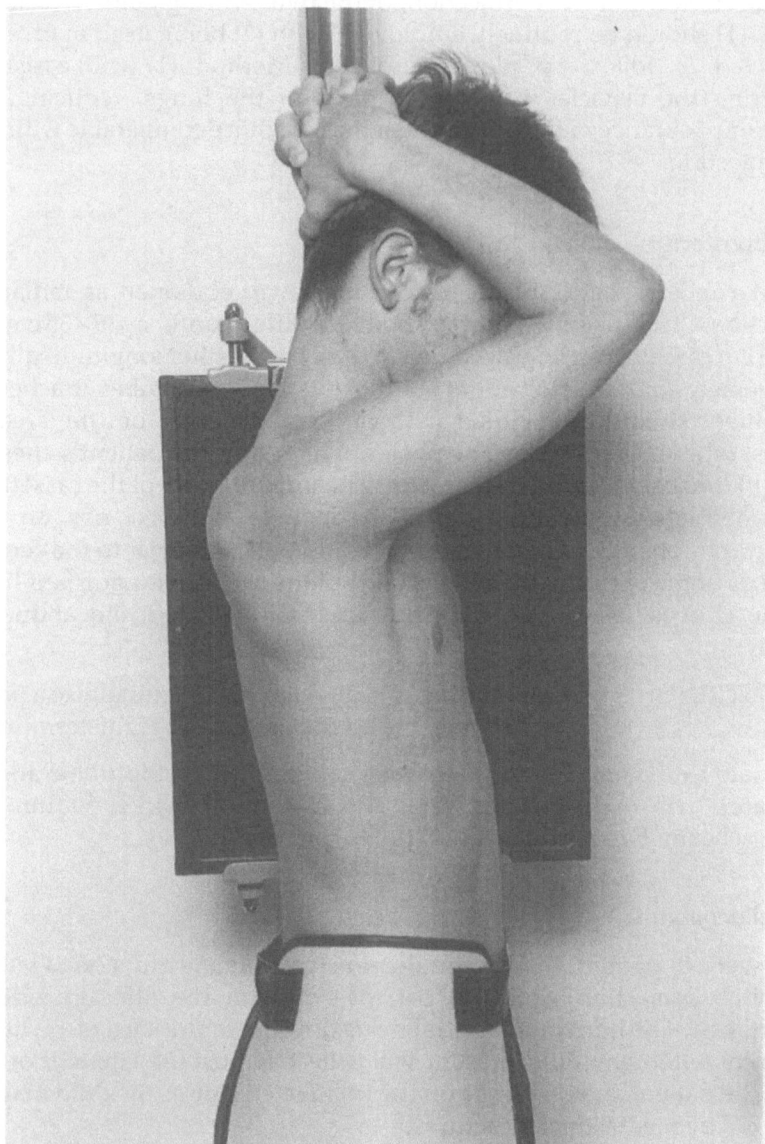

Figure 8.3 Lateral erect chest.

midaxillary line at the level of T6. The arms are raised with the elbows bent and the hands resting on top of the head. The upper arms are positioned parallel to one another so that the lateral aspect of the thorax remains in contact with the cassette.

CENTRING: A horizontal central ray at 90° to the cassette, is directed to a point in the midaxillary line at the level of T6.

Collimate to include apices, diaphragms, posterior costophrenic angles, sternum and posterior rib margins. Apply an AP anatomical marker within the primary beam. Expose on arrested full inspiration.

IMAGE EVALUATION

Correct patient identification and anatomical marker included on the radiograph.

Area of interest

Posteroanterior and anteroposterior

Apices of lungs and C7, costophrenic angles and lateral borders of ribs.

Lateral

Apices of lungs, diaphragms, anterior and posterior chest walls.

Projection

Posteroanterior and anteroposterior

- MSP coincident with midline of film.
- Medial ends of clavicles equidistant about the thoracic vertebral bodies.
- Clavicles projected below level of apices.
- Scapulae projected laterally, clear of lung fields. (NB: They will not be totally cleared in the AP projection.)
- Adequate inspiration assessed by the demonstration of six anterior or nine posterior ribs above the diaphragm.

Lateral

- Superimposition of posterior ribs.
- Superimposition of right and left posterior, superior and inferior borders of vertebral bodies.
- Humeri and soft tissues of upper arms clear of lung fields.
- Left hemidiaphragm lower than the right.

- Adequate inspiration assessed by the demonstration of T12 above the posterior aspect of the diaphragm.

Exposure factors

Posteroanterior and anteroposterior

- kVp sufficient to penetrate the mediastinum, demonstrating the spinous process of T4 through the air-filled trachea (the outline of the lower thoracic vertebrae and intervertebral joint spaces should be just visible through the heart) and lung detail within the costophrenic angles, maintaining contrast between the lung tissue and bony structures.
- mAs to provide adequate image density to demonstrate lung markings throughout the lung fields in contrast to the bones of the thorax and shoulder girdle.

Lateral

- kVp sufficient to penetrate the shoulder masses, demonstrating the heads of humeri within the apices of the chest, maintaining contrast between the lung tissue and bony structures.
- mAs to provide adequate image density to demonstrate lung markings from the apices to the diaphragm in contrast to the thoracic vertebrae and sternum.

No evidence of patient movement or breathing during the exposure.
No artefacts present on the image.

LUNG APICES

RADIOGRAPHIC TECHNIQUE

A 24×30 cm cassette is placed transverely in the erect cassette holder. A lead–rubber apron is applied to the patient's lower abdomen as radiation protection. The patient stands facing the cassette, the centre of which is coincident with the sternal angle. The anterior aspect of the chest is in contact with the cassette and the chin raised, though not resting on the upper border of the cassette. The MSP is perpendicular to the cassette.

> CENTRING: A horizontal central ray is directed 30° caudally to the spinous process of T1, to emerge through the sternal angle.

Collimate to include lung apices between the first and fifth ribs. Expose on arrested full inspiration.

IMAGE EVALUATION

Correct patient identification and anatomical marker included on the radiograph.

Area of interest

Apices of lungs between the first and fifth ribs and lateral rib margins.

Projection

- MSP coincident with midline of film.
- Medial ends of clavicles equidistant about the thoracic vertebral bodies.
- Clavicles projected above the first rib.
- Superimposition of the corresponding anterior and posterior portions of the ribs.

Exposure factors

- kVp sufficient to demonstrate bony trabeculae within the upper five pairs of ribs and the spinous process of T4 through the vertebral body, maintaining contrast between the air-filled lungs and bony structures.
- mAs to provide adequate image density to demonstrate lung tissue in contrast to the ribs.

No evidence of patient movement or breathing during the exposure.
No artefacts present on the image.

LORDOTIC CHEST

RADIOGRAPHIC TECHNIQUE (Fig. 8.4)

A 35×35 cm or 35×43 cm cassette is placed in the erect cassette holder. A lead–rubber apron is applied to the patient's lower abdomen as radiation protection. The patient is erect facing the cassette, with the chin raised and resting on its upper border. The feet are separated for stability. The MSP is coincident with and perpendicular to the central long axis of the cassette. The patient holds on to the chest stand for support and leans backwards from the waist through 30°.

> CENTRING: A horizontal central ray, at 90° to the cassette, is directed through the spinous process of T6 to the centre of the cassette.

Collimate to include clavicles, lung apices, diaphragms, costophrenic angles and lateral rib margins. Apply a PA anatomical marker within the primary beam. Expose on arrested full inspiration.

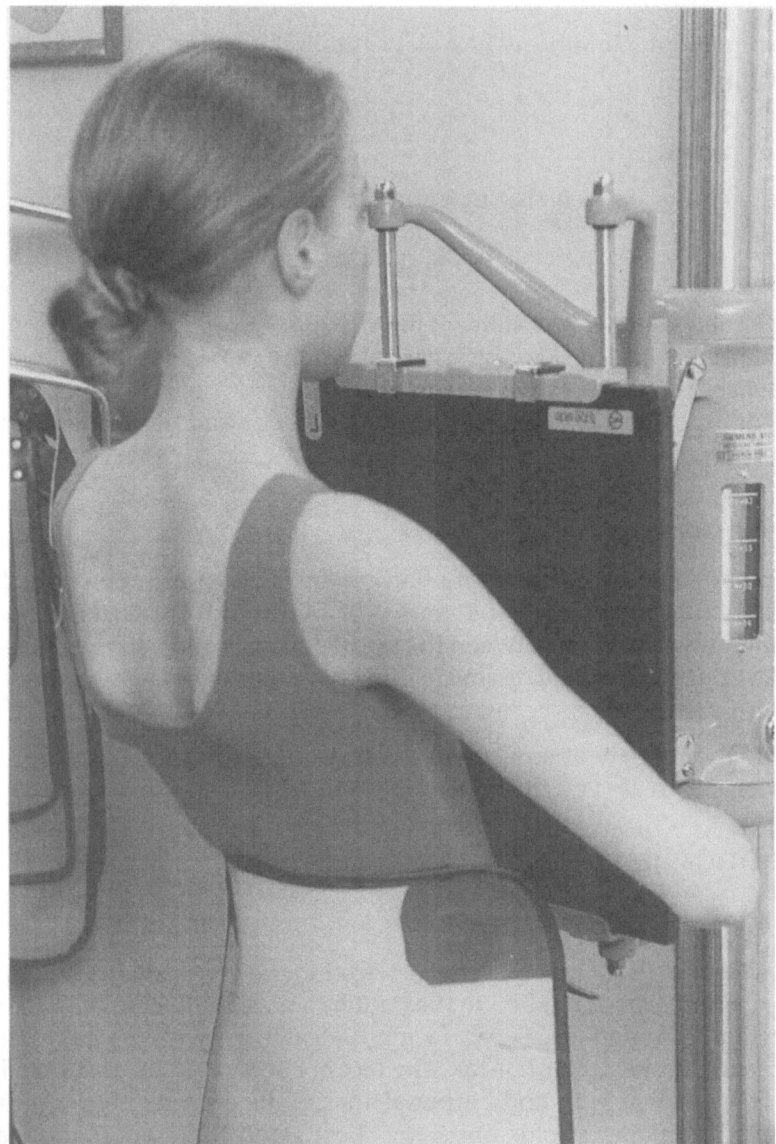

Figure 8.4 Lordotic erect chest.

IMAGE EVALUATION

Correct patient identification and anatomical marker included on the radiograph.

Area of interest

Apices and clavicles, diaphragms and costophrenic angles and lateral rib margins.

Projection

- MSP coincident with midline of film.
- Medial ends of clavicles equidistant about the thoracic vertebral bodies.
- Clavicles projected above the first ribs.
- Anterior and posterior aspects of the ribs almost on the same horizontal plane, with the anterior margins projected slightly below the posterior margins.

Exposure factors

- kVp sufficient to demonstrate bony trabeculae within the ribs and lung detail within the hila and costophrenic angles, maintaining contrast between the air-filled lungs, bony structures and mediastinum.
- mAs to provide adequate image density to demonstrate lung detail in contrast to the bony thorax and mediastinum.

No evidence of patient movement or breathing during the exposure.
No artefacts present on the image.

Exposure factor considerations

In order to minimize the effects of movement unsharpness, usually due to the patient breathing during the exposure, very short exposure times should be used in conjunction with high tube current (mA). This is no problem with modern generators, which allow the selection of exposure times in the region of 0.01–0.02 seconds together with 300–400 mA. A clear explanation of what is expected of the patient, followed by a rehearsal to ensure that they have understood, will reduce the risk of movement/breathing during the exposure.

Whereas traditional kVp values for chest radiography range between 60 and 90, there is now increasing evidence to support the use of kVps in the range of 120–140. Radiographs produced using lower kVps have a higher inherent contrast and tend to accentuate bony detail and mediastinal outlines, at the expense of inner mediastinal structures and pulmonary vascularity (Ravin and Johnson, 1983). Although use of higher kVp values reduces image contrast, it enables a wider range of structures to be demonstrated on the image. Owing to the increase in the amount of scattered radiation produced at high kVp, this method must be used in conjunction with an antiscatter grid or air-gap technique.

Oblique projections of the chest may rarely be requested to demonstrate the lungs fields and mediastinum or a specific pathology, e.g. pleural plaques caused by asbestosis. The degree of rotation of the patient from the PA/AP position will depend on the reason for the examination being undertaken, and advice should be sought from the referring clinician to ensure that the correct projection is produced. As a general rule, anterior/posterior structures are better demonstrated with the patient in the anterior/posterior oblique position, respectively. In all cases, the patient is rotated into the required position and the cassette positioned to include the apices, diaphragms, costophrenic angles and lateral rib margins. A horizontal central beam is directed to the centre of the cassette and the X-ray beam collimated to include the lung fields.

When examining young children, specialized equipment that enables them to be examined erect (sitting) will make positioning easier and lead to greater comfort for the patient, and so less chance of movement during the exposure. The PA projection should be used in preference to the AP when the child's age and behaviour allows. Very young children and babies can be examined in the supine position with the cassette directly beneath them. Using suitable radiation protection measures for the 'holder', the baby's arms should be held by the sides of the head, ensuring that the MSP is perpendicular to the cassette during exposure. The cassette should be raised on a 15° pad, or the X-ray beam directed 15° caudally, to reduce lordosis on the resultant image (Gyll and Blake, 1986).

Although it is preferable to perform chest radiography with the patient erect, Gyll and Blake identify some advantages in using the supine position for young children: it is easier to hold the child still and straight; the child is able to see what is going on and can focus their attention on the light beam; and the radiographer is more able to observe the child's respiration, making the exposure on full inspiration. For inhalation (and ingestion) of foreign bodies, see Chapter 9, Abdomen.

THORACIC INLET

RADIOGRAPHIC TECHNIQUE

Posteroanterior

A 24×30 cm cassette is placed longitudinally in the erect bucky. A lead–rubber apron is applied to the patient's lower abdomen as radiation protection. The patient is erect, anterior aspect of chest in contact with the bucky. The feet are separated for stability. The upper border of the cassette is level with the EAMs. The MSP is coincident with and perpendicular to the central long axis of the cassette. The chin is raised until the occiput and symphysis menti are on the same horizontal plane, and placed in contact with the bucky.

CENTRING: A horizontal central ray, at 90° to the cassette, is directed over the spinous process of T2 to emerge through the sternal notch.

Collimate to include C3, T6 and the lateral soft tissue outlines of the neck. Apply a PA anatomical marker within the primary beam. Expose on arrested inspiration.

Soft tissue lateral neck

The patient position is similar to that for the cervical spine lateral (see Fig. 5.2).

A 24×30 cm cassette is placed longitudinally in the erect cassette holder. A lead–rubber apron is applied to the patient's lower abdomen as radiation protection. The patient is erect, with the MSP parallel to the cassette and their shoulder in contact with it. The feet are separated for stability. The upper border of the cassette is level with the top of the pinna of the ear, its central long axis coincident with the mastoid processes. The chin is raised slightly to clear the angles of the mandible from the larynx, and the shoulders are relaxed.

CENTRING: With an FFD of 180 cm, a horizontal central ray, at 90° to the cassette, is directed to the middle of the neck at the level of the thyroid eminence.

Collimate to include anterior and posterior soft tissues of the neck, nasopharynx and T2. Apply an AP anatomical marker within the primary beam. Expose on arrested inspiration.

Lateral retrosternum (Fig. 8.5)

A 24×30 cm cassette is placed longitudinally in the erect bucky. A lead–rubber apron is applied to the patient's lower abdomen as radiation protection. The patient is erect, with the MSP parallel to the cassette and their shoulder in contact with it. The feet are separated for stability. The centre of the cassette is coincident with the sternal notch. The chin is raised and the shoulders are drawn back to clear the heads of the humeri from the trachea.

CENTRING: A horizontal central ray, at 90° to the cassette, is directed over the sternal notch.

Collimate to include the anterior and posterior soft tissues of the neck, C3 and T6. Apply an AP anatomical marker within the primary beam. Expose on arrested inspiration.

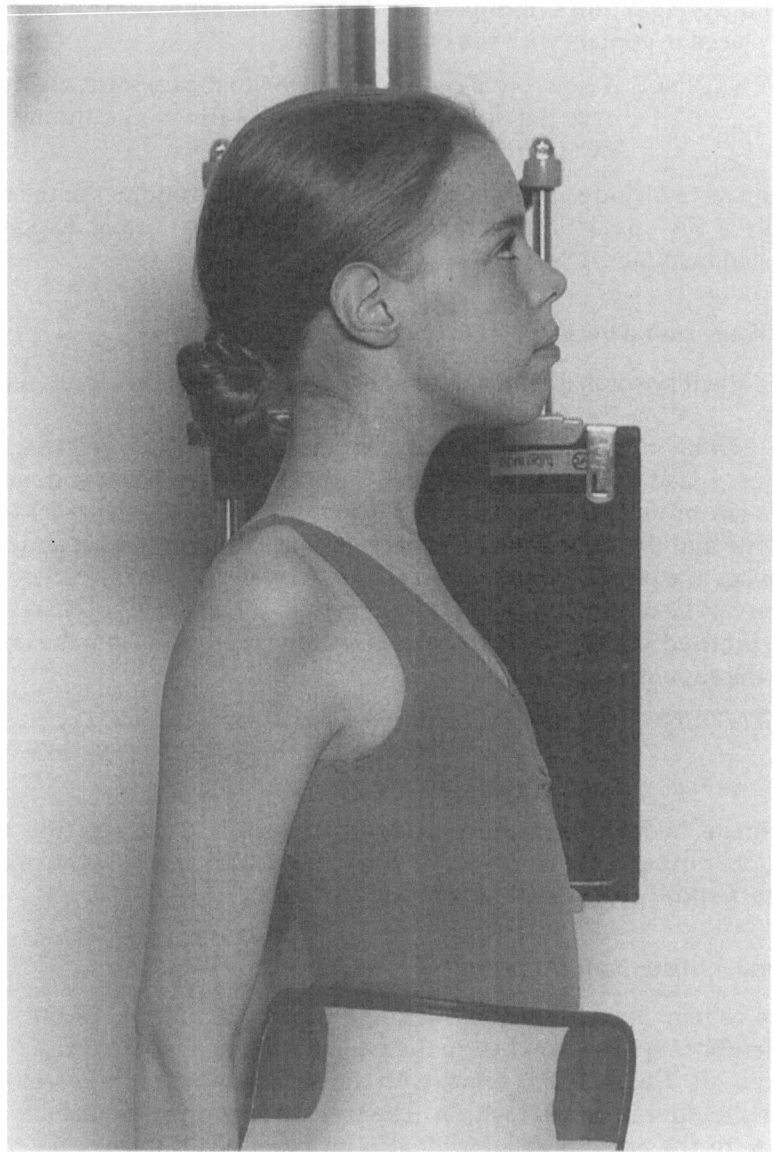

Figure 8.5 Lateral thoracic inlet: lower respiratory tract.

It can be difficult for some patients to pull their shoulders back far enough to clear the humeral heads from the trachea. This situation particularly applies to arthritic, kyphotic or obese patients. An effective alternative is to extend and raise the arms vertically above the head.

Left anterior oblique

A 30×40 cm cassette is placed longitudinally in the erect cassette holder. A lead–rubber apron is applied to the patient's lower abdomen as radiation protection. The patient is erect, facing the cassette holder. The centre of the cassette is coincident with the sternal notch. The patient is rotated towards the right, until the MSP is at 45° to the cassette with the left shoulder in contact with the cassette. The head is rotated a further 45° until its MSP is parallel to the cassette. The feet are separated for stability.

CENTRING: With an FFD of 180 cm a horizontal central ray, at 90° to the cassette, is directed midway between the spinous process of T2 and the right acromion process, to emerge through the sternal notch.

Collimate to include base of skull, carina and lateral soft tissue outlines of the neck. Apply a PA anatomical marker within the primary beam. Expose on arrested inspiration.

IMAGE EVALUATION

Correct patient identification and anatomical marker included on the radiograph.

Area of interest

Posteroanterior

C3, bifurcation of trachea and lateral soft tissue outlines of neck.

Soft tissue lateral neck

Base of occiput and nasopharynx, C7/T1 joint space and clavicle, spinous processes and anterior soft tissue structures of neck.

Lateral retrosternum

Full length of trachea, from clavicle to carina.

Left anterior oblique

Base of occiput and nasopharynx, carina and soft tissue outlines of neck.

Projection

Posteroanterior

• Base of skull superimposed over lower border of mandible.

- Spinous processes demonstrated down centre of vertebral bodies in midline of film.

Soft tissue lateral neck

- Superimposition of right and left posterior, superior and inferior borders of vertebral bodies.
- Angles of mandible cleared from upper cervical vertebrae and pharynx.
- Shoulders dropped below level of C7.

Lateral retrosternum

- Shoulders drawn back so as not to obscure trachea with heads of humeri.
- Superimposition of right and left posterior, superior and inferior borders of vertebral bodies.
- Superimposition of shoulder masses.

Left anterior oblique

- Mandible projected clear of upper vertebrae and air passages.
- Intervertebral foramina demonstrated on opposite side of spine to mandible.
- Trachea demonstrated in its entirety anterior to bodies of vertebrae.

Exposure factors

Posteroanterior

- kVp sufficient to demonstrate spinous processes through the vertebral bodies, maintaining contrast between the vertebrae and air-filled trachea.
- mAs to provide adequate image density to demonstrate detail of trachea in contrast to the vertebrae and soft tissues of the neck.

Soft tissue lateral neck

kVp selected to demonstrate trachea and soft tissue structures in the anterior aspect of neck, increasing the contrast between these structures through their differential absorption of radiation.

- kVp will not be sufficient to demonstrate bony trabeculae within the cervical vertebrae.

- mAs to provide adequate image density to demonstrate trachea in contrast to soft tissue structures in the anterior neck.

Lateral retrosternum

- kVp sufficient to demonstrate trachea down to its bifurcation, maintaining contrast between trachea, air-filled lungs and dense shoulder mass.
- mAs to provide adequate image density to demonstrate detail of trachea in contrast to the lungs.

Left anterior oblique

kVp sufficient to reduce the subject contrast inherent along the length of trachea as it passes down the neck into the thoracic cavity, demonstrating full length of trachea on a single image.

- kVp sufficient to demonstrate the air passages from the nasopharynx down to the carina, maintaining contrast between the air passages, soft tissue structures of the neck, air-filled lungs and vertebrae.
- mAs to provide adequate image density to demonstrate detail of the air passages in contrast to the surrounding soft tissues and vertebrae.

No evidence of patient movement.
No artefacts present on the image.

It is possible to carry out AP and posterior oblique projections of the thoracic inlet rather than the PA and anterior oblique but, in order to reduce the dose to the thyroid gland and breast tissue, they are described here with the patient facing the cassette. Anatomically, the upper airway is closer to the cassette in the PA position, with the lower airway more centrally positioned.

Departmental protocols vary, requiring different combinations of the projections described to be undertaken – PA/AP plus upper and lower lateral projections is the usual routine, but requires the patient to be irradiated three times. Two exposures will suffice if the full length of the trachea can be demonstrated on one lateral image. This will require selection of a relatively high kVp, in conjunction with a lower mAs, in order to reduce the subject contrast along the length of the trachea. A grid may also be necessary to provide adequate image detail of the lower region. However, Wright and Fergusson (1986) advocate the use of the oblique projection to demonstrate the full length of the trachea on a single image. As the patient is not lateral, the subject contrast is not so great along the length of the trachea. At an FFD of 180 cm, the exposure factors selected are the same as those used for the routine lateral projection of the cervical spine, obviating the need for a grid/bucky and producing a quality image with reduced radiation dose to the patient. The most common positional problems – superimposition of the shoulder masses on the air passages, and patient movement during the exposure – are experienced in the lateral projection. In the oblique position, the shoulder masses cause no problem at all and, as the patient does not have to forcibly draw back the arms, there is less risk of patient movement. With particular regard to the radiation dose received by the patient, the single oblique projection of the thoracic inlet would appear to be the examination of choice.

Abdomen

9

RADIOGRAPHIC TECHNIQUE

Supine (Fig 9.1)

A 35×43 cm cassette is placed longitudinally in the table bucky. The patient lies supine on the table, MSP coincident with and perpendicular to its midline. The ASISs are equidistant from the table top. The arms are abducted, resting at the patient's sides. With the FFD set at 100 cm and the bucky tray fully out, the vertical X-ray beam is centred to the middle of the cassette and collimated to its longitudinal and transverse limits. The bucky tray is pushed under the table and the X-ray tube centred to it transversely. The X-ray tube or patient is moved until the superior border of the symphysis pubis is 2.5 cm above the lower border of collimation.

> CENTRING: The vertical X-ray beam, at 90° to the cassette, will be directed over the midline, at the approximate level of the iliac crests, to include the symphysis pubis on the image.

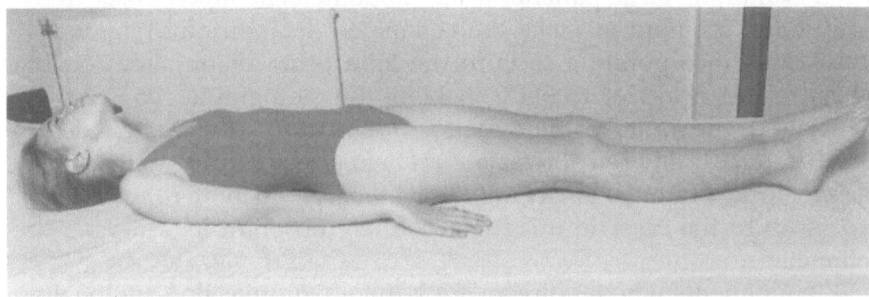

Figure 9.1 Supine abdomen.

The cassette is aligned with the X-ray beam. Collimate to include symphysis pubis, upper abdomen and lateral abdominal walls. Apply an AP anatomical marker within the primary beam. Expose on arrested expiration.

The upper border of the symphysis pubis lies level with the greater trochanters, approximately 10 cm inferior to the ASISs, although this will vary according to patient build and sex. Using either of these as a guide will avoid any embarrassment caused by the radiographer feeling for the symphysis pubis, particularly when X-raying the opposite sex.

Erect abdomen (Fig. 9.2)

A 35×43 cm cassette is placed longitudinally in the erect bucky. With the FFD set at 100 cm and the bucky tray fully out, the horizontal X-ray beam is centred to the cassette and collimated to its longitudinal and transverse limits. The bucky tray is pushed behind the bucky and the X-ray beam centred to it transversely. The patient stands with their back in contact with the bucky, MSP coincident with and perpendicular to its midline. The arms are abducted and the feet separated for stability.

> CENTRING: The horizontal central ray, at 90° to the cassette, is directed over a point in the midline, at the approximate level of the lower costal margins, to include the diaphragm on the image.

The height of the bucky is altered to align the cassette with the X-ray beam. Collimate to include diaphragms, lower abdomen and lateral abdominal walls. Apply an AP anatomical marker within the primary beam. Expose on arrested expiration.

In both projections the collimation is preset for maximum coverage of the cassette and should not be increased, although reducing the area of collimation wherever possible is to be encouraged. This practice represents good radiation protection as it ensures that the area of the primary beam does not exceed the limits of the cassette, and is particularly useful when examining large patients whose abdomens lie much closer to the X-ray tube, seeming to make the collimated area shrink dramatically. Some units incorporate a scale in the light beam diaphragm housing which relates field size to FFD, enabling the radiographer to manually collimate to the limits of the cassette. Others may incorporate a device which automatically sets the maximum field size according to the size of cassette locked into the bucky tray. Remember, if no more primary beam can fit on to the cassette there is absolutely no point in widening the collimation.

Often, patients who require an erect abdomen projection are too ill to stand. In this case the patient can be examined in one of the following ways.

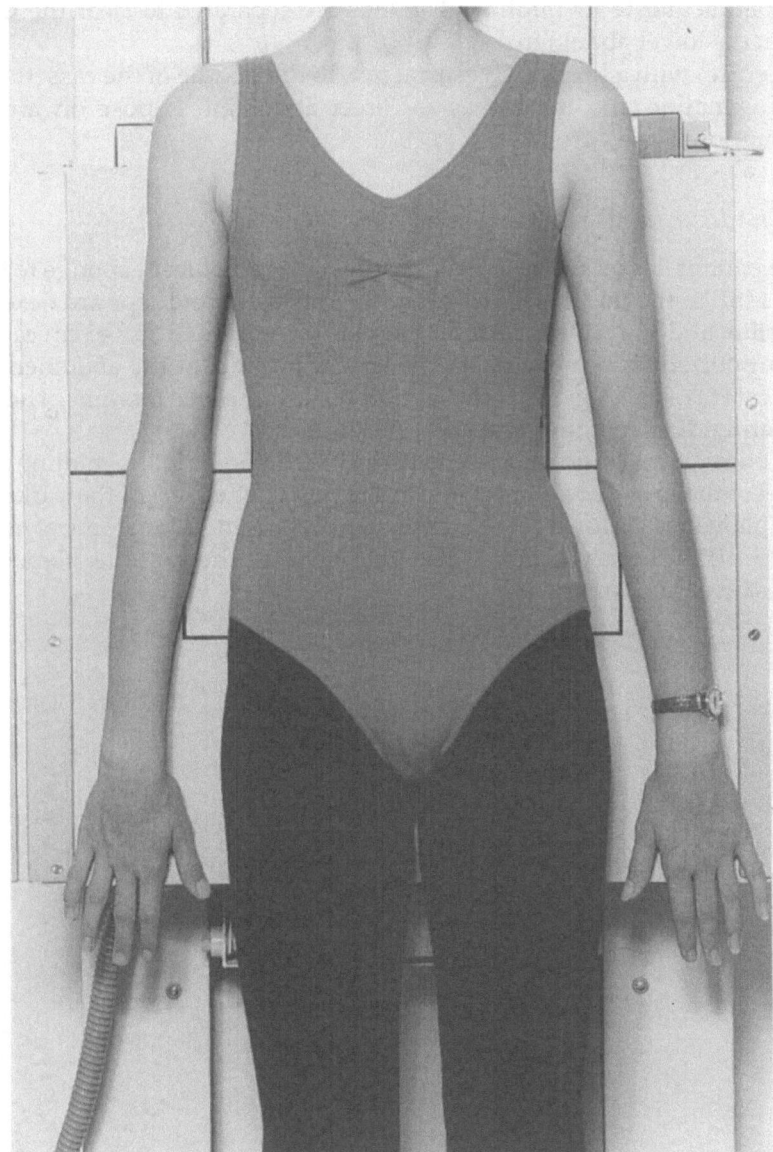

Figure 9.2   Erect abdomen.

Erect sitting

The patient sits on the trolley/bed, with a gridded 35×43 cm cassette supported longitudinally and vertically behind their back, its lower border resting on the trolley top. The MSP is coincident with and perpendicular to its midline. The legs are separated to clear the thighs from the lower abdomen.

Centre, with a horizontal central ray, to the middle of the cassette.

Collimation and marker as for erect abdomen. Expose on arrested expiration.

Lateral decubitus (Fig. 9.3)

The patient lies on their left side, resting on a radiolucent sponge to bring the MSP to the midline of the cassette. The knees and hips are flexed for stability and the arms placed on the pillow. A gridded 35×43 cm cassette is supported vertically against the anterior aspect of the abdomen with the centre of its long axis at the level of the lower costal margins. The MSP is perpendicular to the cassette.

Centre, with a horizontal central ray, over a point in the midline at the level of the lower costal margins on the posterior aspect of the patient.

Collimation as for erect abdomen. Apply a right PA anatomical marker within the primary beam to the long edge of the cassette. Expose on arrested expiration.

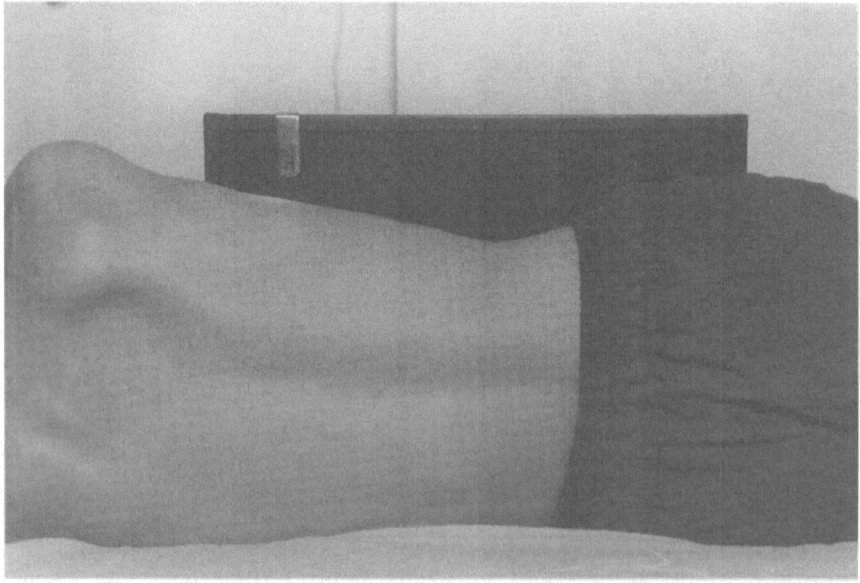

Figure 9.3   Left lateral decubitus.

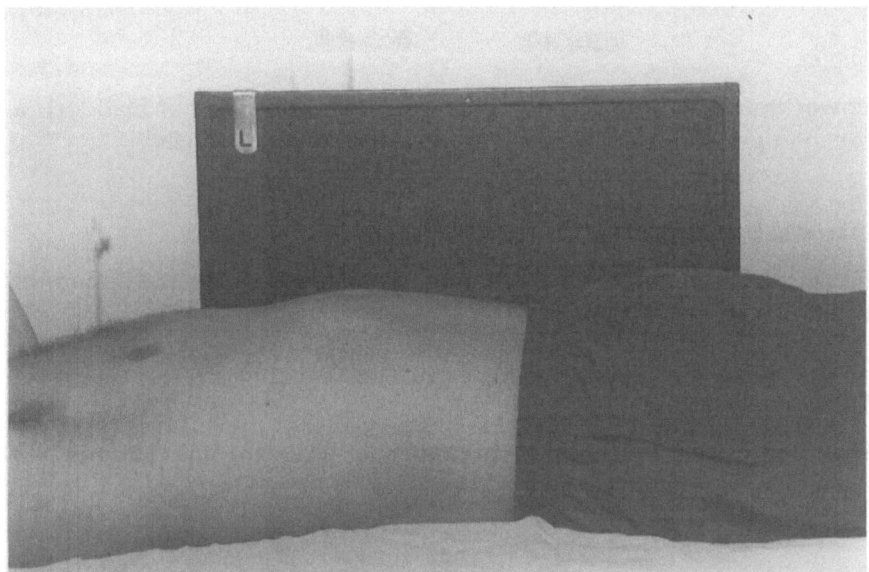

Figure 9.4   Supine decubitus.

Supine decubitus (Fig. 9.4)

The patient remains supine on the trolley/bed. A 35×43 cm gridded cassette is placed, in an erect holder, vertically against the lateral aspect of the abdomen with the centre of its long axis at the level of the lower costal margins. The cassette holder is pushed down into the mattress as far as possible and locked in position. The arms are lifted on to the pillow to clear them from the abdomen. Centre, with a horizontal central ray, at the level of the lower costal margins, midway between the anterior and posterior abdominal walls.

Collimate to include anterior and posterior soft tissues of abdomen, diaphragms and lower abdomen. Apply an AP anatomical marker within the primary beam. Expose on arrested expiration.

For all decubitus projections it is imperative that the X-ray beam is horizontal, i.e. parallel to the floor, if air–fluid levels are to be demonstrated.

IMAGE EVALUATION

Correct patient identification and anatomical marker included on the radiograph.

Area of interest

Supine

Lower border of symphysis pubis (and therefore base of bladder), as much upper abdomen as possible and lateral abdominal walls.

Erect and lateral decubitus

Diaphragms, as much lower abdomen as possible and lateral abdominal walls.

Supine decubitus

Diaphragms, as much lower abdomen as possible and anterior and posterior abdominal walls.

Projection

Supine, erect and lateral decubitus

- Long axis of the spine coincident with the midline of the film.
- Spinous processes demonstrated down the centre of the vertebral bodies.
- Symmetry of the right and left iliac fossae/obturator foramina.
- Diaphragm demonstrated above the level of T10.

Supine decubitus

- Superimposition of right and left posterior, superior and inferior borders of lumbar vertebral bodies.
- Arms raised clear of upper abdomen.
- Diaphragm demonstrated above the level of T10.

Exposure factors

Optimum contrast is essential in order to differentiate between the abdominal viscera.

- kVp sufficient to penetrate bony structures and demonstrate bony trabeculae within them while maximizing image contrast caused by the differential absorption of soft tissue structures at lower kVp.
- mAs to provide adequate image density to demonstrate bony detail of

the pelvis and spine, while not overexposing the soft tissue organs of the abdomen.

No evidence of patient movement or breathing during the exposure.
No artefacts present on the image and no evidence of grid cut-off.

Exposure and respiration

Exposure should routinely be made on arrested expiration, demonstrating the abdominal viscera in their normal relationships. Differences in size, shape and position of individual organs may then be attributed to pathology.

Opacities are frequently demonstrated in the upper abdomen. In order to differentiate between renal calculi and, for example, calcification in the costal cartilages, an additional cross-kidney film may be undertaken (see p. 288), with exposure made on arrested inspiration. As the kidneys change position according to the phase of respiration, the opacities, if in the kidneys, will move accordingly, maintaining the same position in relation to the renal outlines. Opacities that do not appear to move with the kidneys are likely to lie within some other structure.

In some departments it is common practice to expose abdomen films on inspiration, enabling the upper poles of the kidneys to be demonstrated on the same film as the base of the bladder. If opacities are demonstrated in this instance, a cross-kidney film exposed on expiration should be undertaken to confirm/exclude the presence of renal calculi.

THE 'ACUTE' ABDOMEN

In cases of suspected intestinal perforation or obstruction the radiographic examination should consist of a supine abdomen and an erect chest projection (Royal College of Radiologists, 1995), although many departmental protocols still require the inclusion of an erect abdomen.

A supine abdomen is usually sufficient to demonstrate the intestinal gas pattern, and therefore the presence of intestinal obstruction. An erect abdomen should only be considered if the supine abdomen appears normal but there is a strong clinical indication of obstruction.

The erect chest projection is useful in demonstrating subphrenic gas, indicating intestinal perforation, and will exclude chest conditions, e.g. basal pneumonia, as a cause of upper abdominal pain.

The *left* lateral decubitus projection of the abdomen may be necessary to show free abdominal gas in cases where the patient is unable to sit or stand for an erect chest X-ray. The left lateral decubitus position is preferred, as any free gas will be obvious as it collects between the lateral margin of the liver and the right lateral abdominal wall. In the right lateral decubitus position it may not be possible to differentiate between free peritoneal gas and gas naturally occurring within the stomach.

The PA decubitus position is preferred to the AP decubitus as it facilitates compression of the anterior abdomen against the cassette, resulting in the irradiation of a smaller volume of tissue. This leads to less scatter production and therefore a higher-quality image, with reduced dose to the patient. Also, in the PA decubitus position the large bowel is closer to the film, which is appropriate when undertaking these projections during a barium enema examination, achieving dose reduction to the radiosensitive bowel through absorption of the lower enegry radiation by the posterior abdominal structures.

Order of projections for cases of suspected gastro-intestinal perforation

If the patient arrives in the department sitting upright in a wheelchair, the erect chest projection should be undertaken first, followed by the supine abdomen. If it is then felt that an erect abdomen is necessary, the patient should be allowed to sit upright for a minimum of 10 minutes prior to exposure, to allow sufficient time for any free intra-abdominal gas to rise and collect below the diaphragm. If the patient arrives supine on a trolley/bed, the supine abdomen is undertaken first. If the patient is able to sit for an erect chest, exposure is made after the patient has maintained the upright position for a minimum of 10 minutes. If the patient is unable to sit up, a supine chest is taken followed by a left lateral decubitus abdomen, again after allowing the patient to maintain the required position for at least 10 minutes.

Ingestion/inhalation of foreign bodies

In young children it is often not possible to be perfectly certain that a foreign body has been ingested, rather than inhaled, and in this case it is necessary to radiograph the pharynx, chest and abdomen (or upper abdomen if the incident has occurred recently) (Gyll and Blake, 1986).

An adult or eloquent child may be able to indicate to the clinician that a foreign body has been ingested, rather than inhaled, indicating the necessity for abdominal X-ray to demonstrate any opacity. Time of ingestion should be ascertained and indicated on the image; recent occurrence will enable the radiographer to reduce the radiation field to the upper abdomen (from diaphragm to ASIS) and suggest the most likely area for appearance of the object. A chest X-ray may also be necessary if the abdominal radiograph is negative. Since obstruction by foreign body can cause the collapse of a lung, inspiration and expiration films may be necessary to assess inflation/deflation of the lungs. Peanuts are a commonly inhaled foreign body, and as they can cause lung abscess (Gyll and Blake, 1986), the chest X-ray enables the condition of the chest to be ascertained.

Mammography **10**

INTRODUCTION

The use of mammography has greatly increased within the United Kingdom since the Forrest Report (1986) made its recommendations on national breast screening. The number of radiographers undertaking this type of examination has also increased. It is considered to be a specialist area in radiography and this chapter does not aim to offer the full range of information needed by those studying for a certificate of competence in mammography. It does, however, aim to provide an introduction to the topic for students who will gain initial clinical experience in this area.

Mammography is useful in the identification of a range of conditions found in the breast, both benign and malignant, most often being cysts, fibroadenomas, calcification and malignancy. Calcification is generally considered to be benign if large, i.e. >1 mm diameter, single, rounded or scattered throughout both breasts, but suggests malignancy if fine and clustered, in rows in the ducts, short and rod-like or mixed in size (Caseldine *et al.*, 1988). Since microcalcification can be seen in the early stages of malignancy, even before a mass is evident radiologically, these appearances are useful in a screening service which aims to diagnose early enough to improve the chance of a good prognosis.

Mammography is now routinely accompanied by ultrasound of the area, which may be applied for every patient or only those with abnormal (although not necessarily malignant) findings, according to departmental protocol. It does not identify microcalcifications associated with malignancy and cannot currently be used as a replacement for mammography.

Forrest (1986) recommended that projections undertaken for initial screening should be lateral obliques of both breasts, supplemented by other projections if required for further assessment. From 1 August 1995 it became mandatory for all women on their first visit to a breast screening clinic to have craniocaudal and lateral oblique projections carried out. Women referred for symptomatic reasons should have a craniocaudal and lateral oblique of each breast, supplemented by other projections as necessary.

Forrest laid down many specifics for the development and running of a quality breast screening programme, all of which are appropriate for any type of mammography service. In addition to recommendations for suitable age group, population to be served, administration strategies and suitable projections, these specifics included guidelines on equipment specification, film/screen combinations, processing, image quality, patient dose and staff performance (Challen *et al.*, 1990). Forrest also recommended the setting up of an advisory committee on breast cancer screening. This committee sought guidance on quality assurance, which was provided in 1989 by the Pritchard Report (Radiological Advisory Committee, 1989).

Part of the Forrest Report was concerned with protocols for the different stages of patient involvement in breast screening. These are outlined as follows.

- Women aged 50–64 are invited for attendance via computerized lists, information originally being gained from general practitioners, with women over the age of 64 screened on request.
- On attendance the patient supplies information on medical history and undergoes mammographic examination.
- Images are reported and the patient is notified of her result. If the result is negative she will receive her next appointment automatically in 3 years, unless she will be over 64 before the period has elapsed. Patients with suspicious findings are invited for mammographic reassessment at a hospital, which should also offer counselling and access to a surgeon, if appropriate. Assessment may include a combination of further projections, magnified projections, fine-needle aspiration or ultrasound. On attendance the result may be normal and these patients will be counselled and recalled in 3 years.
- Patients with abnormal but benign findings will also be counselled and discuss treatment and further tests, if appropriate, with a surgeon. Patients found to have non-palpable malignancy will go through this procedure and return to the hospital mammography unit for presurgical mammographic localization of the lesion, unless total mastectomy is to be performed.

More specific information can be found in the report itself, or the specialist texts recommended at the end of this chapter.

RADIOGRAPHIC TECHNIQUE

Craniocaudal (C-C) (Fig. 10.1)

The mammography unit is positioned with the cassette horizontal. The patient is erect, facing the mammography unit and the long axis of the cassette holder. The patient is rotated away from the side under examination, until the breast is close to the cassette holder. The degree of rotation will vary from 15 to 30°, depending on breast size and patient build, and will bring more of the upper outer quadrant over the cassette. The arm on the side under examination is flexed at the elbow, to relax the pectoral muscle, and the hand is placed on the patient's lower abdomen or relaxed at the side of the trunk. The radiographer supports the breast, adjusting the height of the unit until the cassette holder is in contact with the inframammary fold and the breast is at approximately 90° to the anterior chest wall. The breast is then carefully placed in contact with the cassette holder, ensuring that no skin folds occur. The unit height is adjusted until the nipple is in profile and positioned to lie at '11 o'clock' (right breast) or '1 o'clock' (left breast). All breast tissue should be included within the boundaries of the cassette and, if possible, the pectoral muscle. The radiographer maintains slight pressure to the back of the patient, to ensure the maximum amount of breast tissue remains in position over the cassette. Compression is applied while the radiographer maintains the position of the breast, eliminating any skin folds.

Apply a craniocaudal anatomical marker, relevant to the breast under examination, within the primary beam and on the axillary edge of the cassette holder.

The projection will indicate the position of any abnormality in relationship to the nipple but will not demonstrate all quadrants of the breast. The slight medial rotation brings more glandular tissue over the film.

Extended craniocaudal – for axillary tail

The unit is positioned as for the craniocaudal projection and then angled 15° towards the side under examination. The patient stands initially as for the craniocaudal projection, with the chest in contact with the edge of the cassette. The radiographer supports the breast, adjusting the height of the unit until the cassette holder is in contact with the inframammary fold and the breast is at 90° to the anterior chest wall. The trunk is rotated 45° away from the side under examination and the breast is maintained at 90° to the chest. The arm of the side under examination is placed along the edge of the cassette holder adjacent to it, and the nipple is at the opposite edge, nearest the medial aspect of the breast. The radiographer pulls the

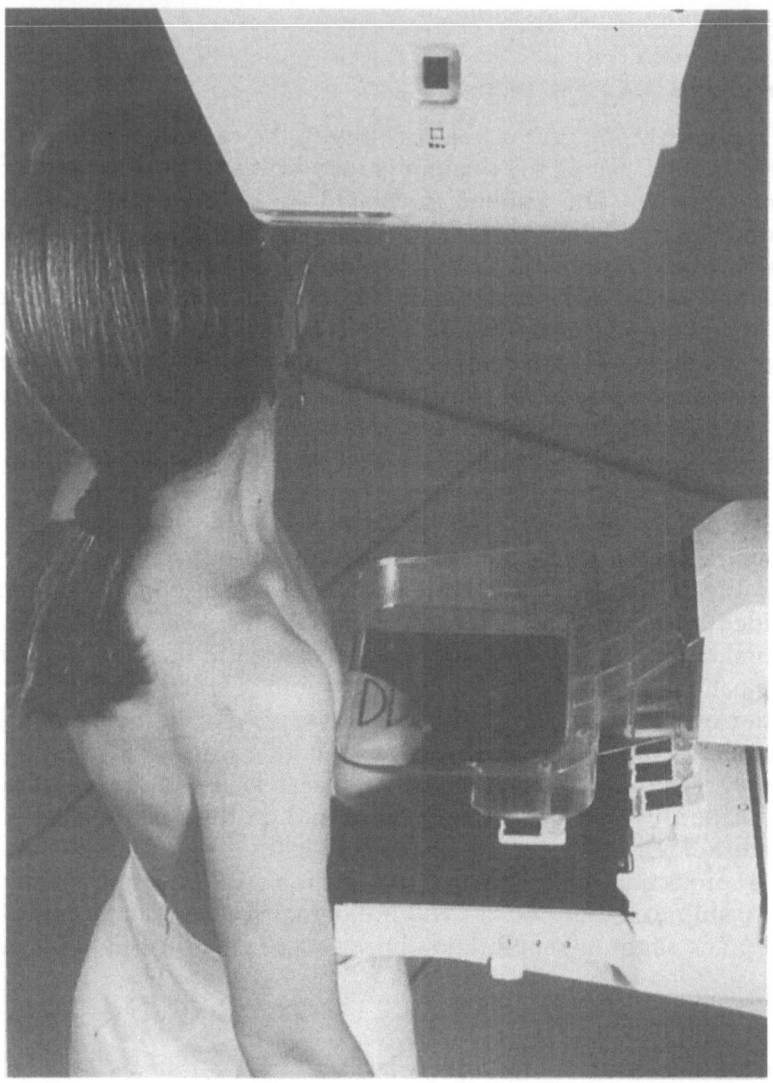

Figure 10.1 Craniocaudal. Courtesy of IGE.

maximum amount of breast tissue possible over the cassette, eliminating any skin folds in the process. The patient leans back towards the shoulder on the side under examination until the axilla and outer quadrants of the breast are in contact with the cassette holder. The patient's hand can now be rested on the vertical support of the unit. The radiographer supports the patient from behind to help keep the breast over the cassette holder, while pulling the breast over the cassette holder during compression. As compression is applied, the fingers continue to pull in this way until compression is complete. If the positioning is correct, the corner of the compression paddle will fill the costohumeral angle.

Apply an extended craniocaudal anatomical marker, relevant to the side under examination, within the primary beam and on the axillary edge of the cassette holder.

This projection demonstrates more of the upper outer quadrant of the breast, tail and axilla than the craniocaudal projection.

Mediolateral oblique (Fig. 10.2)

The mammography unit is initially positioned with the cassette vertical. The patient is erect, facing the mammography unit, with the side under examination next to the cassette. The tube is angled 45° caudally and the height of the unit adjusted until the lower border of the cassette is 2.5 cm below the inferior aspect of the breast. Further height adjustment may be necessary during patient positioning. The patient leans forward towards the unit until the lateral quadrants of the breast under examination lie over the cassette. The patient raises the arm of the side under examination and places the axilla tightly over the corner of the cassette nearest the chest wall. The upper arm rests along the top of the cassette, the elbow is flexed so that the forearm can be placed on the unit for support, and the arm is relaxed. The radiographer lifts the breast, bringing the nipple into profile and eliminating any skin folds. The inframammary fold, nipple, tail of the breast and pectoralis major should all be included within the boundaries of the cassette. The patient rotates the trunk slightly away from the side under examination, to clear the other breast, sternum and ribs from the compression paddle. The radiographer maintains the position of the breast during this movement. Compression is applied while the radiographer maintains the position of the breast, eliminating any skin folds. The trunk is returned to its original position before exposure is made. If the medial aspect of the opposite breast is superimposed over the breast under examination it should be gently moved from the field and held by the patient. Care should be taken not to pull the breast under examination from under the compression paddle, so altering position.

Apply a lateral oblique anatomical marker, relevant to the breast under examination, within the primary beam and on the axillary edge of the cassette holder.

This projection features in mammography referrals of all kinds, since it demonstrates more breast tissue than any other. It is the most effective projection for demonstrating the upper outer quadrant, where most breast carcinomas are found, and also demonstrates the axilla and tail of the breast.

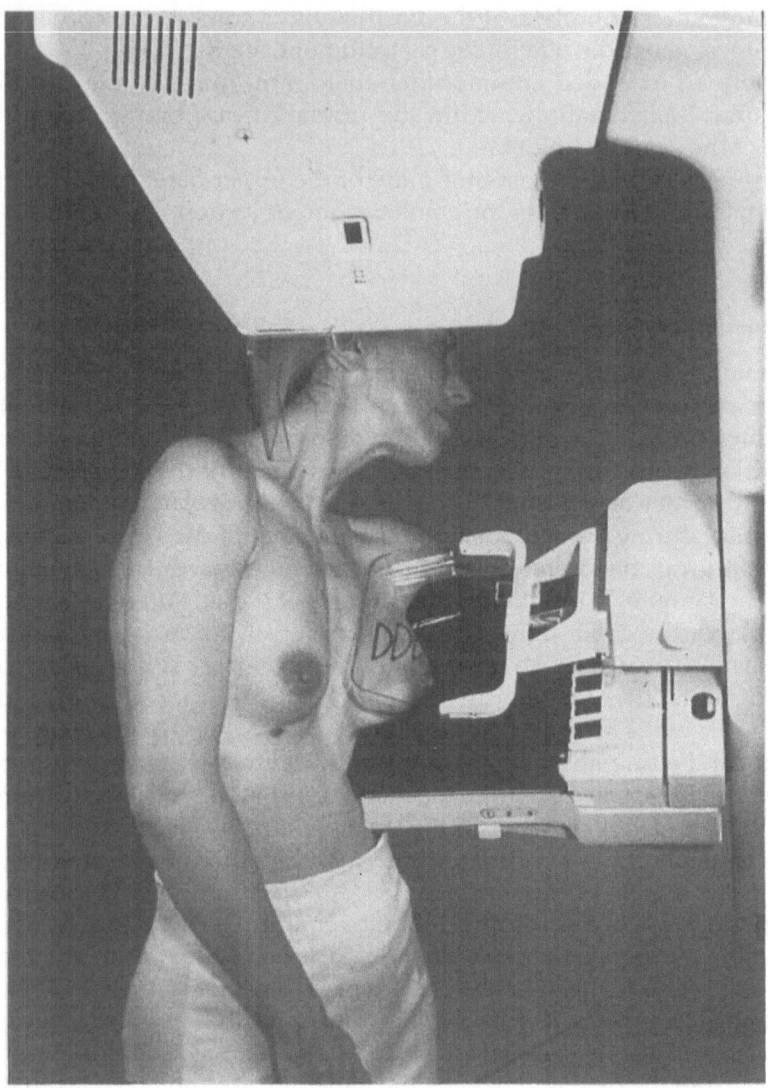

Figure 10.2   Mediolateral oblique. Courtesy of IGE.

Lateral

Laterals (usually the lateromedial) are only undertaken as additional projections, providing information on a suspicious area in relation to the nipple. It is common practice to carry out a lateral projection when a positive malignant finding is noted.

Lateromedial

The mammography unit is positioned with the cassette vertical. The patient initially stands with the unaffected side nearest to the cassette holder and then steps towards it until the edge of the cassette is between the breasts. The lower border of the cassette should be 2.5 cm below the inferior aspect of the breast. The arm on the side under examination is raised and placed across the top of the cassette holder. The medial aspect of the breast is now in contact with the cassette holder. The radiographer lifts the breast to bring the nipple into profile, eliminating any skin folds. The inferior portion of the breast tissue, the main body of the breast and the nipple should all be included within the boundaries of the cassette. Compression is applied while the radiographer maintains the position of the breast, eliminating any skin folds.

Apply a lateral marker, relevant to the breast under examination, within the primary beam and on the axillary edge of the cassette holder.

Mediolateral

The mammography unit is positioned with the cassette vertical. The patient stands with the affected side nearest to the cassette holder and then steps towards it until the lateral aspect of the breast is in contact with the cassette holder. The lower border of the cassette should be 2.5 cm below the inferior aspect of the breast. The arm on the side under examination is raised and placed across the top of the cassette holder. The radiographer lifts the breast to bring the nipple into profile, eliminating any skin folds. The inferior portion of the breast tissue, the main body of the breast and the nipple should all be included within the boundaries of the cassette. The opposing breast is gently cleared from the field by the patient and compression applied while the radiographer maintains the position of the breast, eliminating any skin folds.

Apply a lateral marker, relevant to the breast under examination, within the primary beam and on the axillary edge of the cassette holder.

The key to a successful mammographic examination is a relaxed, cooperative patient. This will only be possible if the radiographer takes time to carefully explain the procedure and demonstrate the basic workings of the equipment.

Anatomical markers used in mammography often have legends which identify the projection and axillary location in addition to the side under examination.

Compression has the effect of pressing the breast into a more uniform density, improving image quality and reducing patient dose. Compression is applied while the radiographer maintains the position of the breast, sliding the fingers away when the paddle has made firm enough contact to support the breast. When compression is adequate, the breast tissue will feel firm.

Centring is not relevant as a separate point, as the central ray is permanently directed to the centre of the cassette. The orientation of the X-ray tube in relation to the breast utilizes the anode–heel effect, i.e. the anode end of the tube is towards the nipple.

Viewing of the images should be undertaken with identical projections of each breast 'back to back' with pectoral aspects touching, no gap between and the nipples at the outer edge. The right breast is displayed on the left side of the viewing box and the left breast on the right side, as though the viewer is looking at the patient from the front. Since an area of bright light around the image will apparently reduce contrast and imply overexposure (Ball and Price, 1989) there should be a facility for masking off the surrounding area on the viewing box.

Magnification is employed to provide additional information over suspicious areas and is useful to demonstrate minute microcalcification. The technique is really a macroradiography technique, and is achieved by inserting a platform over the cassette holder, on which the breast rests. A small compression paddle is often used in conjunction with this technique to offer increased compression over the relevant area, improving image quality. A fine focal spot is selected to reduce the level of geometric unsharpness (Fig. 10.3).

Localization prior to surgery

If a patient is to undergo surgical removal of a malignant area, the radiologist will localize the area with a fine needle and wire. Using the end of the wire as a reference, the surgeon will locate and remove the surrounding area. Localization takes place immediately before surgery. The procedure may vary according to the radiologist's preference. The next section describes one method of localization but other methods include the use of specialized stereotactic units or removal of the compression paddle during needle insertion.

Projections are undertaken with the patient seated and using a compression paddle which has radio-opaque reference marks and large holes or cut-out areas to allow needle insertion (Fig. 10.4). Two projections at 90° are required for this procedure – craniocaudal and lateral.

Images produced during assessment are viewed and the radiologist decides between a lateral or superoinferior needle approach. When this has been decided the patient is first positioned for the relevant projection, e.g. a superoinferior approach will warrant initial positioning for the craniocaudal projection. After the initial exposure is made, the marked compression paddle remains on the breast and the patient is asked to

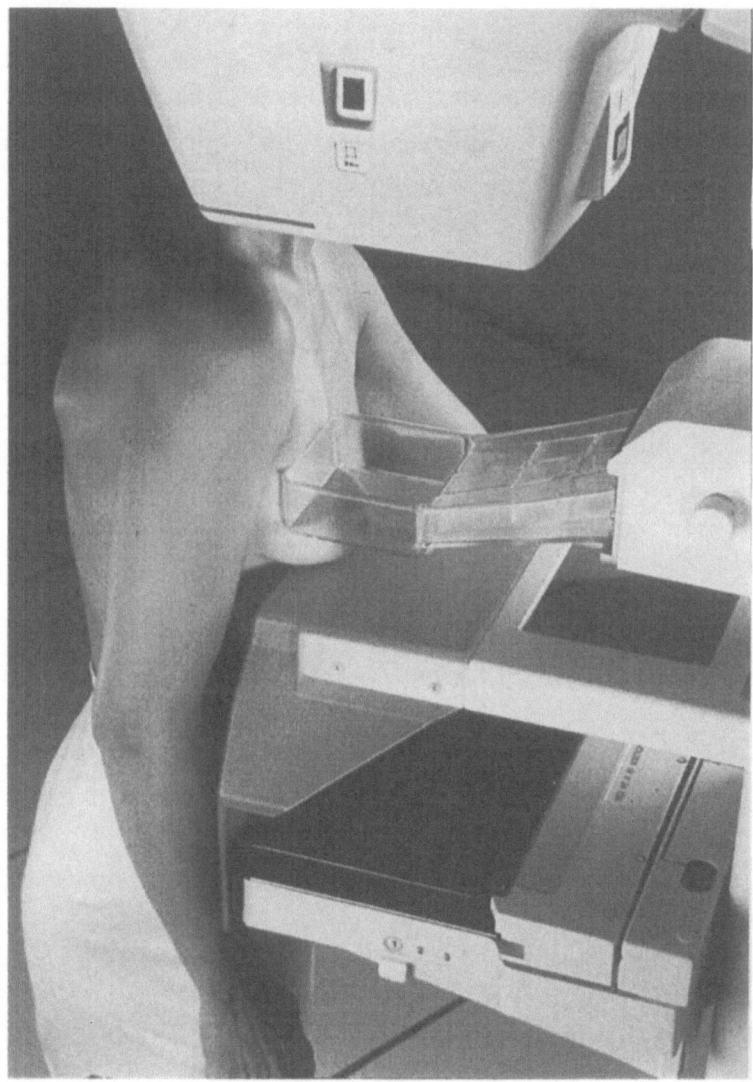

Figure 10.3 Craniocaudal 'magnification'. Courtesy of IGE.

keep very still. A very slight release of the paddle may be allowed if discomfort is intense. The image is viewed and, after reference to the markings on the paddle, skin cleansing and injection of local anaesthetic is followed by needle insertion into the appropriate area. While supporting the breast to avoid dislodging the needle, the unit is turned through 90° in order to carry out the second projection. The compression paddle is again left in place during film processing. The image is viewed to assess

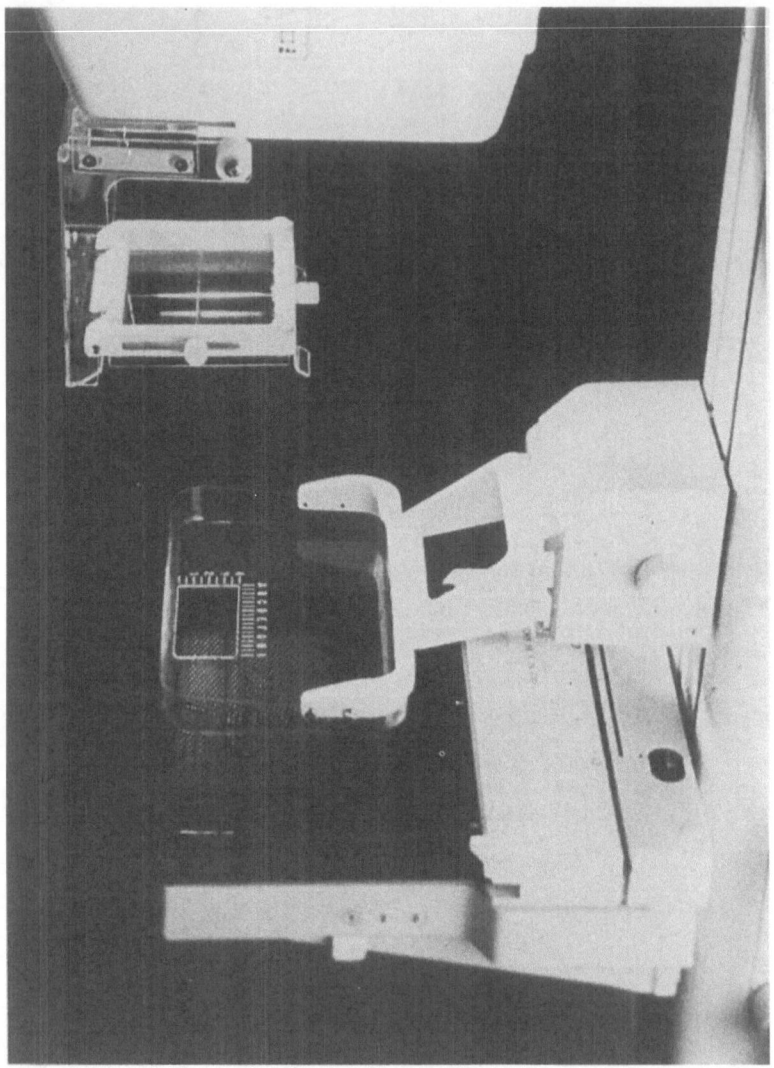

Figure 10.4 Mammography unit with compression paddle for lesion localization. Courtesy of IGE.

the position of the needle tip in relation to the area for excision, and the needle adjusted if necessary.

The fine wire is inserted into the lumen of the needle until the alignment indicator shows that the wire and needle tips are coincident. The needle is then withdrawn, leaving the wire in place. Another exposure is made with the patient in this position and the wire in place. The unit is returned to its original position and the first projection repeated with the wire in place. Care should be taken to ensure that the wire is not compressed by the paddle, but rather sticks out of one of the cut-out areas.

A dry dressing is applied to the area and the films are sent to theatre with the patient.

After surgery the excised area is returned for X-ray, usually a magnified projection. By studying the images of the 'lump', together with the presurgery localization radiographs, the radiologist will assess whether sufficient breast tissue has been removed, relaying the report immediately to the surgeon.

Regular routines for quality assurance

- Equipment service
- Sensitometry (daily)
- Phantom test tool exposure (e.g. LEEDS Test Object)
- Developer temperature check
- Developer and fixer replenishment rate check
- Processor cleaning (weekly)
- Film/screen contact test
- Light leakage test.

IMAGE EVALUATION

Correct patient identification and anatomical marker, indicating projection and position of axilla, included on the radiograph.

Area of interest

Craniocaudal

Nipple, as much breast tissue as possible and pectoral muscle.

Extended craniocaudal

Axillary tail, nipple and as much breast tissue as possible.

Mediolateral oblique

Axilla, axillary tail, pectoralis major and inframammary fold.

Lateral

Inferior and superior aspects of breast back to chest wall.

Projection

Craniocaudal

- Nipple in profile.

- Nipple positioned in 11 o'clock (right breast) or 1 o'clock position (left breast).
- Right and left craniocaudal projections are mirror images when viewed back to back.

Extended craniocaudal

- Nipple in profile.

Mediolateral oblique

- Nipple in profile.
- Pectoral muscle seen at 30° to vertical.
- Right and left pectorals are mirror images when viewed back to back.
- Nipple level with bottom of pectoral muscle.

Lateral

- Nipple in profile.
- Distance between nipple and lateral border of film is equal to that seen on craniocaudal projection.

Exposure factors

- kVp is selected to provide optimum contrast between the differing structures within the breast tissue.
- mAs to provide adequate image density to demonstrate fat, muscle and glandular tissue.

Inadequate compression will result in radiographs of varying density and/or underpenetrated appearance.

No evidence of patient movement.
No skin folds or artefacts present on the image.

FURTHER READING

Challen, V., Kapera, E., Manning, D. *et al*. (1990) *Breast Screening and Mammography*. Postrad.
Caseldine, J., Blamey, R., Roebuck, E. and Elston, C. (1989) *Breast Disease for Radiographers*. Wright, Bristol.
Lee, L., Stickland, V., Wilson, R. and Roebuck, E. (1995) *Fundamentals of Mammography*. Saunders.

Dental radiography 11

To avoid foreshortening/elongation and lateral overlap of tooth images, the angle of the patient's teeth should be assessed before commencing any examination. Although instructions for radiographic examination of the teeth often include guidelines for beam angulation, human dentition can vary immensely and assessment is therefore essential. Examining the interproximal margins between the teeth will give a fairly accurate indication of how to direct the beam in a mesiodistal direction (with the central ray in the horizontal position) in order to pass through the teeth at 90°. However, it is impossible to avoid overlapped images on patients with overlapped teeth. When assessing the angle of the long axis of the tooth, remember to look at the centre of the crown, not the longest cusp, which can cause confusion in premolars.

In September 1994, the NRPB published guidelines stating that there is no justification for the routine use of lead aprons 'in view of the very low effective doses involved in properly conducted dental radiography', and positively discourages their use during panoramic examinations (*BDA News*, 1994). In practice, the artefacts caused by incorrect placement of lead aprons during orthopantomography are a common cause of repeat radiographs, thereby doubling the radiation dose received by the patient. The NRPB also concludes that dental radiography poses no risk to female patients at any stage during pregnancy. While these recommendations should be adopted in all departments undertaking dental radiography, it may be necessary to provide lead aprons for those patients who remain unconvinced, particularly in the case of pregnant women.

RADIOGRAPHIC TECHNIQUE

Bitewings (Fig. 11.1)

Bitewings demonstrate the interproximal areas, crowns and gingival margins of the premolar and molar regions. Two radiographs are usually

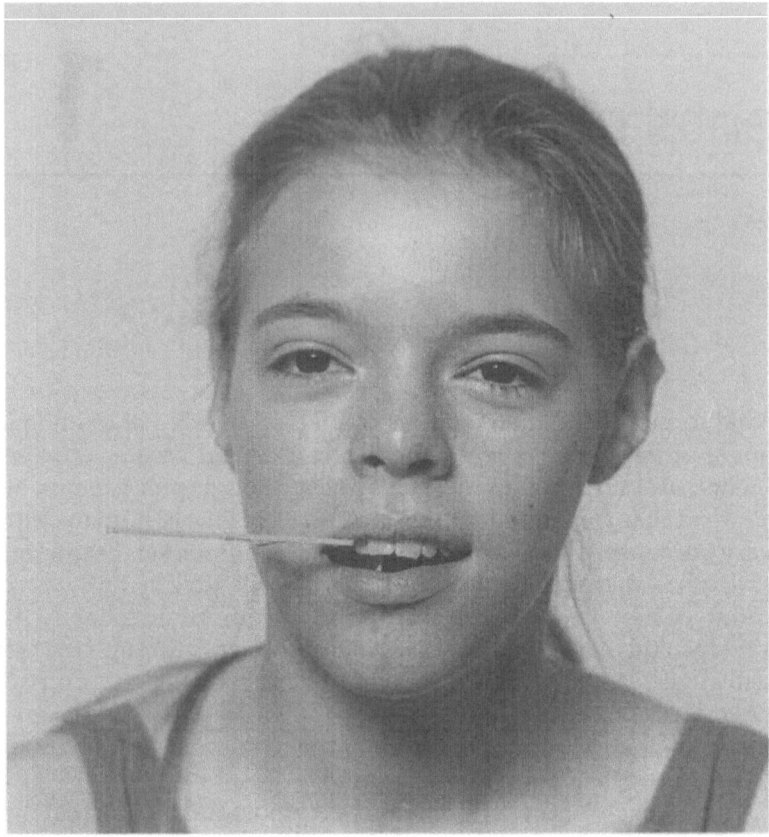

Figure 11.1 Bitewing holder positioned for right premolars. The rod indicates alignment for central ray.

sufficient to demonstrate each side: one to cover the premolars and first molar and the second to cover the three molars.

The patient is seated with their neck leaning on a support. A bitewing film, in a holder, is placed with its tube side in contact with the lingual surface of the teeth under examination as follows.

- for molars the second molars are in the middle of the film;
- for premolars the first premolars are in the middle of the film.

The patient is asked to close their teeth over the bitewing rod. The head is adjusted until the MSP is vertical and the upper occlusal plane horizontal.

CENTRING: A horizontal central ray, 90° to the buccal surface of the teeth and the film, is directed 5° caudally to the centre of the film.

Periapicals

Periapical radiographs demonstrate the crowns, roots and surrounding bone. Because of the gums around the root it is not possible to place the film in contact with the entire length of the tooth. This will unfortunately lead to distortion and magnification of some areas on the image. There are two techniques used for the periapical projection, paralleling and bisecting angle, each with its own advantages and disadvantages.

Paralleling technique (Fig. 11.2)

The patient is seated with their neck leaning on a support. The periapical film is placed in a paralleling film holder, longitudinally for incisors and canines, transversely for all other teeth. The film, in its holder, is placed in the mouth with the tube side facing the lingual surface of the teeth and the

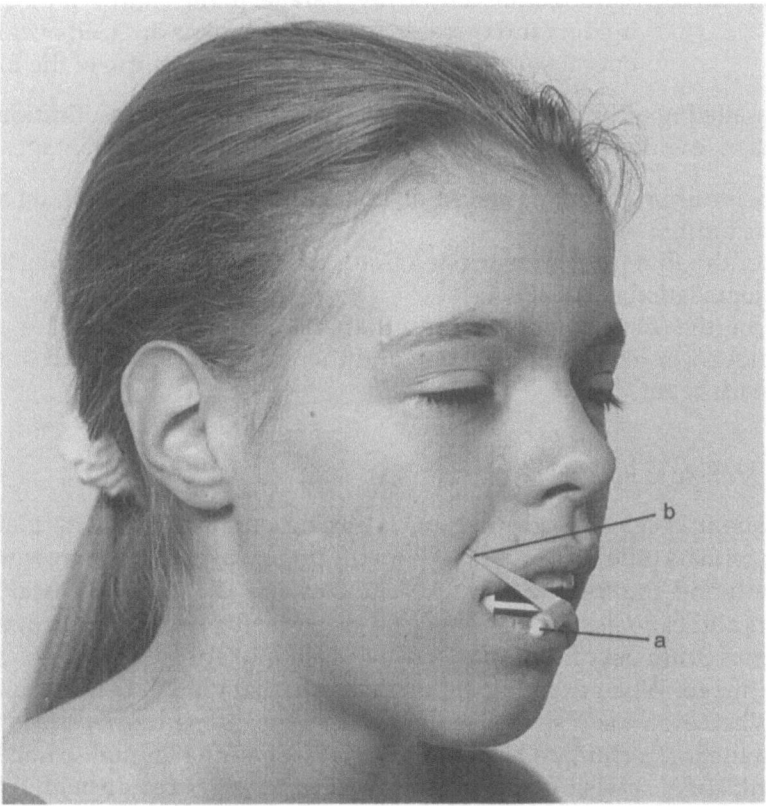

Figure 11.2 Paralleling technique for upper right premolars. The rod (a) indicates alignment for central ray and pointer. (b) indicates the centre of the film.

'pimple' towards the crowns. The film is parallel to the long axes of the teeth under examination, with the upper/lower edge of the film as high/low as possible to ensure inclusion of the roots as well as the crowns. In the case of the upper teeth the film may appear to be almost in the centre of the roof of the mouth. When examining a single tooth, that tooth is centred to the film. When examining several teeth the midline of the film is aligned as follows:

- all incisors – coincident with the MSP;
- second incisor to first premolar – behind the canine;
- first premolar to first molar – behind the second premolar;
- second premolar to third molar – behind the second molar.

The patient is asked to close their mouth over the film holder. The head is adjusted until the MSP is vertical and the upper occlusal plane is horizontal.

> CENTRING: A horizontal central ray, parallel to the handle of the film holder (and therefore 90° to the film), is directed over the buccal surfaces of the teeth and to the centre of the film.

The paralleling technique will unfortunately cause some magnification of the image, owing to increased OFD, but has the following advantages:

- there is minimum image distortion as the film is parallel to the long axis of the tooth;
- use of the film holder ensures accurate beam alignment, centring and immobilization of the film;
- use of the film holder ensures that the patient's fingers are not employed in film immobilization and therefore not in the path of the primary beam.

Bisecting angle technique

The patient is seated with their neck leaning on a support. The film is placed with its tube side in contact with the lingual aspect of the crowns of the teeth and the 'pimple' towards the crowns. The film is vertical for incisors and canines and transverse for other teeth. The occlusal edge of the film is 3 mm beyond the crowns of the teeth to ensure their inclusion on the image. When examining a single tooth, that tooth is centred to the film. When examining several teeth the film is positioned as described for the paralleling technique. The film is held against the lingual surface of the teeth and gum using Spencer–Wells forceps. A gauze pad behind the film will prevent damage by the forceps. The patient holds the forceps during exposure but should avoid excessive pressure, which may bend the film and damage the emulsion. The mouth remains open. The head is adjusted until the MSP is vertical and the occlusal plane relevant to the teeth under examination is horizontal.

CENTRING: A horizontal central ray is adjusted until at 90° to the bisector of the angle formed between the long axis of the tooth and the long axis of the film. It is also 90° to the film in the mesiodistal direction, and is directed over the buccal surfaces of the teeth to the centre of the film.

The following list gives a general guideline for beam angulations needed for the different teeth, but patients should be assessed individually to decide on angulation.

Upper teeth (Upper occlusal plane horizontal)
Incisors   –   55–60° caudally from the horizontal
Canines   –   45–50° caudally from the horizontal
Premolars   –   35–40° caudally from the horizontal
Molars   –   25–30° caudally from the horizontal

Lower teeth (Lower occlusal plane horizontal)
Incisors   –   25–30° cranially from the horizontal
Canines   –   15–20° cranially from the horizontal
Premolars   –   10° cranially from the horizontal
Molars   –   Beam horizontal

Although the bisecting angle technique requires no special equipment and is not so uncomfortable and bulky in the patient's mouth, it does have several disadvanatges.

- There will be some image distortion, as the X-ray beam is not perpendicular to the long axis of either the tooth or film. Bisection of the angle formed between the two will minimize this distortion.
- There is minimal magnification of the crown of the tooth, as the film lies in contact with it, but magnification of the root and neck is greater owing to the increased OFD.
- As the patient supports the film the hand is closer to the primary beam, increasing radiation dose, and as a means of immobilization is unreliable.

As NRPB recommendations (Royal College of Radiologists, 1994) state that film holders incorporating beam-aiming devices should be adopted by the year 2001, the technique of choice is paralleling.

Occlusals

Occlusals are taken to demonstrate the following.

70° Maxillary	Hard palate
	Upper incisors and canines
Oblique maxillary	Upper canines (unerupted)
	Premolars
Oblique mandibular	Lower canines (unerupted)
	Premolars
45° Submandibular	Symphysis menti
	Lower incisors
Submental	Submandibular ducts

The patient is seated with their neck leaning on a support. An occlusal film is placed in the mouth, transversely with tube side uppermost for maxillary teeth and down for mandibular teeth. (It may be necessary to use the film longitudinally for children, or when the mouth is narrow.) The film is pushed back as far as possible and at least to the first molars, with the incisors included anteriorly. The short axis of the film is coincident with the MSP. The mouth is closed on to the film and the head adjusted until the MSP is vertical. For maxillary and mandibular occlusals the occlusal plane is horizontal (Fig. 11.3a); for submental occlusal the

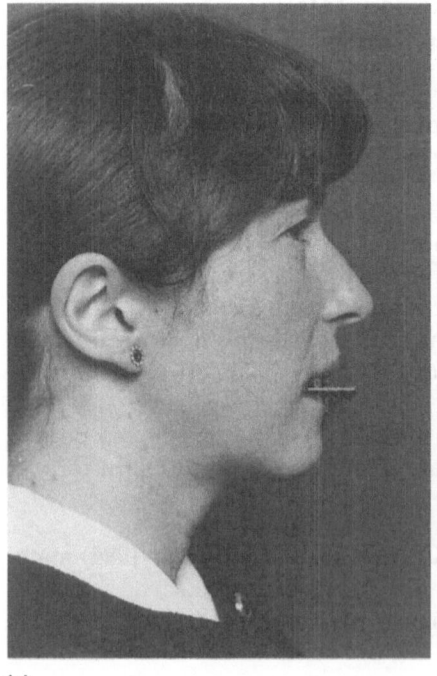 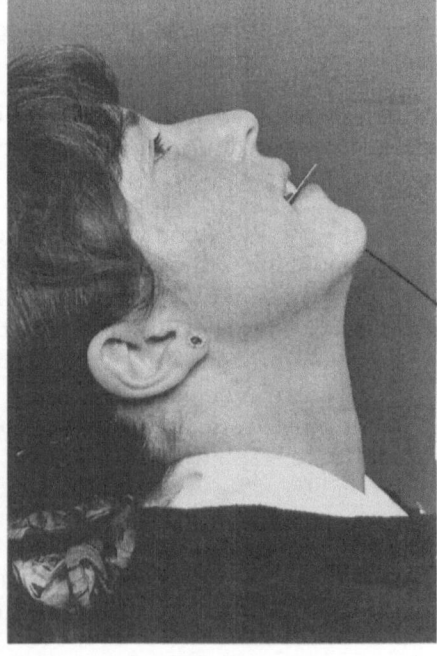

(a)   (b)

Figure 11.3 Positions for (a) maxillary and mandibular occlusals. (b) Submental occlusal.

neck is extended as far as possible to bring the occlusal plane towards the vertical, and the head and neck are supported in this position (Fig. 11.3b).

CENTRING: *70° Maxillary occlusal*

With the X-ray tube in front of the patient the vertical central ray is angled 20° towards the nose to make an angle of 70° to the film. The beam is directed over the superior aspect of the nose to emerge through the nasal septum over the centre of the film.

Oblique maxillary occlusal

The X-ray tube is opposite the outer canthus of the eye on the side under examination, the horizontal central ray parallel to the MSP. The X-ray beam is then angled 65° caudally and rotated 45° towards the MSP, and directed just lateral to the ala of the nose on the side under examination, to emerge over the centre of the film.

Oblique mandibular occlusal

The X-ray tube is opposite the corner of the mouth on the side under examination and the horizontal central ray is parallel to the MSP. The X-ray beam is then angled 45° cranially and rotated 45° towards the MSP, and directed over the inferior aspect of the mandible, below the corner of the mouth, to emerge over the centre of the film.

45° submandibular occlusal

With the X-ray tube in front of the patient, the horizontal central ray is angled 45° cranially through the symphysis menti to the centre of the film.

Submental occlusal

A horizontal central ray is adjusted until at 90° to the film and centred 3 cm behind the symphysis menti, to emerge over the centre of the film.

Extraoral oblique mandible

These projections require the use of cassettes and intensifying screens and can be carried out with a conventional X-ray tube as an alternative to dental equipment. The area covered lies from the canine to the third molar, and this examination is only carried out if orthopantomography equipment is not available. Both sides are examined for comparison.

An 18×24 cm cassette is placed transversely on the table top. The left-hand half of the cassette is masked off with lead–rubber. The patient is seated facing the table and a lead–rubber apron applied to the lower abdomen and legs as radiation protection. The patient leans over the table and places the left side of the face in contact with the right-hand side of the cassette. The neck is extended slightly to clear the ramus of the mandible from the cervical vertebrae. The chin, nose and cheek are in contact with the cassette, the nose and chin aligned with its right-hand edge. The lips are coincident with the centre of the short axis of the cassette.

CENTRING: A vertical central ray is angled 10° cranially, parallel to the line of the lips, to a point 7.5 cm behind the symphysis menti.

If the specific region of interest is the third molars, from the position described above the head is rotated slightly to bring the tip of the nose approximately 1 cm away from the cassette.

Orthopantomography

Figure 11.4 shows the OPT unit at rest. Using the 'test' setting, movement of the unit is demonstrated to the patient before the examination commences. The unit is then returned to the start position.

An OPT cassette is placed in the cassette holder and a disposable bite rod/cover is inserted. The patient is seated or standing with their chin resting well forward on the support. The patient is instructed to place their incisors into the notches on the bite rod and bite gently. The head is adjusted until the MSP is vertical and perpendicular to the bite rod. The chin rest/height of the unit is adjusted until the occlusal plane is horizontal. The patient is asked to step forward slightly to bring the cervical spine vertical (if seated, they are pulled forward by the radiographer). Head clamps are applied for immobilization. The patient is asked to press their tongue against the roof of the mouth and to maintain this during tube movement. Exposure is made with constant reminders to the patient to keep still.

Many units are fitted with slit light devices which are aligned to the MSP, occlusal plane and canines to ensure that the patient is positioned correctly within the OPT machine.

Cephalometry

For faciomaxillary surgery and orthodontics it is necessary to examine the soft tissues of the face, facial bones and teeth simultaneously. After initial radiographs assessment is made at regular intervals during treatment, and therefore it is essential that all images are comparable. To minimize variation, equipment is designed to ensure that consistent images are produced. Facilities include a fixed FOD (minimum 150 cm to minimize magnification and geometric unsharpness) and head clamps with ear plugs which fit into the EAMs to ensure accurate and consistent positioning. On some units the OFD can be altered, and in these cases a

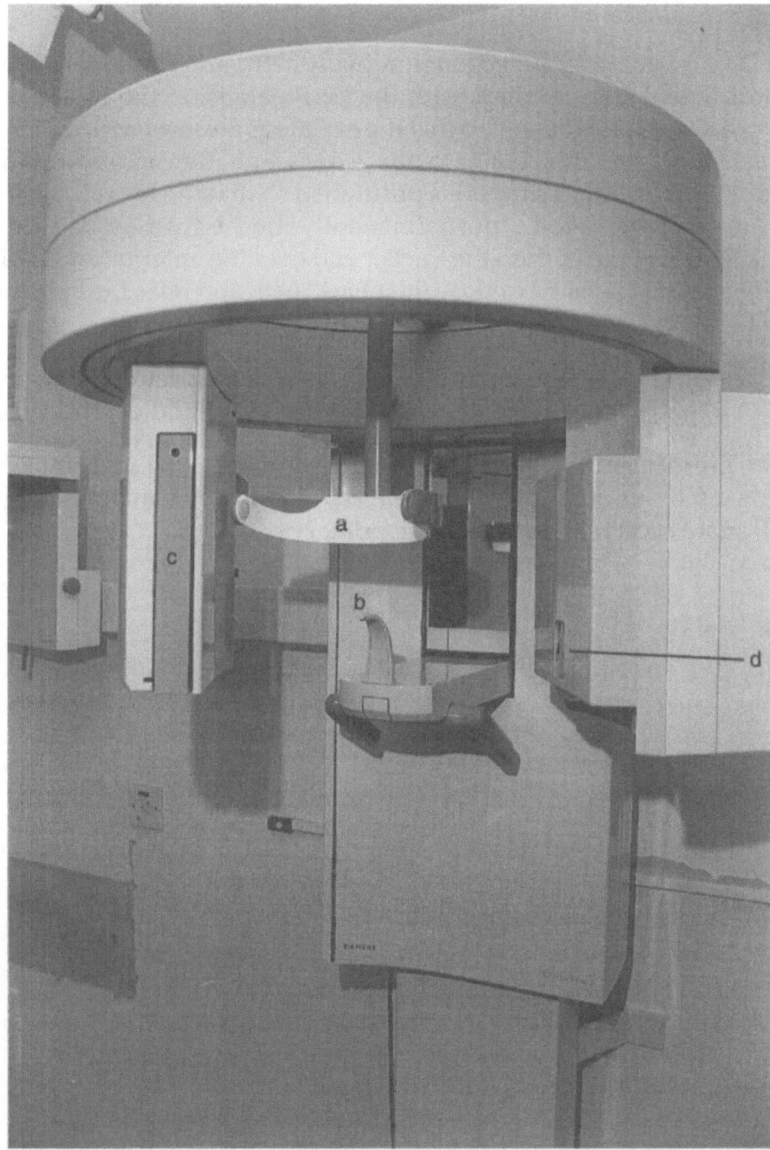

Figure 11.4   OPT unit at rest. a, forehead rest; b, bite rod; c, cassette holder; d, slit beam diaphragm.

marked nasion support (an inverted L-shaped support, marked at 1 mm intervals for accurate reference during assessment) should be used.

To compensate for the range in density from facial soft tissue to facial bones, a filter is used. This can be an aluminium wedge attached to the light beam diaphragm or may be inherent within the tube head.

Lateral cephalogram

A 24×30 cm cassette is placed longitudinally in the erect cassette holder on the unit. The patient is erect, with the MSP parallel to the cassette. The height of the unit is adjusted so that the ear-plugs are level with the EAMs. The ear-plugs are inserted into the EAMs and the occlusal plane is horizontal. The nasion support is positioned so that the horizontal line of the 'L' rests on the nasion. If not permanently attached to the tube head, the wedge filter is inserted with the thicker end over the anterior aspect of the face. The patient is asked to close their back teeth and relax the lips during exposure.

CENTRING: The horizontal beam, at 90° to the cassette, is directed to the centre of the ear-plugs, over the middle of the cassette.

Unless preset, as may be the case with specialized units, collimate to include soft tissue outlines of the forehead, face/nose and mandible. Apply an AP anatomical marker within the primary beam.

IMAGE EVALUATION

Film(s) correctly orientated and mounted and marked with the patient's details.

Area of interest

Bitewings

Crowns of teeth and alveolar crests between them.

Periapicals

Full length of tooth from crown to apex, and surrounding alveolar bone and periodontal membrane.

70° maxillary occlusal

Anterior arch of maxillary teeth back to first molars.

Oblique maxillary occlusal

Full length of incisors, canines and premolars, including crowns, apices and surrounding alveolar bone.

Oblique mandibular occlusal

Canines and premolars of side under examination.

45° submandibular occlusal

Symphysis menti and anterior mandibular arch back to first molars.

Submental occlusal

Mandibular arch, including incisors and first molars.

Extraoral oblique mandible

Mandibular teeth from canines to third molars on side under examination.

Orthopantomogram

Full mandible, including symphysis menti, rami, bodies and temporomandibular joints, palate and inferior border of maxillary sinuses.

Lateral cephalogram

Frontal sinus, symphysis menti, soft tissue outline of face, including nose and posterior border of ramus of mandible.

Projection

Bitewings

- No evidence of elongation or foreshortening of teeth.
- No overlap of adjacent teeth.
- Slight separation of occlusal surfaces of opposing teeth.

Periapicals

- No evidence of elongation or foreshortening of tooth.
- No overlap of adjacent teeth.
- Tooth under examination centralized on film.

70° maxillary occlusal

- Foreshortening of incisors and canines, with premolars and molars demonstrated axially.
- Symmetry of maxillary arch about MSP.

Oblique maxillary occlusal

- Elongation of incisors, canines and premolars of side under examination.
- 'Flattening out' of dental arch on side under examination, demonstrating area from incisors to premolars.
- Superimposition of teeth of opposite side, from incisors backwards.

Oblique mandibular occlusal

- 'Flattening out' of mandibular arch of side under examination.
- Superimposition of teeth of opposite side, from incisors to premolars.
- Elongation of incisors and canines, with foreshortening of premolars.

45° submandibular occlusal

- Demonstration of symphysis menti, with foreshortening of lower incisors.
- Superimposition of teeth over mandible, from canines to molars.

Submental occlusal

- Mandibular arch demonstrated in profile, with foreshortening of incisors and canines.
- Distal premolars and molars projected over lingual aspect of mandible.

Extraoral oblique mandible

- Side remote from film projected anterior and superior to side under examination, demonstrating area from canines to third molars.
- Ramus of mandible and distal teeth projected clear of cervical vertebrae.

Orthopantomogram

- Occlusal surface between upper and lower teeth horizontal.
- Bite block seen between upper and lower central incisors, ensuring slight separation of occlusal surfaces of teeth.
- Tongue resting against palate and not casting an image over upper teeth.
- All teeth of both arches in focus.

- Central teeth slightly obscured by superimposition of image of cervical vertebrae.
- Outline of mandible smooth, with no 'steps'.

Lateral cephalogram

- Superimposition of images of right and left ear-plugs and of right and left facial structures.
- Anthropological baseline horizontal.

Exposure factors

All projections except lateral cephalogram

- kVp sufficient to demonstrate the roots of the teeth within the alveolar bone, maintaining contrast between the pulp cavity, enamel, lamina dura and surrounding bone.
- mAs to provide adequate image density to demonstrate detail of all areas of the teeth in contrast to the surrounding membranes and bone.

Lateral cephalogram

- kVp sufficient to demonstrate bony trabeculae within the mandible, maintaining contrast between the bony structures, air-filled sinuses and soft tissues. The use of the filter facilitates the demonstration of bony detail and soft tissue outlines of the face on the same image.
- mAs to provide adequate image density to demonstrate bony detail in contrast to the soft tissue outlines of the face.

No evidence of patient movement.

In dental radiography metal fillings are common, unavoidable artefacts, as is the film holder, which may be seen on the film when employing the paralleling technique. Only those artefacts which are not removable should be visible.

Positional faults

Bitewings and periapicals:

- Elongation or foreshortening of the tooth/teeth under examination indicates that the occlusal plane was not horizontal, or that the vertical angulation of the X-ray beam in relation to the teeth/film was incorrect.

- Overlap of adjacent teeth indicates that the X-ray beam was not perpendicular to the buccal surface of the dental arch and film.

Orthopantomogram:

- The commonest fault on OPT radiographs tends to be caused by incorrect positioning of the occlusal plane – a 'smiling' image indicates that the chin was positioned too low, while an 'inverted smile' indicates that the chin was raised too high.
- Narrow, unsharp incisors indicate that the patient was too far forward into the machine; broad, unsharp incisors indicate that the patient was too far back.
- An irregular, 'wavy' outline to the mandible indicates that the patient has moved during exposure.

Contrast examinations 12

INTRODUCTION

The following five points must always be checked prior to administering any contrast agent to a patient.

Type – Water-soluble or oil-based. Water-soluble contrast agents should be non-ionic low osmolar compounds, as with ionic high osmolar compounds the risk of adverse patient reaction is considerably increased, a consequence that should no longer be tolerated in light of the range of 'safer' contrast agents now available.

Concentration – The iodine content 'strength' of the solution, measured in mg/ml.

Dosage – The amount of contrast agent to be administered, measured in ml.

Temperature – Warming contrast agents intended for intravascular use reduces their viscosity, making them physically easier to inject. Warming the contrast to body temperature prior to injection reduces the risk of adverse reaction caused by introducing a cold solution into the warm bloodstream. Mixing barium enema solutions with warm water will reduce the likelihood of bowel spasm as the contrast agent is introduced.

Condition – The contrast agent should only be used if the tamperproof seal is intact and the label can be clearly read. Water-soluble agents should be clear fluids containing no foreign articles and with no evidence of crystallization.

Expiry date – All contrast agents are marked with the date of manufacture, batch number and the date of expiry; they should not be used beyond the expiry date.

Patient preparation for abdominal contrast examinations varies according to departmental protocol. Commonly, the patient has nil by mouth for 6–12 hours before the examination, e.g. for biliary, renal and upper gastrointestinal procedures. In the case of the barium enema the patient is given laxatives to clear the large bowel and instructed to follow a low-residue diet for 2 days prior to the examination. For the oral cholecystogram the patient ingests the contrast agent 12 hours before attending for examination.

INTRAVENOUS UROGRAPHY

Radiographic examination of the urinary tract following the intravenous injection of a radio-opaque contrast agent.

Contrast agent: 50 ml water-soluble non-ionic low osmolar compound, 300/370 mgI/ml. 1.5 ml/kg body weight for a child, up to a maximum of 50 ml.

Trolley setting:
50 ml syringe
Contrast agent
Tourniquet
Alcohol-impregnated swabs
19G butterfly needle
Adhesive tape
Sticking plaster.

RADIOGRAPHIC TECHNIQUE

Supine – kidneys, ureters and bladder (KUB)

A 35×43 cm cassette is placed longitudinally in the table bucky. The patient lies supine on the table, MSP coincident with and perpendicular to its midline. The ASISs are equidistant from the table top. The arms are abducted, resting at the patient's sides. With the FFD set at 100 cm and the bucky tray fully out, the vertical X-ray beam is centred to the middle of the cassette and collimated to its longitudinal and transverse limits. The bucky tray is pushed under the table and the X-ray tube centred to it transversely. The X-ray tube or patient is moved until the superior border of the symphysis pubis is 2.5 cm above the lower border of collimation.

> CENTRING: The vertical X-ray beam, at 90° to the cassette, will be directed over the midline, at the approximate level of the iliac crests, to include the symphysis pubis on the image.

The cassette is aligned with the X-ray beam. Collimate to include symphysis pubis, bladder, renal outlines and lateral abdominal walls. Apply an AP anatomical marker within the primary beam. Expose on arrested expiration.

The upper border of the symphysis pubis lies level with the greater trochanters, approximately 10 cm inferior to the ASISs, although this will vary according to patient build and sex.

Upper tract ('cross-kidney')

A 24×30 cm or 30×40 cm cassette is placed transversely in the table bucky. The patient lies supine as above. A lead–rubber sheet is placed over the patient's lower abdomen as radiation protection. The centre of the short axis of the cassette is level with a point midway between the xiphisternum and the lower costal margins.

> CENTRING: A vertical central ray, at 90° to the cassette, is directed over the midline midway between the xiphisternum and the lower costal margins.

Collimate to include renal outlines and upper third of ureters. Apply an AP anatomical marker within the primary beam. Expose on arrested expiration.

Bladder

An 18×24 cm or 24×30 cm cassette is placed longitudinally in the table bucky. The patient lies supine as for the KUB projection.

> CENTRING: A vertical central ray is directed 15° caudally over the midline midway between the ASISs and the upper border of the symphysis pubis.

The cassette is displaced so that its centre coincides with the central X-ray beam. Collimate to include lower ends of ureters, bladder and symphysis pubis. Apply an AP anatomical marker within the primary beam.

Posterior oblique kidney (Fig. 12.1)

An 18×24 cm cassette is placed longitudinally in the table bucky. The patient lies supine as for the KUB projection and is rotated through 30°, towards the side under examination. The arm of the side under examination rests on the pillow and radiolucent pads support the raised side under the shoulder and pelvis. The leg on the raised side is flexed at the knee, with the foot resting on the table for comfort and stability. A lead–rubber sheet is placed across the lower abdomen as radiation protection. The centre of the long axis of the cassette is level with the midpoint between the xiphisternum and lower costal margins.

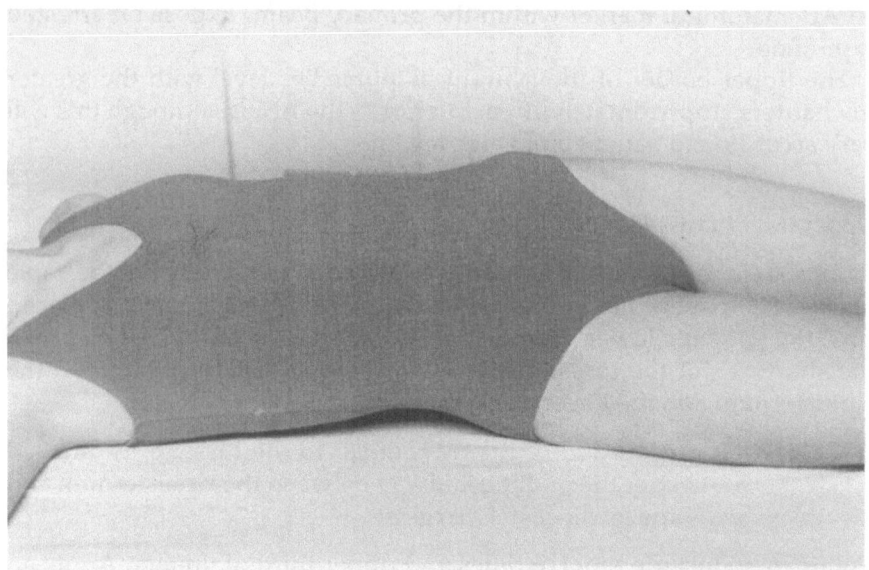

Figure 12.1   Right posterior oblique – renal tract.

CENTRING: A vertical central ray, at 90° to the cassette, is directed over the midline, midway between the xiphisternum and the lower costal margins.

Collimate to include the renal outline of the side under examination and upper third of the ureter. Apply an AP anatomical marker within the primary beam. Expose on arrested expiration.

Prone abdomen (Fig. 12.2)

A 35×43 cm cassette is placed longitudinally in the table bucky. The patient lies prone, with the MSP coincident with and perpendicular to the long axis of the table. The PSISs are equidistant from the table top. The head is turned to one side and the arms raised on to the pillow for comfort. With the FFD set at 100 cm and the bucky tray fully out, the vertical X-ray beam is centred to the middle of the cassette and collimated to its longitudinal and transverse limits. The bucky tray is pushed under the table and the X-ray tube centred to it transversely. The X-ray tube or patient is moved until the coccyx lies within the lower border of collimation.

CENTRING: The vertical X-ray beam, at 90° to the cassette, will be directed over the midline, at the approximate level of the iliac crests, to include the symphysis pubis on the image.

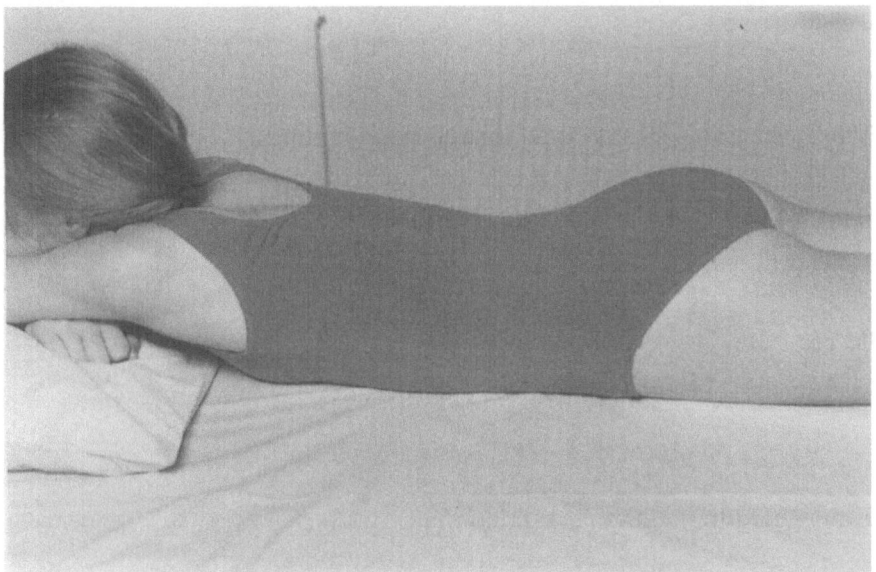

Figure 12.2 Prone abdomen.

The cassette is aligned with the X-ray beam. Collimate to include symphysis pubis, bladder, renal outlines and lateral abdominal walls. Apply a PA anatomical marker within the primary beam. Expose on arrested expiration.

Posterior oblique bladder/lower end of ureter (Fig. 12.1)

A 24×30 cm cassette is placed transversely in the table bucky. The patient lies supine as for the KUB projection and is rotated through 30°, away from the side under examination. Radiolucent pads support the raised side, under the trunk and thighs. The leg on the raised side is flexed at the knee, with the foot resting on the table for comfort and stability.

CENTRING: A vertical central ray is directed 15° caudally to a point midway between the upper border of the symphysis pubis and the ASIS on the raised side.

Collimate to include lower ends of ureters, bladder and symphysis pubis. Apply an AP anatomical marker within the primary beam.

The cystoureteric junction of the raised side will be demonstrated.

IMAGE EVALUATION

Correct patient identification and anatomical marker included on the radiograph.

Area of interest

Supine and prone abdomen

Symphysis pubis, base of bladder and renal outlines.

Upper tract

Renal outlines.

Bladder

Symphysis pubis, base of bladder and sacrum.

Posterior oblique kidney

Outline of kidney under examination.

Posterior oblique bladder/lower end of ureter

Symphysis pubis, base of bladder and lower ends of ureters.

Projection

Supine and prone abdomen and upper tract

- Long axis of spine coincident with midline of film.
- Spinous processes demonstrated down centre of vertebral bodies.
- Diaphragm demonstrated above level of T10.
- Inclusion of appropriate timing and patient orientation legend.

Bladder

- Spinous tubercles projected down centre of sacrum.
- Ischial spines prominent on circumference of pelvic inlet.
- Superimposition of superior and inferior pubic rami with associated narrowing of obturator foramina.
- Symmetry of left and right halves of pelvic inlet.
- Inclusion of appropriate timing legend.

Posterior oblique kidney

- Spinous processes projected towards side of spine opposite to that of kidney under examination.
- Ribs on side under examination 'flattened out'.

- Kidney under examination demonstrated in profile close to spinal column.
- Inclusion of appropriate timing legend.

Posterior oblique bladder/lower end of ureter

- Ilium of side closer to table demonstrated *'en face'*.
- Superimposition of pubic rami and ischium of side closer to table.
- Obturator foramen of side closer to table 'closed', with that on raised side demonstrated *'en face'*.
- Inclusion of appropriate timing legend.

Exposure factors

Optimum contrast is essential in order to differentiate between the abdominal viscera.

- kVp sufficient to penetrate bony structures and demonstrate the bony trabeculae within them, while maximizing image contrast caused by the differential absorption of soft tissue structures at lower kVp. The introduction of the intravenous contrast agent will enhance contrast between the organs of the urinary system and the other abdominal viscera.
- mAs to provide adequate image density to demonstrate the organs of the urinary system in contrast to the bony pelvis and spine and the other soft tissue structures within the abdomen.

No evidence of patient movement or breathing during exposure.
No artefacts present on the image.

Typical series

A typical series of projections for a routine IVU, together with reasons for inclusion, is as follows.

Prior to contrast

Control (full length renal tract):

- to assess the exposure factors prior to injection of the contrast agent;
- to demonstrate the presence of any radio-opaque renal calculi which may be obscured following the introduction of the contrast agent;

- to identify the position of the kidneys to ensure the demonstration of the complete renal outlines on the post contrast images;
- to demonstrate any gross pathology within the abdominal cavity.

If the full length of the renal tract – upper poles of kidneys and base of bladder – is not demonstrated on the control radiograph, it will be necessary to carry out a separate cross-kidney or bladder projection.

Post-contrast

Immediate ('cross-kidney'):

- The 'renal blush'/nephrogram, as the contrast agent first reaches the renal cortex, demonstrates the contours of the renal outlines and the comparative rate of excretion of both kidneys.

5-minute ('cross-kidney'):

- a second chance to demonstrate the renal outlines if not clearly visualized on the immediate film;
- visualization of the renal calyces and pelvises, allowing a comparison of the excretion rates of the kidneys.

If the 5-minute radiograph does not adequately demonstrate the calyces, a compression device is applied on either side of the midline, at the level of the ASISs, in order to compress the ureters against the pelvic brim, preventing the flow of contrast agent into the bladder.
  5 minutes following application of compression ('cross-kidney'):

- Demonstrates the anatomy and relative physiology of the pelvicalyceal collecting systems and proximal ureters distended with contrast agent.

15 minutes/compression release abdomen:

- This demonstrates the collecting systems, full length of ureters and bladder enhanced with contrast agent.

Full bladder (collimated):

- Demonstrates the anatomy of the bladder.

Post-micturition (collimated bladder or full abdomen):

- Demonstrates any residual volume or reflux of contrast into the ureters after emptying the bladder.
- Emptying the bladder causes the upper tracts to drain, demonstrating

parts of the ureters not seen on the *15 minutes/compression release* radiograph.

Additional projections may be necessary for a complete examination.
Oblique kidney:

- Demonstrates the kidney free of overlying gas or faecal matter.
- Allows the differentiation of renal calculi within the collecting system or renal cortex.

Oblique bladder:

- Demonstrates the cystoureteric junction clear of the overlying bladder – a common site of ureteric obstruction.
- Demonstrates irregularities in the outline of the bladder.

Prone abdomen:

- May demonstrate the exact site of ureteric obstruction and aid emptying of the upper renal tract.

Certain conditions/situations dictate a change to this routine. Typical examples are as follows.
Renal colic/emergency IVU/trauma

- full-length control, immediate cross-kidney, no compression applied, 10-minute full length, full-length post-micturition;

Delayed excretion of one or both kidneys

- full-length control, immediate and 5-minute cross-kidney, no compression applied, 15-minute full-length, full-length post-micturition once contrast reaches the bladder, delayed films at 0.5–1 hour intervals for as long as necessary;

Spina bifida

- full-length control, immediate and 5-minute cross-kidney, no compression applied, 20-minute full-length, post-micturition;

Post-renal transplant

- full-length control, immediate, 10-minute and post-micturition collimated to the transplanted kidney, no compression applied;

Children

- patient given a fizzy drink during the injection to take their mind off the needle, counter any feeling of warmth due to the contrast and produce a 'gas window' for clearer visualization of the kidneys, particularly the left. Full-length control, 5-minute cross-kidney, no compression applied, 10-minute full-length, post-micturition (Gyll and Blake, 1986).

Respiration and radio-opaque opacities

The full-length and 'cross-kidney' radiographs should be exposed on arrested expiration in order to demonstrate the kidneys in their normal position in relation to the other abdominal viscera. If the full-length control demonstrates opacities within the renal outlines, a separate cross-kidney projection in the opposite phase of respiration will be necessary to differentiate between renal calculi and calcification within the costal cartilages or other areas of the abdomen. Opacities within the kidneys will appear to move with the kidneys on inspiration, maintaining the same position in relation to the renal outlines, whereas calcification elsewhere will appear in a different position in relation to the kidneys. An oblique projection of the suspect kidney will also demonstrate whether calcification lies within or outside the renal outline, although as this entails a complete change in patient position it is more time-consuming and less convenient.

Tomography

Tomography of the kidneys may be carried out at any stage of the examination following the introduction of the contrast agent to demonstrate the kidneys more clearly, free of overlying bowel gas and faeces. The patient is positioned for a 'cross-kidney' projection and the tomography equipment prepared.

Pivot height = 8–11 cm above the table top for an average-sized adult.
Movement = 20° circular or linear.

Zonography, i.e. tomography using an exposure angle of <10° to produce relatively thick layers, lends itself particularly well to the renal tract. It is most commonly used to demonstrate the renal area in a single cut, blurring out the overlying bowel shadows.

BILIARY SYSTEM

ORAL CHOLECYSTOGRAPHY

Radiographic examination of the gallbladder and biliary ducts following the ingestion of a radio-opaque contrast agent.

Contrast agent: An oral biliary contrast agent in capsule or powder form. Although the numbers of referrals for cholecystography have fallen over the last 10–15 years, they are still carried out in some centres. It is for this reason that they are included in this text.

Prior to booking the examination it should be ascertained that the patient has not previously undergone cholecystectomy or, where records are available, that their serum bilirubin level is not too high to allow concentration of the contrast agent. Chapman and Nakielny (1993) indicate that bilirubin levels in excess of 34 μmol/l will cause the examination to be unsuccessful.

RADIOGRAPHIC TECHNIQUE

Prior to irradiating the patient the radiographer should check that the instructions relating to diet and taking of the contrast agent have been followed.

Left anterior oblique – prone (Fig. 12.3)

A 24×30 cm cassette is placed longitudinally in the table bucky. The patient lies prone, MSP perpendicular to the table top, with their head turned to the right, the right arm placed on the pillow and the left arm resting at the side of the trunk. The patient is rotated to raise the right side through 20°. Radiolucent pads support the raised side and the right leg is flexed slightly at the knee and hip for support. The centre of the long axis of the cassette is 5 cm above the level of the iliac crests. A lead–rubber sheet is placed across the patient's lower abdomen, below the level of the ASISs, as radiation protection.

> CENTRING: A vertical central ray, at 90° to the cassette, is directed midway between the spine and right flank, 5 cm above the level of the lower costal margin.
>
> Gallbladder position, and therefore centring point, will vary according to patient build:
> *thin patients* – centring will be lower and closer to the midline;
> *large patients* – centring will be higher and closer to the flank.

Collimate to include right lateral abdominal wall, spine, right iliac crest and 11th rib. Apply a right PA anatomical marker and a 'prone' legend within the primary beam. Mark the centring point with a cross as a reference point for when examining the gallbladder and ducts after the patient has been given a 'fatty meal'. Expose on arrested expiration.

For oral cholecystography an erect version of this projection is also carried out. Although the patient is standing, positioning is as for the

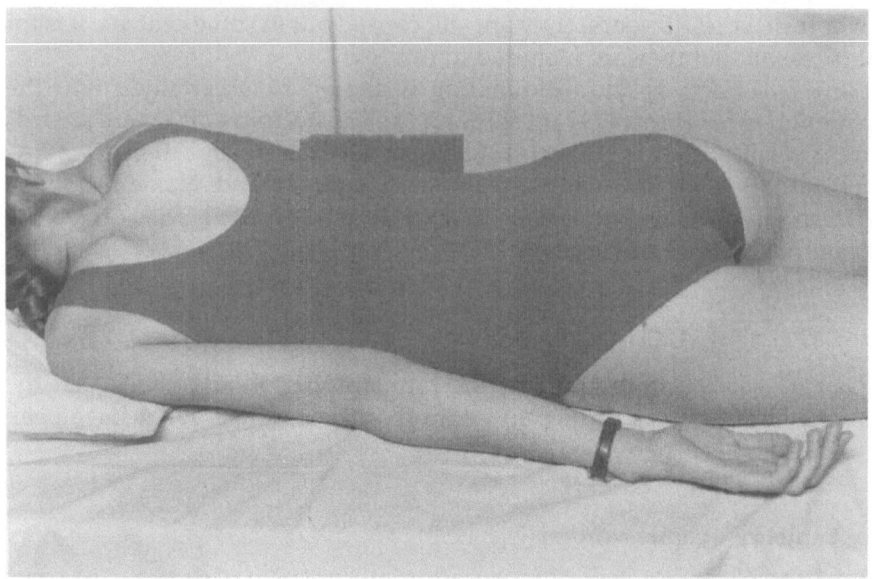

Figure 12.3   Left anterior oblique – biliary system.

prone anterior oblique projection. However, the gallbladder will drop slightly from its original position in the abdomen. Lowering the centring point by 5 cm from the prone oblique projection will compensate for the change in gallbladder position. An 'erect' legend is applied within the primary beam.

Right posterior oblique – supine (Fig. 12.4)

A 24×30 cm cassette is placed longitudinally in the table bucky. The patient lies supine on the table, MSP perpendicular to the table top. The patient is rotated, raising the left side through 20°. The right arm rests on the pillow and radiolucent pads support the left side under the pelvis and shoulder. The left leg is flexed at the hip and knee, with the foot resting on the table for stability. The centre of the long axis of the cassette is 5 cm above the level of the iliac crests. A lead–rubber sheet is placed over the patient's lower abdomen, below the level of the ASISs, as radiation protection.

> CENTRING: A vertical central ray, at 90° to the cassette, is directed midway between the midline and right flank, 5 cm above the level of the lower costal margin. As for the LAO projection, the centring point will vary according to patient build.

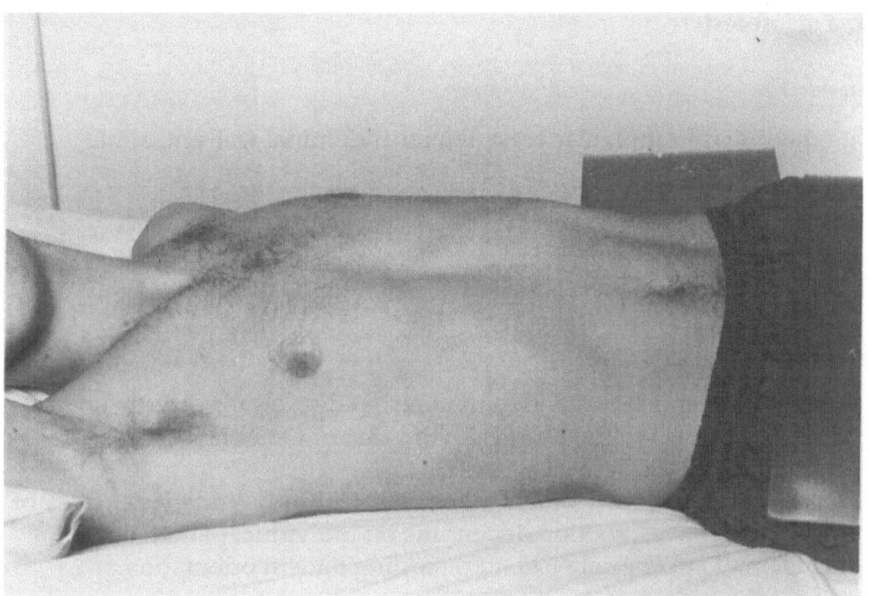

Figure 12.4 Right posterior oblique – biliary system.

Collimate to include right flank, spine, right iliac crest and 11th rib. Apply an AP anatomical marker and 'supine' legend within the primary beam.

As for the LAO projection, mark the centring point with a cross for reference for the 'after fatty meal' image. Expose on arrested expiration.

'After fatty meal'

After viewing initial projections with contrast, the projection(s) which most adequately demonstrate(s) the gallbladder is/are selected for 'after fatty meal' image(s).

The gallbladder may not fall in the centre of the initial radiographs and centring for the 'after fatty meal' film(s) should be revised, if necessary, by viewing the LAO/RPO projections and using the cross marked on the patient's skin as a landmark. By centralizing the gallbladder on this image it is possible to use an 18×24 cm cassette and collimate accordingly.

IMAGE EVALUATION

Correct patient identification and anatomical marker included on the radiograph.

Area of interest

Left anterior and right posterior obliques

Right hemidiaphragm, iliac crest, lateral abdominal wall and spine.

'After fatty meal'

Gallbladder and cystic duct.

Projection

- Vertebrae demonstrated down medial edge of film, with spinous processes projected towards left-hand side of vertebral bodies.
- 'Flattening out' of right ribs.
- Opacified gallbladder should be visible within boundaries of area of interest, the exact position depending on individual patient build.
- Inclusion of appropriate legend regarding patient orientation.

'After fatty meal'

- Gallbladder and cystic duct are demonstrated in centre of image.
- Inclusion of 'AFM' and appropriate patient orientation legend.

Exposure factors

Optimum contrast is essential in order to differentiate between the abdominal viscera.

- kVp sufficient to demonstrate bony trabeculae within the iliac crest and spine, while maximizing image contrast caused by the differential absorption of soft tissue structures at lower kVp. Opacification of the ingested contrast agent will enhance contrast between the biliary system and other abdominal viscera.
- mAs to provide adequate image density to demonstrate the gallbladder and cystic duct in contrast to the bony pelvis and spine and other soft tissue structures within the abdomen.

No evidence of patient movement or breathing during the exposure.
No artefacts present on the image.

INTRAVENOUS CHOLANGIOGRAPHY

Radiographic examination of the gallbladder (if present) and biliary ducts following the introduction of a radio-opaque contrast agent.

Contrast agent: An intravenous biliary contrast agent for infusion (50–85 mgI/ml) or bolus injection (175–180 mgI/ml).

Trolley setting:
Contrast agent for infusion or injection
Connecting tube and air inlet for infusion technique
Syringe for bolus injection technique
Tourniquet
Alcohol-impregnated swabs
19G butterfly needle
Adhesive tape
Sticking plaster.

Techniques used for intravenous cholangiography do not need to be described separately, as the projections used are either the right posterior oblique or left anterior oblique as described for oral cholecystography.

Initially, a 'control' LAO or RPO projection is taken. This is repeated after intravenous infusion or bolus injection of the contrast agent. Frequently the biliary system shows poor concentration of the contrast agent, and conventional tomography may be selected as a supplementary technique. The patient is positioned as for the RPO or LAO projection, with the height of the tomographic axis in relationship to the table top set at 12 cm for the RPO and 9 cm for the LAO. These heights are approximate, for patients of 'average' build, and will vary according to patient thickness. A circular movement is the tube movement of choice in order to avoid the linear streaking effect, with a minimum of 20° angle of swing selected in order to provide image 'slices' narrow enough to provide detailed demonstration of the area. If a circular movement is not available then a 20° linear movement is acceptable.

Exposure is made on arrested expiration and the initial tomogram viewed to assess accurate selection of pivot height. Further exposures are made, with the pivot height set at 0.5 cm intervals, to demonstrate the entire biliary system, a range of approximately 3–4 cm.

Optimum image contrast is essential in order to differentiate between the abdominal viscera. As the objective constrast in a tomographic image is inherently less than that of a conventional radiograph (image contrast reducing with decreasing layer thickness), the lowest possible kVp that will achieve the required penetration should be used. The exposure time will be dictated by the length of time taken for the X-ray tube to complete the selected movement, leaving the tube mA as the factor for change in order to obtain a correctly exposed image.

IMAGE EVALUATION

As the projections used are the same as those for oral cholecystography, the criteria for image evaluation are also the same. Exposure times may be longer than in conventional radiography of the biliary system, allowing the X-ray tube to complete its movement, but there should be no evidence of breathing/movement unsharpness.

PEROPERATIVE CHOLANGIOGRAPHY

Radiographic examination of the biliary ducts following the introduction of a radio-opaque contrast agent during cholecystectomy.

Contrast agent: 20ml water-soluble compound with low iodine content (140–150 mgI/ml) so as not to obscure residual calculi.

Conventional projections used for demonstration of the biliary system cannot be used during sterile procedures. The mobile X-ray unit and two 30×40 cm gridded cassettes are cleaned and taken to theatre, where the radiographer changes into suitable clothing and footwear.

RADIOGRAPHIC TECHNIQUE

The surgeon indicates the centring point for the X-ray beam in relation to the incision site and the position of the bile ducts.

Most modern operating tables have a cassette tray or space under the table top for cassette positioning. The position for the centre of the cassette is assessed by one of the following methods.

Cassette tray opening at the side of the table
The centre of the long axis of the gridded cassette is aligned with the centring point as indicated by the surgeon, and the edge of the cassette is placed level with the patient's right flank.

Cassette tray inserted at the top of the table
Cassette trays used for this method are removable and have a long handle attached to the end of the tray. This gives the tray an appearance likened to a large rectangular 'frying pan', and is often nicknamed thus. The handle has a movable marker which is used as a landmark for positioning the tray. The longitudinal distance between the incision site and the top end of the table is measured, and the distance between the centre of the tray and the marker on the handle is set to equal the measurement taken. The gridded cassette is placed longitudinally in the centre of the tray and the tray slid under the table so that, transversely, the cassette is aligned with the centring point indicated by the surgeon and, longitudinally, the marker on the tray handle coincides with the top end of the table.

If the operating table is tilted it is returned to the horizontal position before the X-ray beam is centred, in order to prevent grid cut-off.

The vertical X-ray beam is centred over the indicated centring point and the surgeon prepares for injection of the contrast agent.

Once the radiographer and anaesthetist are wearing lead–rubber aprons, all other non-protected personnel are asked to leave the theatre. The anaesthetist is asked to suspend respiration, the surgeon commences injection and indicates the moment for exposure. Two exposures are usually made: one after injection of 10 ml of contrast agent and one after a further 10 ml. Two separate exposures will demonstrate that any filling defects are constant and not caused by air bubbles. The second image should show the flow of contrast agent into the duodenum, indicating no obstruction of the ducts.

Processing and delivery of the images to the surgeon is carried out immediately, enabling the removal of residual calculi, if present, prior to suturing of the operation site.

IMAGE EVALUATION

Correct patient identification and anatomical marker included on the radiograph.

Area of interest

Right hemidiaphragm, flank, iliac crest and spine.

Projection

- Long axis of spine parallel to long axis of film.
- Spinous processes demonstrated down centre of vertebral bodies.

Exposure factors

- kVp sufficient to penetrate bony structures and demonstrate bony trabeculae within them, maintaining contrast between the contrast-filled biliary ducts and other abdominal viscera.
- mAs to provide adequate image density to demonstrate the contrast-filled biliary ducts in contrast to other soft tissue structures within the abdomen, demonstrating any filling defects within them.

No evidence of patient breathing during the exposure.
No artefacts present on the image and no evidence of grid cut-off.

BARIUM ENEMA

Fluoroscopic examination of the large bowel following the introduction of a radio-opaque contrast agent and air.

Contrast agent: Barium sulphate suspension, 125% w/v, minimum 500 ml.

The undertaking of barium enema examinations by radiographers is a classic example of the acceleration of role development within the profession in recent years. Research published in 1995 showed that of the 333 diagnostic imaging departments who responded to a survey on role development, just under 50 employed radiographers who undertook barium enema studies (Paterson, 1995). Although this figure represents only approximately 14% of the sample it is by no means insignificant, and the numbers of radiographers specializing in this technique will probably have increased in the period between data collection for the study and publication of this text, continuing to do so in the future.

As in other chapters which cover more specialized areas, this section does not aim to provide information to the standard of certificate level, nor does it discuss the paediatric barium enema, but rather is intended as an introduction to the skill.

The examination demonstrates the large bowel from caecum to rectum, using barium sulphate and air as contrast agents. The barium is run into the large bowel and subsequently run out again before air is introduced, providing a fine barium coating over the mucosa.

Conditions demonstrated by this technique include diverticular disease, ulcerative colitis, neoplasm, polyps and fistulae. Indications for the examination include change in bowel habit, rectal bleeding or melaena, abdominal pain or a palpable mass.

The colon must be 'clean' so that the examination is successful, and patients are given instructions for appropriate bowel preparation. This includes the taking of laxatives accompanied by a minimal-intake low-residue diet over the 2-day period leading up to the examination, with fluids only allowed on the day of examination. Patients with inflammatory bowel diseases are not supplied with laxatives.

The barium enema is a fluoroscopic examination which requires a fluoroscopy suite with undercouch tube and tilting table, in addition to overcouch tube with table bucky, since images may be required. Images may be produced using large-format film, 100 mm cut film or a laser system.

PREPARATION

As with all radiographic procedures, equipment should be prepared in advance to ensure smooth running of each individual procedure and the session as a whole. Lead aprons must be clean and available, equipment switched on and assessed for safety, table turned into the horizontal position and the appropriate imaging method selected. The mattress is removed from the table and replaced with incontinence pads.

Trolley setting:
Disposable barium enema bag prefilled with barium paste/powder
Large measuring jug containing warm water
Antibubble agent (if required)
Enema connecting tube
Disposable enema tip
Enema tip with inflatable cuff for patients who cannot retain the catheter
Disposable rubber gloves
Lubricant jelly-covered gauze swabs
Adhesive tape
Sponge forceps to clamp the enema tube
Balloon insufflation pump
Paper roll.

Before the patient enters the room the tube leading from the enema bag is clamped off and 500 ml of warm water added to the contents. The barium solution is mixed thoroughly and the bag sealed and hung on the drip stand, which has been placed at the foot of the table. The disposable enema tip is attached and barium run down to the end of the enema bag tubing, which is then clamped off.

Smooth muscle relaxants may be needed and should be set out in readiness:

Buscopan 20 mg or Glucagon 1 mg
2 ml syringe
25G needle
Tourniquet
Alcohol-impregnated swabs
Sticking plaster.

Buscopan will reduce peristalsis immediately and usually for the duration of the examination. It is contraindicated for patients with a medical history of glaucoma or cardiovascular disease, Glucagon being the recommended alternative. Glucagon acts almost immediately, but the effects will last for approximately 3 hours (Chapman and Nakielny, 1993). Patients should be advised not to drive home until their eyesight has returned to normal.

PROCEDURE

One of the most important aspects of this examination is the establishment of good communication with the patient. This will help ensure maximum cooperation, essential to a successful examination, and assist in making the patient feel as comfortable and well cared-for as possible.

Careful explanation of the procedure in advance and at each stage of the examination will augment any written information which may have been supplied in advance, and provide the basis for good communication throughout.

Screening time must be kept to a minimum and should not exceed 5 minutes in total.

After a full identity check the patient is asked to lie on their left side on the table with their knees drawn up towards the chest. The radiographer/nurse puts on a pair of rubber gloves, applies lubricant jelly to the enema tip and carefully inserts the tip into the rectum, fixing it in place with adhesive tape over the buttocks. At this stage intravenous muscle relaxant may be administered.

DEMONSTRATING THE COLON

Unfortunately, the bowel does not follow an identical pattern for each individual. If each patient's bowel appeared as represented in textbook illustrations then it would be easy to describe a set number of projections, like those for general radiographic examinations! In fact, each patient's bowel differs in its loops and convolutions, and as a result individual radiologists have traditionally devised their own method to thoroughly and systematically produce the required images. This has resulted in a variety of ways in which this examination can be successfully completed. Since most radiographers who undertake this examination still produce images for report by a radiologist, they often have to conform to the system preferred by that radiologist. In a small imaging department which employs only one radiologist this is acceptable, but larger establishments will require radiographers to work with several radiologists, potentially complicating working practices by forcing the radiographer to perform a different technique according to the radiologist who will provide the report. Some departments have addressed this by discussion among the teams who carry out barium enema examinations, in order to establish a protocol for projections which will provide the information needed. This is no small task, considering the variation in routines studied by the authors: numbers of images produced ranged from seven to 18, and overcouch projections either totalling three or four in number or being omitted completely. Even the routine for running in the barium and air insufflation varies, as does when to record images, which can be done after the colon is totally coated by air and barium, or as each bowel section is demonstrated.

All routines have methods to ensure mucosal coating with barium, with adequate distension of the bowel with air. These include:

1. tipping the patient slightly head-down to aid initial running in of barium;

2. tipping the patient head-down in the supine position to clear barium from the caecum;
3. tipping the patient head-down while they are lying on the left side, turning them prone, returning them to the left side and then over into the supine position to also clear barium from the caecum;
4. standing the patient erect to allow air to fill the flexures, superior aspects of bowel loops and rectum;
5. turning the patient through 360° to coat the mucosa.

Bearing in mind these variations, the routine described in this chapter can be considered to be an example of a working technique and is not implied to be the only way of providing a complete examination of the large bowel.

SUGGESTED ROUTINE

When using an undercouch tube the patient position described will be opposite to that for overcouch techniques. For example, a supine oblique with the right side raised for overcouch technique is normally described as a left posterior oblique (LPO), but is referred to as a *right* anterior oblique (RAO) for undercouch techniques.

Following injection of the bowel relaxant, the patient lies on their left side and the barium is run in, the flow controlled by releasing or reapplying the clamp to the enema tubing. The column of barium is monitored by intermittent screening and the rectosigmoid region, sigmoid loops and distal descending colon are assessed. With the patient in this position, a *lateral rectum* image is recorded.

The patient rolls slowly towards supine until the sigmoid loops are separated and an exposure is made in this position – *right anterior oblique of sigmoid*.

The patient is turned prone and the clamp released to allow the barium to reach the mid-transverse colon; intermittent fluoroscopy will allow assessment of the area. The enema bag is dropped on to the floor and the barium is now drained back out of the colon. The tubing is reclamped and the balloon insufflator attached to the enema tube. The patient is informed that the air is to be introduced, and air is pumped in to distend the rectum and rectosigmoid region during intermittent fluoroscopy.

The *lateral rectum* and *right anterior oblique* of sigmoid region are taken again, this time with the double contrast. If there are multiple loops of sigmoid colon it may be necessary to make further exposures with varying degrees of obliquity in the right anterior oblique position. The patient is then turned to the supine (PA) position.

Air continues to be introduced, during intermittent fluoroscopy to allow assessment of the bowel and progress of the barium, until the barium reaches the caecal region. The enema tubing is clamped once again.

The patient is informed that the table will tilt until upright and they are asked to move their feet down the table towards the step, which will support them once erect. Handles are attached to the table, level with the patient's hands, and they are instructed to hold on to them for support. While tilting the table, the radiographer offers reassurance by placing a hand against the patient's shoulder. It may help to warn the patient that they will feel as if they are tipping forward, when in fact the table will stop in a vertical position. The patient is observed to ensure that those who feel faint can quickly be returned to a horizontal position. The patient is allowed to shift their feet to gain a steady position.

In the erect position, the patient is screened while turning to each side in turn to separate out the hepatic (*right anterior oblique*) and splenic flexures (*left anterior oblique*) in turn. Spot films are taken in each position.

The patient is turned to the lateral position, with their left side in contact with the table top, and a *right lateral* image of the rectum is taken.

With the patient still in the lateral position, the table is tilted back to the horizontal position. To successfully empty the caecum of barium, the patient is turned prone and then returned to the right lateral position, left side in contact with the table, before turning supine (PA). The right side is raised slightly, the caecum is screened and an image recorded in the *right anterior oblique* position. If the barium has passed through the ileocaecal valve a film may be taken of the terminal ileus.

The patient is turned on to their left side to allow air to float to the right side, followed by dropping the right side until the loops of colon are opened; an image of the hepatic flexure and right side of the bowel is recorded (*right anterior oblique*). This sequence is repeated for the opposite side, to demonstrate the splenic flexure – *left anterior oblique*. A supine projection (PA) is taken to demonstrate the flexures and transverse colon.

The fluoroscopic section of this examination is now complete and may be supplemented by additional overcouch projections. At this stage the enema tip may be removed from the rectum and the patient instructed to squeeze the anal muscles tight to retain the barium.

Alternatively, the enema tip may be left in place until the overcouch projections are completed. This will help the patient retain the barium and air but may hinder movement.

Overcouch projections which may be used to supplement fluoroscopic examination:

Prone abdomen with 30° caudal angulation ('Hampton's view')
Positioning is as far as the prone abdomen featured in the IVU section of this chapter, with the vertical central ray directed 30° caudally to a point

midway between the PSISs. The oblique central ray will separate the loops of sigmoid on the image.

Left lateral decubitus
Positioning is as for the left lateral decubitus described in Chapter 9, with the patient lying on their left side and a right PA marker placed on the uppermost long edge of the cassette.

Air rises and lies on the fluid level of the barium in the raised right side, to demonstrate the right aspect of the bowel, hepatic flexure, and sometimes the caecum. Loops of bowel may be separated as the patient turns through 90°.

Right lateral decubitus
Positioning is as for the lateral decubitus, with the patient lying on their right side.

Air rises and lies on the fluid level of the barium in the raised left side, to demonstrate the left aspect of the bowel and splenic flexure. Loops of bowel may be separated as the patient turns through 90°.

Descriptions of the lateral decubitus projections may be confusing, since the *left* lateral decubitus actually demonstrates the *right* aspects of the bowel, and the *right* lateral decubitus demonstrates the *left* aspects of the bowel. The projectional name refers to the side upon which the patient lies, not the side demonstrated. Markers should be attached to the cassette to indicate the raised side.

Some radiographers prefer to carry out one lateral decubitus projection AP and the other PA, to avoid excessive movement of the patient (in order to carry out both projections in a PA position the patient is asked to sit up and place their head at the opposite end of the table between projections. This is often an unreasonable request for the catheterized patient, especially if elderly or infirm). If one projection is to be carried out in the AP position, it should be remembered that the bowel will be more magnified than in the PA projection and that radiosensitive areas (bowel, breast, gonads) will be anteriorly positioned.

When the examination is complete the patient is immediately taken to the toilet to empty the bowel of as much barium as possible. They are warned that their stools will be white for a few days following the procedure, and encouraged to take in plenty of fluid to avoid constipation.

Arrangements for a follow-up appointment with the referring clinician are checked and the patient instructed to dress and go home.

Elderly patients

Many patients who may be regarded as 'elderly' will be perfectly capable of undergoing a routine examination: the radiographer should avoid prejudging their ability. However, a high proportion of barium enema examinations are carried out on elderly patients who may require some modification of technique owing to infirmity, disability or lack of control over the retention of the catheter and/or barium.

With careful use a balloon catheter will help retain both catheter and barium, but must not be used in cases of inflammatory bowel disease or if there is any possibility of a tight stricture/obstruction in the bowel. Since it will not necessarily be known that a stricture or obstruction is present, the balloon should never be inflated until barium has been seen to reach well into the descending colon, with no evidence of narrowing or obstruction.

Special care should be given to the fragile skin of the elderly, which can be easily damaged in the seemingly simple task of turning over on an unyielding table top. Foam elbow guards should be used to protect this particularly vulnerable area.

The addition of 1000 ml of warm water to the barium enema bag will promote a more free-flowing mixture which will reach the caecum more easily, demonstrating any gross pathology or obstruction, the main concerns when examining the elderly patient. Mucosal coating may be less effective but a double-contrast effect can be obtained with the introduction of less air, this having the added advantage of being less uncomfortable for the patient.

Suggested routine for the elderly patient

Horizontal table
Lateral rectum, single contrast
RAO sigmoid, single contrast
Introduction of air
Lateral rectum, double contrast
RAO sigmoid, double contrast
Introduction of more air

Erect table (if possible)
PA upper abdomen
PA lower abdomen
Right lateral rectum

Horizontal table
Caecum emptied of barium as in routine series
Oblique caecum (RAO or LAO according to whichever demonstrates the caecum best on the fluoroscopic image)
RAO abdomen
LAO abdomen

Overcouch projections
Supine abdomen with 30° cranial angulation, centred in the midline, midway between the upper border of symphysis pubis and ASISs.
Post-evacuation full abdomen if any suspicious areas have not been adequately demonstrated previously.

SALIVARY GLANDS AND SIALOGRAPHY

Demonstration of the salivary glands following the introduction of a radio-opaque contrast agent.

Contrast agent: 2 ml water-soluble (200–240 mgI/ml) or oil-based (480 mgI/ml) compound.

Trolley setting:
2 ml syringe
Contrast agent
Lacrimal dilator
18G blunt needle with polythene catheter.

Use of an oil-based contrast agent will theoretically ensure maximum concentration, since it cannot be diluted by the saliva, but may lead to the obscurement of small calculi. However, water-soluble contrast agent is widely used and neither type is considered to be more advantageous (Chapman and Nakielny, 1993).

RADIOGRAPHIC TECHNIQUE

Required projections vary according to the salivary glands under examination:
Parotid: Anteroposterior, lateral, lateral oblique.
Submandibular: Lateral, lateral oblique, occlusal.
Sublingual: Occlusal, although these glands are rarely examined with contrast agent as they are difficult to cannulate.

Symptoms which warrant referral for sialography include pain and/or swelling in the region of the salivary glands, particularly related to eating.

These examinations may be carried out with the patient erect or supine. However, the supine position is more comfortable for the patient and there is less chance of dislodging the cannula. This is therefore the method described.

Anteroposterior

An 18×24 cm cassette is placed longitudinally in the table bucky. The patient lies supine on the table. A lead–rubber sheet is placed over the trunk as radiation protection. The occiput is in contact with the table top, the MSP and OMBL perpendicular to the cassette. The long axis of the cassette is coincident with a sagittal plane through the middle of the orbit of the side under examination. The upper border of the cassette is level with the upper border of the orbit.

> CENTRING: A vertical central ray, at 90° to the cassette, is directed to a point midway between the symphysis menti and the angle of the mandible, on the side under examination.

Collimate to include soft tissues of the neck and face, symphysis menti and zygoma of the side under examination. Apply an AP anatomical marker within the primary beam.

Lateral

An 18×24 cm cassette is placed longitudinally in the bucky. From the supine position the patient turns 45° towards the side under examination. Pads are placed under the raised side to aid immobilization. The head is turned through a further 45° until its MSP is parallel to the cassette and the cheek is in contact with the table top. The middle of the cassette is coincident with the angle of the mandible.

> CENTRING: A vertical central ray, at 90° to the cassette, is directed over the angle of the mandible remote from the cassette.

Collimate to include soft tissues of the neck, symphysis menti, angles and rami of mandible and zygomas. Apply an AP anatomical marker within the primary beam.

Lateral oblique

An 18×24 cm cassette is placed longitudinally in the table bucky. The patient is positioned as for the lateral projection. The vertex of the skull is then tilted 15° towards the cassette, resting on the table top for stability. The chin is raised to clear the mandibular condyles from the neck.

> CENTRING: A vertical central ray, at 90° to the cassette, is directed 10° cranially to a point midway between the angles of the mandible.

The cassette is displaced cranially until its centre is coincident with the central ray. Collimate to include soft tissues of the neck, symphysis menti, angles and rami of mandible. Apply an AP anatomical marker within the primary beam.

Submental occlusal

The patient lies supine with the shoulders raised on a pillow. The neck is extended over the pillow as far as possible. An occlusal film is placed in the mouth, tube side (dimple) facing the floor of the mouth, with its long axis coincident with the MSP. The film is then displaced as far back in the mouth as possible and towards the side under examination. The patient gently closes their mouth to hold the film in place. The MSP is vertical.

CENTRING: A vertical central ray is directed at 90° to the occlusal plane and film, to the centre of the film.

Collimate to include symphysis menti, soft tissues of the floor of mouth, submandibular duct under examination and alveolar margin of that side.

IMAGE EVALUATION

Correct patient identification and anatomical marker included on the radiograph.

Area of interest

Anteroposterior, lateral and lateral oblique

Ramus, angle and body of mandible and surrounding soft tissue outlines of face and neck.

Submental occlusal

Arch of mandible, including symphysis menti and first molars.

Projection

Anteroposterior

- Sagittal plane through centre of orbit coincident with midline of film.
- Superior border of petrous ridge coincident with supraorbital margin.
- Parotid gland projected lateral to ramus of mandible within soft tissues of face.

Lateral

- Superimposition of right and left inferior and posterior borders of mandible.

- Posterior borders of mandibular rami and salivary glands projected clear of cervical vertebrae.

Lateral oblique

- Side remote from film projected superiorly, enabling clear visualization of salivary glands and ducts in region of ramus and angle of mandible of side in contact with cassette.
- Posterior borders of mandibular rami and parotid area projected clear of cervical vertebrae.

Submental occlusal

- Teeth superimposed on body of mandible.
- Symmetry of arch of mandible about MSP.
- First molars included on radiograph.

Exposure factors

kVp is selected so as not to overpenetrate any small calcifications, maximizing contrast between the gland, the overlying mandible and soft tissues of the face.

- kVp sufficient to demonstrate the opacified gland and ducts following the introduction of a contrast agent, maintaining contrast between the salivary gland and mandible.

mAs selected so as not to overexpose the soft tissue area of the gland.

- mAs to provide adequate image density to demonstrate detail of the gland and ducts in contrast to the adjacent bone and soft tissues.

No evidence of patient movement.
No artefacts present on the image.

SIALOGRAPHY PROCEDURE

Prior to introduction of contrast agent the relevant projections described are carried out as 'controls' to demonstrate any radio-opaque calculi. They are then repeated following administration of the contrast agent. Before commencing the examination the procedure is explained to the patient and instructions given on remaining still. A signal should be agreed for the patient to use when they experience a tight feeling in the contrast-filled salivary gland.

The patient is given a sialagogue to initiate dilatation of the duct: sucking a fruit drop or sipping lemon juice will achieve this.

The patient lies supine with their head supported on a sponge pad during cannulization. The relevant duct is located, the parotid duct being adjacent to the crown of the second upper molar and the submandibular duct adjacent to the base of the frenulum linguae. The duct is then opened further with a lacrimal dilator.

An 18G blunt needle connected to a polythene catheter is attached to a 2 ml syringe containing the contrast agent. The catheter is flushed through with contrast to avoid introducing air into the duct. The needle is inserted into the duct and contrast injected slowly until the patient indicates that the gland feels tight (and is therefore filled with contrast agent). The plunger is taped in position to avoid backflow of contrast into the syringe, and the patient asked to gently close their lips over the catheter.

Handling the syringe carefully to avoid dislodging the needle, the patient is positioned for the required projections. The catheter should be placed so that its does not obscure the gland or duct. Once the initial post-contrast images have been checked and accepted, an additional lateral projection may be required in examination of the submandibular glands, with the patient depressing the tongue and floor of the mouth with a spatula/spoon during exposure. This will demonstrate the glands below the overlying mandible.

One or more of the projections may be repeated following the administration of a sialagogue in order to demonstrate how effectively the glands drain.

The normal salivary gland will resemble a finely branching tree, whereas the obstructed gland will not demonstrate the finely branching network of ducts. Obstruction by calculus can cause dilatation of the ducts – sialectasis – which appears as fine mottling of the contrast medium, which has entered the minute ruptures within the gland. This will only be apparent if the contrast has been able to pass around the calculus or the calculus has recently cleared. Tumours will be demonstrated by a soft-tissue opacity, accompanied by any combination of distortion, destruction or displacement of the duct's branches and erosion of adjacent bone, depending on the tumour type.

DACROCYSTOGRAPHY

Radiographic examination of the lacrimal system following the introduction of a radio-opaque contrast agent.

Contrast agent: 0.5–2 ml per side of an oil-based compound, 480 mgI/ml.

Trolley setting:
2 ml syringe
Contrast agent

Lacrimal dilator
18G blunt needle with polythene catheter.

The contrast agent is oil-based, since a water-soluble one would be dissolved by the tears; 2 ml are drawn into the syringe, but as little as 0.5 ml may be injected.

Dacrocystography is most frequently requested for patients suffering from epiphora, commonly caused by obstruction of the lacrimal duct, occasionally due to malignancy.

RADIOGRAPHIC TECHNIQUE

A lead–rubber cape is applied to the patient's shoulders as radiation protection.

Occipitomental

An 18×24 cm cassette is placed longitudinally in the erect bucky. The patient is seated facing the bucky. The chin is raised until the OMBL is at 45° to the horizontal, resting against the bucky. The middle of the long axis of the cassette is level with the inferior orbital margins. The MSP is perpendicular to and coincident with the central long axis of the cassette.

> CENTRING: A horizontal central ray, at 90° to the cassette, is directed to the midline of the occiput to emerge midway between the inferior orbital margins.

Collimate to include orbits and maxillary sinuses. Apply a PA anatomical marker within the primary beam.

Lateral

An 18×24 cm cassette is placed longitudinally in the erect bucky. The patient is seated facing the bucky, their head turned through 90° to bring the side under examination into contact with it. The MSP of the head is parallel to the cassette and the interpupillary line perpendicular to it. The centre of the cassette is coincident with a point 2.5 cm below the outer canthus of the eye.

> CENTRING: A horizontal central ray, at 90° to the cassette, is directed to a point 2.5 cm below the outer canthus of the eye.

Collimate to include orbits and maxillary sinuses. Apply an AP anatomical marker within the primary beam.

IMAGE EVALUATION

Correct patient identification and anatomical marker included on the radiograph.

Area of interest

Outline of bony orbits and maxillary sinuses.

Projection

Occipitomental

- MSP coincident with midline of film.
- Equidistance of lateral borders of orbits to outer tables of skull.
- Superior border of petrous ridge coincident with inferior margin of maxillary sinuses.

Lateral

- Superimposition of right and left facial structures and floor of anterior cranial fossa.

Exposure factors

- kVp sufficient to demonstrate the floor of maxillary sinuses and areas of overlap of the zygoma on the bones of the skull in the OM projection, and areas of overlap of the right and left facial structures in the lateral, maintaining contrast between the facial bones and air-filled sinuses.
- mAs to provide adequate image density to demonstrate the contrast agent within the lacrimal ducts in contrast to the adjacent bony structures.

No evidence of patient movement.
No artefacts present on the film.

Prior to introduction of contrast agent the projections described are carried out as 'controls', to demonstrate possible (rare) calcification within the gland or bony involvement in tumour development. The projections are then repeated after administration of contrast agent.

CANNULATION OF THE LACRIMAL DUCT

The patient is seated with their back resting against the erect bucky or skull unit and the area over the lacrimal sac gently pressed to express tears. The lacrimal duct is dilated to facilitate cannulization. An 18G blunt needle attached to a polythene catheter is inserted into the inferior canaliculus and the patient is turned to face the erect bucky.

The patient is positioned for the OM projection and contrast agent is injected. When the patient feels the sensation of the contrast agent in the nose, the injector retires and exposure is made. This sequence is repeated for the lateral projection.

If the duct is obstructed contrast will not be felt in the nose and will overspill from the canaliculus. OM and lateral projections are undertaken.

Radiographically, a normal duct will appear as a streak of contrast agent travelling from the medial aspect of the orbit down the lateral aspect of the nasal cavity. The obstructed duct will show as a pool of contrast agent over the medial aspect of the orbit, or will not be seen at all.

As for the facial bones, OM and lateral projections can be undertaken with the patient supine on the table of an isocentric skull unit, although the radiologist may prefer to introduce the contrast medium with the patient sitting up, before lying them down. Macroradiography is a technique which lends itself well to dacrocystography, and is easily achieved on isocentric skull units by simply leaving the cassette holder at the end of the C-arm (maximum OFD), rather than sliding the cassette close to the face as in routine examinations. In this case, 24×30 cm cassettes will need to be used in order to accommodate the magnified image. Alternatively, in the absence of an isocentric unit, a mento-occipital projection may be carried rather than the OM, although this will only produce a slight degree of image magnification at the expense of increased radiation dose to the radiosensitive lenses of the eyes.

LOWER LIMB VENOGRAPHY

Fluoroscopic examination of the lower limb venous system following the intravenous injection of a radio-opaque contrast agent.

Contrast agent: 50 ml water-soluble, non-ionic compound per leg, 200/240 mgI/ml.

Trolley setting:
50 ml syringe
Contrast agent
10 ml syringe
0.9% saline for injection
Tourniquets
Alcohol-impregnated swabs
19G butterfly needle
Adhesive tape
Dressing for injection site.

Lower limb venography is commonly used in the diagnosis of deep vein thrombosis, causes of leg oedema, and to demonstrate incompetent imperforate veins. The examination requires a fluoroscopy suite with tilting table and image recording system.

Like the barium enema examination, lower limb venography is slowly showing itself as another area where radiographers are developing their role.

PREPARATION

Equipment preparation should follow that described for barium enemas, with the fluoroscopy unit programmed to split the films longitudinally if using large-format film; 35×35 cm cassettes can be split to take three images and 24×30 cm cassettes split to take two images.

No specific patient preparation is required, although patients with cold feet or narrow veins may need to warm their feet in a bowl of warm water immediately prior to the examination. Patients with oedematous legs should rest in bed with their feet elevated for several hours beforehand. If the patient still presents with gross oedema of the foot, it may not be possible to cannulate a vein. Pressing over the metatarsophalangeal joint may demonstrate a vein for injection, as may sitting the patient with their feet in warm water as described above.

PROCEDURE

The foot-step is placed on the end of the table and a large sandbag placed in contact with it on the side of the *unaffected* limb. When the table is tilted vertically, the step will enable the patient to stand and take weight on the unaffected limb while not placing any weight at all on the limb under examination.

The patient lies supine on the table with the unaffected foot resting on the sandbag. The table is tilted foot-down 30–45° and the patient's full body weight borne on the unaffected limb. A tight tourniquet is placed around the ankle, just above the level of the malleoli, and the injection site cleaned with the alcohol-impregnated swab. The vein over the first metatarsophalangeal joint (part of the dorsal venous arch) is usually selected for introduction of the contrast agent. If this is not suitable or successfully demonstrated, all visible veins on the dorsum of the foot are examined and the most distal vein possible is selected for injection. The patient is warned that they will feel some discomfort as the needle is inserted, and the radiographer must be prepared for the foot to be jerked away. When the needle is successfully inserted into a vein, it is taped in position to prevent it being dislodged. The cap is removed from the needle tubing and blood allowed to flow back to the end. The 10 ml syringe containing 0.9% saline is connected and the syringe plunger drawn back until a little blood enters the syringe. Saline is flushed through to ensure that the needle is positioned correctly, with no extravasation around the tip.

The 50 ml syringe containing the contrast agent replaces the 10 ml syringe and the contrast agent is slowly injected, the radiographer screening intermittently to check for extravasation. If the needle appears to be correctly sited but the patient complains of pain in the area of the needle during injection, the foot should be screened to exclude extravasation of the contrast agent.

When the deep calf veins are full, after approximately 25–30 ml of contrast have been injected, three exposures are made over the calf on one 35×35 cm cassette or separate 100 mm films (remembering that an undercouch tube is being used): *PA, oblique with internal rotation*, and *oblique with external rotation*.

As the contrast reaches the popliteal vein the table is taken to the horizontal position. Injecting continues until all 50 ml of contrast agent has been injected. Three exposures are made on a second 35×35 cm cassette or separate 100 mm films as the relevant veins fill:

PA – popliteal vein;
PA lower femur including knee joint – distal femoral vein;
PA upper femur and hip joint – proximal femoral vein.

The tourniquet is released at the ankle and, while screening, the leg is raised and one or two films are taken on a 24×30 cm cassette or 100 mm film(s) as the contrast agent flows towards the inferior vena cava: *PA – iliac veins.*

The 50 ml syringe is replaced with the 10 ml syringe containing 0.9% saline and the line is flushed through.

Films are reviewed before removing the needle as it is possible to identify an area of clot on the hard images when it has been missed during fluoroscopy. The needle is removed when the examination is complete and a dry dressing applied to the puncture site.

In total: 30 seconds – 1 minute fluoroscopy time plus 8×100 mm spot films
OR
2×35×35 cm films each with three images plus 1×24×30 cm films with one/two images.

References

Badr, I., Thomas, S.M., Cotterill, A.C. *et al.* (1996) X-ray pelvimetry: What is the best technique? *Clinical Radiology* (in press).

Ball, J. and Price, T. (1989) *Chesney's Radiographic Imaging*, Blackwell Scientific Publications, Oxford.

Ballinger, P.W. and Merrill, V. (1991) *An Atlas of Radiographic Positioning and Radiological Procedures*, C.V. Mosby, St Louis.

Beamer, J. (1994) *The Radiological Examination of the Scaphoid Following Trauma: A Suggested Protocol.* BSc Thesis, Kingston University.

Bell, G. and Finlay, D. (1986) *Basic Radiographic Positioning and Anatomy.* Baillière Tindall, London.

Caseldine, J., Blamey, R., Roebuck, E. and Elstone, C. (1988) *Breast Disease For Radiographers*, Wright, London.

Challen, V., Kapera, E., Manning, D., *et al.* (1990) *Breast Screening and Mammography*, Postrad, Lancaster.

Chapman, S. and Nakielny, R. (1993) *A Guide To Radiological Procedures*, Saunders, London.

Colleran, C. (1994) PA lumbar spines: a future concept. *Radiography Today*, **60**(681), 17–20.

Day, A. (1994) Radiation doses to radiosensitive organs during two different chest radiography techniques. *Radiography Today*, **60**(690), 17–20.

Forrest, P. (1986) *Breast Cancer Screening*, HMSO, London.

Francis, C. (1993) Centring techniques for posterior obliques of lumbar vertebrae. *Radiography Today*, **59**(669), 20.

Gallagher, D. (1993) Current practices in skull radiography. *Radiography Today*, **59**(673), 21–4.

Grech, P. (1981) *Casualty Radiology – a Practical Guide for Radiological Diagnosis*, Chapman & Hall, London.

Greenspan, A. and Norman, A. (1986) The radial head capitellum view: a useful technique in elbow trauma. Cited by Jack, L.M. and Grundy, A. Radial head views – an alternative. *Radiography*, **57**(605), 246–7.

Groocock, S. (1995) *The Radiological Examination of the Scaphoid Bone: Are Five Projections Really Necessary?* BSc Thesis, Department Of Radiographic Studies, Keele University.

Gyll, C. and Blake, N. (1986) *Paediatric Diagnostic Imaging.* Heinemann, Oxford.

Lewis, S. (1984) Cephalic index and how it may be of relevance in radiography of the petrous temporal bone. *Radiography*, **50**(592), 180–4.

Lewis, S. (1988) New angles on the radiographic examination of the hand. *Radiography Today*, **54**(617), 44–5; (618), 20–30; (619), 47–8.

Paterson, A. (1995) *Role Development – Towards 2000. A Survey of Role Developments in Radiography*. College of Radiographers, London.

Ponsford, A. and Clements, R. (1991) A modified view of the facial bones in the seriously injured. *Radiography Today*, **57**(646), 10–12.

Radiological Advisory Committee (1989) Guidelines on the establishment of a *Quality Assurance System For the Radiological Aspects of Mammography* used for Breast Screening, (The Pritchard Report) DoH, London.

Ravin, C.E. and Johnson, G.A. (1983) The 'optimal' chest radiograph. *Seminars in Respiratory Medicine*, **5**(1). Thieme-Stratton Inc.

Richmond, B. (1995) A comparative study of two radiographic techniques for obtaining an AP projection of the thumb. *Radiography Today*, **61**(696), 11–15.

Robinson, C. (1995) The elimination of a moving anti-scatter grid in the radiographic imaging of the AP cervical spine. *Radiography Today*, **61**(697), 13–16.

Royal College of Radiologists Working Party. (1995) *Making The Best Use Of A Department Of Clinical Radiology – Guidelines For Doctors*, 3rd edn, RCR, London.

Royal College of Radiologists NRPB (1994) Guidelines on radiology standards for primary dental care. *Documents of the NRPB*, **5**(3). NRPB.

Swallow, R.A., Naylor, E., Roebuck, E.J. and Whitley, A.S. (1986) *Clark's Positioning In Radiography*, Heinemann, Oxford.

Wallace, W.A. and Hellier, M. (1983) Improving radiographs of the injured shoulder. *Radiography*, October, Vol **49**(586), 229–33.

Webb, W., Brant, W. and Helms, C. (1991) *Fundamentals Of Body CT*, WB Saunders, Philadelphia.

World Health Organisation (1985) *Manual Of Radiographic Interpretation For General Practitioners*, WHO, Geneva.

Wright, I. and Fergusson, P. (1986) Supplementary projection to demonstrate the thoracic inlet. *Radiography*, **52**(601), 52–3.

Index